'Alderman's analysis of deconstruction is meticulous and riveting. He also persuasively highlights its archetypal repetition in the mythology of the eternal youth. But his argument is not merely polemical; it is a nuanced reworking of its gifts into a synthesis which will engage readers across the field of contemporary thought'

**Roger Brooke**, *Professor Emeritus, Duquesne University.*

'In prose reminiscent of Hillman, Alderman illuminates the myth of our era - the rejection of our embodied origin in matter that leaves us in the Neverland of Eternal Youth. This book offers a powerful corrective to the rootless inflation so present in our current cultural moment.'

**Lisa Marchiano**, author of *Motherhood.*

'At last, a vigorous collision of Jung and deconstruction that superbly illuminates both. *Eternal Youth and the Myth of Deconstruction* succeeds in capturing what these vital perspectives share and how profoundly they diverge. Alderman philosophizes Jung, psychologizes Derrida, and mythologizes Butler. Essential reading for the twenty-first century transdisciplinary era.'

**Susan Rowland, PhD**, author of *Jungian Arts-Based Research and the Nuclear Enhancement of New Mexico* (2021).

# ETERNAL YOUTH AND THE MYTH OF DECONSTRUCTION

In *Eternal Youth and the Myth of Deconstruction*, Bret Alderman puts forth a compelling thesis: Deconstruction tells a mythic story. Through an attentive examination of multiple texts and literary works, he elucidates this story in psychological and philosophical terms.

Deconstruction, the method of philosophical and literary analysis originated by Jacques Derrida, arises from what Carl Jung called "a kind of readiness to produce over and over again the same or similar mythical ideas." In the case of deconstruction, such ideas bear a striking resemblance to a figure that Jungian and post-Jungian writers refer to as the *puer aeternus* or eternal youth. To make his case, in addition to a careful analysis of numerous Derridean texts, he offers readings of literary works by Milan Kundera, J. M. Barrie, Dante, Apuleius, and others. These texts help illustrate that deconstruction's preoccupations over questions of presence, deferral, authority, limits, time, and representation are also recurrent issues for the eternal youth as described by Marie-Louise von Franz and James Hillman. Judith Butler's deconstruction of sex and gender reflects similar patterns, and she features in this work as a contemporary exemplar of the deconstructive approach.

*Eternal Youth and the Myth of Deconstruction* will be a compelling read for both students and teachers of depth psychology and continental philosophy. The clarity of its style will be appealing to advanced scholars and educated laypersons alike.

**Bret Alderman** is an author who received his PhD in depth psychology in 2013 from the Pacifica Graduate Institute in Carpinteria, California. His recent interests include ideological possession, deconstruction, gender, and the interface between psychology and philosophy.

## Philosophy & Psychoanalysis Book Series

Jon Mills
Series Editor

*Philosophy & Psychoanalysis* is dedicated to current developments and cutting-edge research in the philosophical sciences, phenomenology, hermeneutics, existentialism, logic, semiotics, cultural studies, social criticism, and the humanities that engage and enrich psychoanalytic thought through philosophical rigor. With the philosophical turn in psychoanalysis comes a new era of theoretical research that revisits past paradigms while invigorating new approaches to theoretical, historical, contemporary, and applied psychoanalysis. No subject or discipline is immune from psychoanalytic reflection within a philosophical context including psychology, sociology, anthropology, politics, the arts, religion, science, culture, physics, and the nature of morality. Philosophical approaches to psychoanalysis may stimulate new areas of knowledge that have conceptual and applied value beyond the consulting room reflective of greater society at large. In the spirit of pluralism, *Philosophy & Psychoanalysis* is open to any theoretical school in philosophy and psychoanalysis that offers novel, scholarly, and important insights in the way we come to understand our world.

Titles in this series:

**Archetypal Ontology**
New Directions in Analytical Psychology
*Jon Mills and Erik Goodwyn*

**Eternal Youth and the Myth of Deconstruction**
An Archetypal Reading of Jacques Derrida and Judith Butler
*Bret Alderman*

For more information about this series, please visit: www.routledge.com/Routledge-Handbooks-in-Religion/book-series

# ETERNAL YOUTH AND THE MYTH OF DECONSTRUCTION

## An Archetypal Reading of Jacques Derrida and Judith Butler

*Bret Alderman*

Routledge
Taylor & Francis Group
LONDON AND NEW YORK

Designed cover image: © Getty Images

First published 2024
by Routledge
4 Park Square, Milton Park, Abingdon, Oxon OX14 4RN

and by Routledge
605 Third Avenue, New York, NY 10158

*Routledge is an imprint of the Taylor & Francis Group, an informa business*



*British Library Cataloguing-in-Publication Data*
A catalogue record for this book is available from the British Library

ISBN: 978-1-032-45533-4 (hbk)
ISBN: 978-1-032-45532-7 (pbk)
ISBN: 978-1-003-37743-6 (ebk)

DOI: 10.4324/b23321

Typeset in Times New Roman
by Apex CoVantage, LLC

# CONTENTS

# ACKNOWLEDGMENTS

This book could not have come into being without the insight and encouragement that I received from many people. Lisa Marchiano, Colette Colfer, and Xavier Bonilla read drafts of the introductory chapters and offered valuable feedback. Gary Accord improved the text considerably with his careful proofreading and commentary. Donovan Cleckley helped me immensely with formatting citations. Enrique Aguilar offered encouragement and advice in the final stages of the book's production. By helping to create a vibrant intellectual community in Critical Therapy Antidote, Val Thomas provided an invaluable source of support and encouragement that helped me bring this project to full fruition. Many years ago, when these pages were little more than a vague intuition, Alexandra Fidyk heard the initial vision, which at the time I imagined manifesting as a short chapter or article, and encouraged me to move forward. I would like to thank all of them. I would also like to thank the editorial staff at Routledge, most notably the Editorial Assistant Alice Maher, Commissioning Editor Katie Randall, and Series Editor Jon Mills, all of whom I peppered with numerous and sometimes unnecessary questions that they patiently answered.

# INTRODUCTION

## The Present Deferred

### I

*Life Is Elsewhere* is the title of Milan Kundera's (1976 [1986]) second novel, an ironic epic lampooning the spirit of youth, poetry, and revolution. It is also the thesis statement of deconstruction, the method of philosophical and literary analysis originated by Jacques Derrida. This assertion is perhaps hyperbole or caricature, but not without warrant: For deconstruction, the *Lebenswelt* as Edmund Husserl called it, the world of lived experience,[1] is not quite here, in the present, as one might have thought (Derrida, 1973). It is elsewhere. In this regard, Jaromil, the tragic adolescent hero of Kundera's novel, and Derrida, the inimitable French philosopher, share a common thesis and are kindred spirits. For both, real life, if there is such a thing, is to be found in another place at another time. There is a set of existential themes they have in common that coalesce around terms like *life*, *presence*, and *distance* among many others. Jungian and post-Jungian writers have a name for such spirits. The name is *puer aeternus* or *puella aeterna*, Latin for *eternal youth*. This book portrays deconstruction as a manifestation of this youthful spirit, one present in myth and literature, but also one potentially present everywhere.

For such writers, it is this ubiquity—the fact that it can be found in so many iterations at so many times and places—that makes the eternal youth an archetypal figure, that is to say, one that is archaic and typical. Despite the differences in its multiple manifestations, it remains essentially the same over time. Carl Jung (1953) said that "the archetype is a kind of readiness to produce over and over again the same or similar mythical ideas" (p. 69) and when I say that Jaromil and Derrida share a common thesis and are kindred spirits it is with such a statement in mind. The two are quite different of course: One is a literary protagonist and poet

DOI: 10.4324/b23321-1

born of a novelist's imagination and the other is an immensely influential and erudite philosopher of prodigious intellect. You will not find the statement 'life is elsewhere' in Derrida's writing. Yet you will find arguments that bear a striking family resemblance if you are willing to take the time to discern their basic contours. Such a resemblance suggests, to use Jung's phrasing, a kind of readiness to produce over and again the same or similar mythical ideas.

Derrida and deconstruction reflect a certain character type, a fundamental disposition that is perennial. Deconstruction is a story we have seen before. How this is possible and why it would even matter are two questions the responses to which will unfold slowly throughout the present text. The first, regarding how such a singular genius might reflect a rather ordinary type, will require a thorough, informed reading of Derrida that does justice to his prolific, perplexing brilliance and satisfies the expectations of philosophically minded readers. It will also require, with the help of Jungian and post-Jungian scholars, the unearthing of parallels in mythic and literary texts that, at first glance, may seem far afield.

Regarding the second question as to why it might matter that deconstruction reflects a perennial disposition or type, it matters because deconstruction in the strict sense of the word—a form of textual hermeneutics originated by Derrida—is also something that has expanded well beyond this strict sense. Look no further than the term *deconstruction* itself, which has become commonplace in both academic and popular vernacular and is used by people who know little or nothing of its origins. The term's prevalence bespeaks Derrida's cultural impact, perhaps far more than the innumerable citations of his works. Some critics, like Michele Lamont (1987), have suggested that this impact has little to do with the intrinsic value of his work and more to do with a rather opportune institutional legitimation resulting from his appeal to the intellectual public as a status symbol. This appeal resulted from a rather innovative approach to the politics of the late 1960s. Such a thesis suggests that the term's widespread adoption satisfies a preexisting imperative or desire. Deconstruction gives voice to something that was already there, something that wanted to be expressed and found its proxy.

The term deconstruction conjures different definitions and associations in each of us. For some, it is a careful dismantling of an argument, idea, or narrative that makes us privy to all its latent biases and preconceptions. It is a means to demythologize a text to reveal its falsehoods and unwarranted assumptions. Others might simply associate it with a rather esoteric vocabulary, including words like *logocentrism* and *phonocentrism*, *trace* and *supplement*, *signifier* and *signified*, *undecidability* and *sous rature*, *metaphysics of presence*, and, most notably, *différance*. For some individuals, these words hold considerable cachet. They are like shibboleths that demonstrate a person's intellectual bona fides. For others, they are trendy buzzwords wielded as weapons to quickly disarm an opponent, weapons, one might add, that require no license or permit and are often wielded with little acumen. Yet others might associate the term deconstruction with the idea of gender, which in recent years has come to be one of its primary targets.

Deconstruction in a broad sense has become, or perhaps always has been, more than merely a doctrine or a technique. It is an intellectual style, and currently a very popular one. It is an attitude, a disposition, a psychological pattern, one forever eager to point out the contradictions of accepted wisdom, dispel commonly held beliefs, point out the absurdity of received ideas, and topple every well-established edifice of understanding. It is a mindset that seeks to erode tradition in the name of the new, to undermine norms or 'normativities,' with the often-unspoken assumption that doing so is a liberating endeavor. In a quest to dismantle all prejudices and reveal their corruption, it points out the apparent arbitrariness and even insidiousness of conventional beliefs. This dispeller of illusion, the spirit of deconstruction exists well beyond the texts or techniques that bear its name. You can hear its echo in every assertion that something seemingly self-evident is, in fact, just a social construct, something quite flimsy and ephemeral, not as substantial or real as one had previously thought. Deconstruction as perennial type matters precisely because it is so present, so contemporary, yet so perennial. It is both current and recurrent. This suggests that it springs from a readiness to produce over and again the same or similar ideas as those that have been produced in ages prior.

The word *archetype* merits further attention at the outset. Deconstruction has been at the forefront of an anti-essentialist fervor that views with a highly astute and semiotically sophisticated skepticism any talk of essential structures, innate characteristics, or transhistorical human nature. Such structures, characteristics, and natures are, in fact, precisely what it attempts to reveal as illusory. They are the sorts of fundamentals or principles that Derrida called into question, and in so doing, he called into question the entire heritage of Western philosophical thought (Derrida, 1967 [1978]). And *archetype*—perhaps more than any other word in the Western philosophic tradition—gives off a rather pungent waft of essentialist rot, even from the far-off and far-fetched realm of eternal Platonic forms. Deconstructive critics will immediately point out the jarring contradiction and blatantly oxymoronic character of the paired adjectives *eternal* and *Platonic*, noting that such forms are the inventions of a particular philosopher living at a particular place and time which, in and of itself, belies their eternal provenance. This is the nub of the issue, part of the logical impasse that defines what Derrida calls a metaphysics of presence—a generalized system of schemata with all of its assumptions, biases, and baggage that is foundational to the Western philosophic tradition.

The same holds for Jungian archetypes. Though by no means identical to their Platonic forebears, they nevertheless allude to the sort of target that Derrida takes aim at—an abiding presence, the heart of which he seeks to split with his analytic quiver. So construing deconstruction in terms of the archetypal means starting from premises that are antithetical to its fundamental critical thrust, which seeks to undermine any reference to any such structure, pattern, or type, anything that might be considered as a metaphysical substance (Derrida, 1973). An archetypal reading of a discourse that is anathema to the archetypal is simultaneously an implicit challenge *to*, and implicitly challenged *by*, the subject matter it addresses.

## II

Who is the eternal youth? The short answer is that he is someone for whom life is elsewhere and time is a problem. The former theme I have already spoken of in terms of Husserl's *Lebenswelt*, the world of lived experience, a world that is for deconstruction not quite here, in the present, as one might have thought. The latter theme is perhaps best epitomized by Derrida's assertion that time itself is "an impossible possibility" (1982 [1986], p. 55). A longer answer might include a list of mythic figures like Hermes, Cupid, Phaeton, Icarus, Dionysus, Attis, Adonis, Osiris, Adam, Corybas, Pan, and Bacchus (Hillman & Slater, 2005; Jung, 1959, 1969; Yeoman, 1998 [1999]). Tristan from the chivalric romance of Tristan and Iseult might be added to the list, as well as Lucius from the ancient Roman novel *The Golden Ass* (Von Franz, 1970 [1992]). In more contemporary times, he has appeared as Peter Pan, as well as the aforementioned Jaromil of Kundera's satiric novel. But within this list, we might include any living person who seems to have fallen under the sway of a mentality or a psychological disposition that resembles these figures from literature and myth. These are individuals enthralled by the archetype of the eternal youth, with its readiness to produce over and over again the same or similar mythical ideas.

What exactly these mythical ideas are will be addressed throughout the present work. Those conversant in Jungian and post-Jungian thought may already be quite familiar with them and quite familiar with the *puer aeternus*. For those less acquainted with this archetypal figure, we will begin here a preliminary sketch of him and, in so doing, also introduce the thought of both Marie-Louise von Franz and James Hillman, two authors who loom large in the literature on this figure yet conceive the youth in somewhat different terms. The two represent contrary yet complementary poles of thought within the Jungian tradition. The former might be thought of as representing the Preoedipal aspect of the youth's problematic while the latter is more focused on Post-Oedipal aspects. In the process of sketching the silhouette of this youth, we will also begin to draw parallels with deconstruction and in so doing hopefully help readers who are less conversant in this style of thought to get a clearer picture of its primary tenets. This is, upon first glance, a daunting task. Derrida is a difficult writer and although many readers may feel familiar with a style of thought that can be called deconstruction, they may have never read primary texts of deconstruction *sensu stricto*. Even a careful reading of these primary sources is a challenge in itself. But if it is true that the mythical ideas that constitute the eternal youth are also, in their basic contours, those that constitute deconstruction, this is perhaps not quite the challenge that it appears to be. In commencing our sketch, we simply need to proceed one pencil stroke at a time.

To begin, consider two simple words: *not yet*. These two words are central to puer's dilemma and, as we will see, they are also central to deconstruction. Men and women who see through the eyes of the eternal youth and have become bewitched by this particular psychological pattern suffer from temporal displacement: *not yet, not yet, not yet* is their refrain. At the same time, nostalgia—that sentimental yearning for the erstwhile and the elsewhere—is their malady (Hillman & Slater, 2005). Filled with future plans, panged with hungers for an imagined past, they are never quite present, never quite here, never quite now. *Pueri aeterni* live provisional lives. This is a phrase often associated with them. Everything about them is provisional because they are haunted by the peculiar feeling that they are not yet in real life (Von Franz, 1970 [2000]), though they could be, some day. They should be, and would be, and may be, and perhaps once were, and will be, but *are* not, at least not now. Somehow, their very being is not quite in the present.

Yet this displacement is not merely temporal; it is spatial as well: For such an individual, the greatest dread is to be bound and pinned down, thereby "*entering space and time* completely" (emphasis added) (Von Franz, 1970 [2000], p. 8). The *modus vivendi* is to be not here, not now, and thus not *present*, in the dual sense of this word—not of this particular place, not of this particular moment. As regards place, the eternal youth "never quite touches the earth. He never quite commits himself to any mundane situation but just hovers over the earth, touching it from time to time, alighting here and there" (p. 11). He is not grounded but fleet-footed, so that his footfall leaves only traces, or traces of traces, that are erased almost before they are even formed. He flies, metaphorically, propelled perhaps by the firm conviction that somewhere beyond his present location there is another place, a better place, where he needs to be. Distant and dreamy, ponderous and pensive, he longs for what is far off. He yearns for what is absent.

As James Hillman has shown in his seminal work *Senex and Puer* (Hillman & Slater, 2005), the ancient Greeks had a word to describe this penchant for the "not yet": the word is *pothos*. One of many possible manifestations of eros, pothos refers to a particular form of desire, a desire for that which is absent (Stewart, 1993). It is the longing for that which is elsewhere (Illbruck, 2012). On Hillman's reading, pothos is, in fact, the insatiable yearning that characterizes the puer aeternus (Hillman, 1975a; Hillman & Slater, 2005). This desire is at the heart of his displacement, his conflict with both space and time. This desire is also, by another name, at the heart of deconstruction's critique of the metaphysical underpinnings of Western thought.

Pothos has its correlate in deconstruction and it goes by the name of différance. This assertion is fundamental to the argument being made herein and I will return to it again and again. Without this term there is no deconstruction and without pothos there is no eternal youth. There is an isomorphic parallel between différance—Derrida's conception of semiotic deferral—and puer's *not yet*. Both are expressions of *the present deferred* and an ambivalent desire for that which is absent. By way of this quasi-philosophical notion, couched in ornate sophistry and circuitous prose, Derrida has cleverly mastered the art of postponement in a way that is not dissimilar to the eternal youth's penchant for procrastination, delay, dithering, and general dillydally. Just like the eternal youth, différance and the thought inspired by it do not enter space and time completely. On the contrary, they seem to inhabit something like a mythic isle, call it Neverland, that exists outside time's passing.

The opening chapter of the present text is a discussion of différance, one that is hopefully carried out with a diligence and rigor that will satisfy those familiar with Derrida's work, yet also with a clarity that will satisfy those who are not. Another related correlate should be mentioned at the outset: What is desired, the far-off person, place, or thing that is the object of pothos is what, in deconstructive parlance, is known as the *transcendental signified*, another key term to be explicated in greater detail as we slowly paint, brushstroke by careful brushstroke, the portrait of deconstruction as a variant of the myth of the eternal youth.

Imagined through this myth, both différance and the transcendental signified are not what Derrida says they are, or more precisely, they are that and so much more. They reflect a voracious yet ambivalent yearning for what is both absent and unattainable. Envisioning deconstruction as myth is, as Hillman would have it, a way to "remove the discussion of ideas from the realm of thought to the realm of psyche" (1975b, p. 121). This is a resonant phrase that contains a primary conceit of the present work. Herein we attempt to do just that—elucidate deconstructive ideas and then place them in the realm of psyche, and more precisely, the mythic or archetypal psyche, because "it is their appearance in the psyche, their significance as psychic events, their psychological effect and reality as experiences relevant for soul, that demand our attention" (Hillman, 1975b, p. 121).

This relocation of the discussion of ideas might also be described as a simple act of recontextualization, a consideration of deconstruction not only within the context of academic and philosophic discourse but also within a broader psychological one. A primary reason behind this recontextualization is the understanding that ideas and ideologies "are hardly independent of their complex roots; so ideas can be foci of sickness, part of an archetypal syndrome" (Hillman & Slater, 2005, p. 120). Addressing the psyche requires that we attend to images in ideas and symptomatic dimensions in abstractions. Removing the discussion of ideas from the realm of thought to the realm of psyche is an acknowledgment that not only is it the case that "symptoms are unconscious metaphors" but also that "this is so for individuals, cultures, and epistemologies" (Romanyshyn, 2007, p. 213). A similar intuition is expressed by Hillman (1997) when he writes in *The Myth of Analysis* that "the mythic appears within language, observations, and theories even of science" (p. 6). These are not new ideas, merely ones that some, following in Jung's footsteps, have continued to develop. Jung, following the path laid out by Theodore Ziehen's work on word association, understood complexes to be clusters of emotionally charged representations, ideas laden with affect, and such ideas can show up just about anywhere (Stevens, 2001).

As a result of recontextualizing in this way and a desire to get at this archetypal syndrome, there is a certain rhythm to the forthcoming chapters that moves between explicating the *logos* of deconstruction, on the one hand, and describing its *mythos* on the other. Put differently, there is an ebb and flow between a more philosophic register and one that is more properly depth psychological.

The thematic content of deconstruction lends itself to a reading in terms of the eternal youth not only in relation to différance and the transcendental signified. The readiness to produce over and over again similar ideas, as Jung claims that archetypes do, is in no way limited to these two terms. On the contrary, similarities are abundant: The deconstruction of textual authority by way of the critique of *logocentricism* and a *metaphysics of presence*—terms that will be explored at greater length further on—shares an undeniable family resemblance with a certain youthful anti-authoritarianism typical of this mythic character. The free play of signifiers that, for deconstruction, precludes any definite, fixed, rigid interpretation, and thereby liberates a multiplicity of heterogeneous readings—this too bears witness to the eternal youth's spirit of transgression and desire for absolute, limitless freedom. Neither the eternal youth nor deconstruction is what they are without limitless play, it is so important and central to their outlook. Both also appear to struggle at times with confusion as to play's relation to a world that is *not* mere play—a world of real-life consequences, subject to certain laws of causality, where empirical truths can be demonstrated or refuted. Both revel in a certain ecstasy, what might be called a pleasure of displacement, that appears to have no limiting principle. Adding to the list, eternal youths are often quite convinced of their own exceptionalism: They are not ordinary people with ordinary talents, although such a belief often resides in simply never having put their talents to the test of time. This too has its correlate in deconstruction, most notably perhaps as regards its central term *différance*, which in a strange way is also spared the test of time.

The eternal youth is there to see within the works of Derrida, and those who have followed in his footsteps. The thematic content of the philosopher's writings more than lends itself to such a statement: Its preoccupations over questions of temporality, displacement, presence, authority, limits, and structure are also recurrent issues for puer and figure prominently in the literature about him (Bly, 1990 [2004]; Greene & Sasportas, 1987; Hillman, 1979; Hillman & Slater, 2005; Porterfield et al., 2009; Yeoman, 1998 [1999]). All of these themes, in one form or another, are to be found in abundance in Jungian and post-Jungian descriptions of the eternal youth. The very term *deconstruction* testifies to an attitude toward structure that is resonant with the eternal youth's antipathy to fixity, order, and rigidity. Puer, like deconstruction (Wood & Bernasconi, 1988), strives toward the decomposition and desedimentation, the unraveling and undoing of structures. Derrida's notion of *undecidability* mirrors the eternal youth's notorious indecision and speaks to their shared desire to undermine binary logic. His seeming reduction of everything to a matter of representation also echoes a theme common to this youth. Even issues of erudite speculation that might seem far afield and unrelated—like Derrida's assessment of Aristotle's thinking on potentiality and actuality—reveal themselves to be, on closer inspection, yet another iteration of a theme typical of this figure; making the potential actual is his recurrent insurmountable challenge, part of the 'not yet' motif that forms his existential dilemma. The dilemma, as one might imagine, is also evidenced by the utopic quality of his desire, which is yet another aspect of his displacement. Utopia, as often noted and as its etymology attests, is no place. It is nowhere. The aforementioned cluster of themes all point in the same direction, to the same readiness to produce over and over again similar mythical ideas. They are the mythical ideas typical of the puer aeternus.

## III

Von Franz and Hillman offer two differing visions of the eternal youth and where they differ is, first and foremost, regarding who they view as the youth's primary antagonist. For von Franz it is the Great Mother, whose mythic expressions find form in figures like Ereshkigal, Maya, Ishtar, Astarte, Atargatis, Cybele, Mary, and Kali. For Hillman, it is the Senex, the aged patriarch, whose mythic forms are, among others, those of Yahweh, Chronos, Daedalus, Saturn, Zeus, Phoebus, and Jehovah. With a certain poetic license that remains faithful to both Hillman's and von Franz' writings, I have rechristened these two antagonists as the *primordial mother* and the *temporal father*.

These two figures are at the core of the eternal youth's problematic, and they are at the core of deconstruction's as well. In one venue, the mythic, they are expressed in the archaic idiom of the imagination, while in the other, the philosophic, they take the form of abstractions bolstered by rather difficult, labyrinthine arguments, and for this reason, the parallels may seem forced but on closer inspection are not. Beginning with Derrida's most foundational and influential texts, *Speech and Phenomena* (1973) being perhaps the most foremost among them, he calls into question the very concept of *primordiality*, and he does so by way of claims regarding *temporality*. He takes aim at the idea of the primordial—a first beginning, an origin—and what may seem like unrelated notions that are in fact quite essential to it, like *phenomena* and *perception*. Derrida's argument is one regarding sequence, that is to say, temporal unfolding. He challenges the ideas of primordiality and perception *through* a critique of time as traditionally understood, specifically a critique of what is understood as *the present, the now*. His qualm, translated into mythic terms, is with the primordial mother and the temporal father, and like many youths faced with parental difficulties, he seems to pit one parent against the other.

Derrida's critique of the present or the now and its relation to issues of primordiality and perception, as well as many others, will be addressed from multiple perspectives throughout the present work, as will its relation to the aforementioned mythic figures. However, in the interest of giving the reader a schematic preview of the pages to follow, so that he or she does not hit the ground too flat-footed, a few more words on some key elements of his analysis of time, his critique of a 'metaphysics of presence' and its mythic parallels are warranted.

For Derrida, time is the name of an "impossible possibility" (1982 [1986], p. 55) and the question of truth is never dissociable from the question of time

(Currie, 2013). The impossibility involves a logical impasse or *aporia* regarding time's continuity and divisibility, a disjuncture between two conceptions of the now, two conceptions of the present—one that is continually abiding and one that is of potentially infinite divisibility. Time, when considered through these dueling conceptions of the present, is an impossible possibility because it "is continuous according to the now and divided according to the now" (Derrida, 1982 [1986], p. 54). The latter conception comprehends time as a series of discrete moments, while the former does not. For one, the present moment always is. It is eternal in the sense of being continuous. For the other, it is but one moment in a succession of infinitely divisible moments. For Derrida this is a great problem, and it affects how we understand what truth is.

In laying bare this aporia, he sheds light on a particular conception of the present that, on his telling, has bedeviled Western thought at least since Aristotle (Derrida, 1976). But this laying bare does more than shed light, it shakes the very foundations of an entire ontology, on Derrida's account, one that has defined our historical epoch and the entire edifice of Western metaphysics (1973, 1982 [1986]). In the last analysis, he tells us, what matters is this equivocal conception of the present, the now. And the revelation of this duplicitous conception acts like an epistemic earthquake, leaving no discipline on firm footing—not science, not philosophy, not the humanities—so profound are its implications. Another way of framing this critique of the now is to say that the living present, as Husserl would call it, can no longer serve as a source of certitude. It cannot be an origin of sense. It has been emptied of sense. It has become *a hollowed now*, one that is of no significance, lacking all substance, a vacuous form.

Another name for this aporia of divisibility and continuity is the conundrum of time and eternity. We know that the dual and sometimes dueling concepts of time and eternity have occupied philosophers for millennia and elicited contrary views: the pre-Socratic school of philosophers known as the Eleatics conceived of being as eternal and immutable, while change was an illusion; Heraclitus took a contrary view and held that relentless temporal flux was real and stasis illusory; Aristotle merged the two concepts, conceiving the eternal as everlasting time, without beginning or end; and Plato considered time to have, in fact, a beginning, in contrast to a realm of eternal forms that did not. The debate, of course, did not, and does not, end or begin there. Like Ariadne's thread in the Minotaur's labyrinth, it runs forward in time, through the speculations of medieval scholastics and Enlightenment philosophers to, and through, the German idealism of Hegel, who conceived of eternity as a form of absolute presence. It winds through Nietzsche's idea of an eternal return—infinite time coupled with a finite number of possible events—and coils its way through Heidegger's interrogation of philosophy's relationship to the question of time. Moving ever forward, its gossamer path leads us to, and even through, Derrida's critique of a metaphysics of presence. Yet if the riddling route of Derrida's prose is any indication, we are not out of the labyrinth and may even be more lost than ever. It is clear that Derrida knows the terrain quite well, yet what is not clear is whether he has led us out of the labyrinth or simply presented us with a sort of philosophical tangle: We seem to be as deep in the minotaur's maze as ever, yet find Ariadne's thread now hopelessly wadded in our hands.

Perhaps, then, it is an opportune moment to tease apart the tangle and to retrace our steps, mindful of the fact that Ariadne's thread is *both* a mythic allusion to a gift bestowed to Theseus as an aid in a heroic journey of confusing complexity *and* a technical term within philosophy, one that refers to a particular, algorithmic application of logic. This fact serves as a reminder that while philosophers have perplexed over their abstractions, storytellers have vexed over these same issues, albeit by way of more arcane, symbolic language. Perhaps by following the thread that they have gifted us we can find our way out of the labyrinth. Perhaps by discerning the mythic dimensions of philosophical issues, we can clarify them a bit and see them from a slightly different perspective.

The logical impasse regarding time and eternity, or the now's divisibility and continuity, viewed with an understanding of the mythic, archetypal psyche represents much more than an intellectual conundrum. In light of Hillman's reading, it suggests a psychological dissociation or conflict between two mythic figures: the eternal youth and father time. In a similar vein, deconstruction's seemingly revolutionary critique that purports to shake the very foundations of Western thought is less the result of philosophical insight and more the result of psychological conflict, as well as a rather overweening pretension that is a response to this conflict.

Such a reading that envisions a story of mythic dimension and import conceives this seeming irreconcilability of temporal continuity and divisibility not simply as something that needs to be resolved solely with an effort of the analytical intellect, argued for or against, and accepted or rejected only by virtue of the plausibility of an argument. Such an approach would only serve to further entrench the sterile conflict that is in need of resolution. Rather, this irreconcilability is between two archetypal sensibilities that share a common root. From this perspective, the enigma of time and eternity is but one aspect of a psychological conflict, as is the apparent irreconcilability of the finite with the infinite and the immanent with the transcendent—philosophical binaries that also play implicit and explicit roles in this archetypal conflict within Derrida's work.

The aporia of time's continuity and divisibility is more than a logical puzzle. Seen from a perspective informed by depth psychology, it stems from a fissure at the level of experience, an alienation of archetypal dispositions intrinsic to the human condition. It is in service of a therapy of ideas (Hillman, 1997) that the present work moves the discussion of such philosophic abstractions from the realm of thought to the realm of psyche. In so doing, it follows in Hillman's footsteps insofar as he was always relentlessly questioning abstracted and abstruse principles divorced from their human context. He always insisted on returning them to their original, experiential ground.

Because the archaic idiom of the imagination is not mere allegory, the figures of senex and puer are not just stand-ins substituting for philosophic abstractions.

On the contrary, they represent the fundamental attitudes, dispositions, styles of consciousness, and psychological patterns that give rise to these abstractions. Time and eternity, in a sense, are lived as percepts before they are thought as concepts, or, at the very least, the perceptual and conceptual are inseparably entwined and to consider one without the other is mistaken. We see through the eyes of time, and we see through the eyes of the eternal. They represent two perspectives that bring with them a panoply of associations, experiential matrices, and recurrent motifs.

Puer and senex are relevant for a discussion of time and eternity and finding our way out of a philosophical labyrinth, or at least understanding its perplexing contours, because they help bring into clearer view the psychological, experiential background before which these concepts arise. My intention in writing this book is to do just that: to situate Derrida's critique of time in such a way as to reveal its psychological provenance and relevance. My intention is not to deconstruct myth but rather to mythologize deconstruction and situate it within an archetypal context. This may also, in turn, help shed new light on difficult philosophical issues that Derrida, to his credit, relentlessly draws our attention to.

Just as senex, or the temporal father, is relevant for a discussion of Derrida's critique of time and a metaphysics of presence, so is the primordial mother or what might also be called mother matter. For this latter figure we turn to the writings of Marie-Louise von Franz. More than any other author within the classical Jungian tradition, including Jung himself, she helped form the discussion of the puer personality. For her, in contrast to Hillman, the essential conflict at the heart of the eternal youth's turmoil does not involve father time, but rather mother matter. Referencing Jung's *Psychology and Alchemy* and *Mysterium Coniunctionis* (1970), she (1970 [1992]) describes the youth's adversarial relationship as one involving "the mother goddess Materia," which is also understood as a feminine anima mundi, a soul in cosmic matter (Von Franz, p. 209).

Such a mother refers to a sense of the maternal that extends far beyond the personal mother to include the archetypal. In other words, it speaks to "the mother" in a much greater and much more metaphorical sense that includes any being, any force or dynamic that might serve as an origin, a source. Mother Earth is a great example of this archetypal sense insofar as the earth is our site of origin, the creative, living matrix from which we are all born. Any originating presence, any source, has something maternal about it. Any term that echoes a sense of the primordial does as well. The term *primordial* refers to a first beginning and, because of this, finds itself within the grasp of the metaphorical tendrils of 'the mother,' which also holds within it, by implication, all that is primal, primeval, and primitive.

To some readers, such a description may appear to merely trade in tired gender stereotypes or outworn tropes, seeming naively essentialist and hopelessly anachronistic by today's standards. But these standards are to a great degree the result of the very deconstructive critique that is at issue here. More importantly, I would note that the term *primordial*, with all of the aforementioned connotations of primal, primeval, primitive, and primary, plays a critical role in Derrida's (1973) critique of Husserl's phenomenology. And just as one can see in the aporia of time and eternity a conflict between senex and puer, one can read a mythic drama at work in deconstruction's particular approach to terms like *primordiality* and *origins*, as well as *perception* and *phenomena*, all of which have historic, mythic, and etymologic ties to the idea of 'mother.' This reading lends itself nicely to an interpretation by way of von Franz's work, particularly when it comes to her understanding of the eternal youth's deep ambivalence toward the beloved yet dreaded mother, which seems to parallel deconstruction's equivocal attitude toward primordiality and closely related ideas. In short, the critical thrust that relies on claims of naive essentialism and anachronism as regards *the mother* is not itself beyond the mythic reading being offered here.

Such an assertion offers a convenient segue to another philosopher whose name is often linked with deconstruction, specifically as regards gender. That philosopher is Judith Butler. Though often associated with Michel Foucault, Butler draws upon Derrida a great deal for her deconstruction of the gender binary and, perhaps more importantly, one can read a similar mythic drama at work in her particular approach to issues like gender performativity, normativity, identity, (mother) matter, and many others. Gender as performance in particular suggests a reading in terms of the eternal youth's penchant for conflating pretend worlds with real ones. It also suggests a kinship with the sort of gender confusion that manifests itself throughout a work like J. M. Barrie's *Peter Pan* (2011), which is in many ways the quintessential text that epitomizes the eternal youth's attempt to escape time. The mythic drama underlying Butler's work is that of the *puella*, and so it should come as no surprise that her argument, in typically deconstructive style, is one regarding sequence, that is to say, temporal unfolding, and it results in her taking issue with mother matter, or more specifically, the *materiality* of sexed bodies (1996 [2011]).

Butler's cameo appearance in a work largely dedicated to deconstruction's founder provides an opportunity to discern the present-day effects of ideas put forth decades ago—by a leading figure, perhaps *the* leading figure, of postmodernism's first generation—ideas that nevertheless continue to resound throughout contemporary culture, finding expression in the current generation of more 'applied' postmodernism. Such effects are both evidence of Derrida's lasting impact and, as mentioned earlier, suggest that deconstruction in its current iteration continues to satisfy a preexisting need or desire. It gives voice to something perpetually present that seeks expression and finds its proxy in our particular historical moment in the form of deconstruction.

In Von Franz's (1970 [2000]) reading, one of the eternal youth's maladaptive responses to his conflict with the archetypal mother is to avoid decisive action by drawing action back into the realm of fantasy and theory. In lieu of action, he opts for reflection. He flees the mother, flies into the stratosphere of ideas and imagination, and "escapes into the intellect where generally she cannot follow him" (Von Franz, 1970 [1992], p. 22), but at the cost of his relationship with the earthlier plane of phenomenal reality. Preemptively, as a defense against the immediacy of perception and feeling, he converts this immediacy into its representation, in the form of fantasy or idea. One might say that he puts life in quotes, so that it becomes "life"—something safely enclosed within punctuation, prophylactically reduced to the merely textual or symbolic. Puer conflates life with its representation and subsumes the former under the latter. He assimilates intellectually that which would best be assimilated otherwise, through feeling or action. This form of assimilation results in a dangerous conflation between representation and reality: Like Antoine de Saint-Exupéry's little prince, he "thinks the design [of sheep] is as good as real sheep. Everything remains in the world of mental activity" (Von Franz, 1970 [2000], p. 47). Everything remains in Wonderland where he can wonder endlessly while another life—in some sense more real—slowly passes him by. It is as if he walks through a magic portal and later is unsure which side of the portal he is on, the one of consensus reality or the one that is beyond time and space, in a place called Neverland. Through this defensive maneuvering, he thinks his way out of the immediacy of living in a world that demands action and one in which actions have consequences. In his avoidance of entering space and time completely, he turns the present into the *re-presented.* All of these themes can be found in deconstruction. They form fundamental aspects of its primary content.

## IV

> It always seems to us as if meaning—compared with life—were the younger event, because we assume, with some justification, that we assign it ourselves, and because we believe, equally rightly no doubt that the great world can get along without being interpreted. But how do we assign meaning? From what source, in the last analysis, do we derive meaning? The forms we use for assigning meaning are historical categories that reach back into the mists of time—a fact we do not take sufficiently into account. Interpretations make use of certain linguistic matrices that are themselves derived from primordial images. From whatever side we approach this question, everywhere we find ourselves confronted with the history of language, with images and motifs that lead straight back to the primitive wonder-world.
>
> (Jung, 1969, pp. 32–33)

For Jung, the forms we use for assigning meaning, our linguistic matrices, the weblike systems of associations solidified into words, grammar, and syntax, are not arbitrary; rather, they are rooted in the same soil as the primordial images and motifs that he spent a lifetime trying to discern. In other words, they are rooted in experiences that, through repetition, have coalesced into linguistic categories, just like mythic images tend to coalesce into certain repetitive motifs or patterns. In the same way that myth provides a sort of evolving record of perennial human experience that is simultaneously changing and changeless, so do languages. They arise from the same substructure of sensemaking, the substratum that Jung referred to as the collective unconscious, the realm of the archetypes, which arrange the human psyche into associative, affective clusters, organizing images and ideas (Jung, 1983). Although they cannot be represented in and of themselves, they allow for the possibility of representation.

Jung's understanding of the derivation of language and the way in which we view its history is important to mention at the outset for a few different reasons, the first of which is that it offers a stark contrast with Derrida's. Simply put, for the latter figure, there can be no sense in which something called 'life' can have much say in the creation of meaning conveyed in language. From the beginning of his critique of phenomenology, Derrida takes aim at what Husserl called the 'life world' or *Lebenswelt*, a world immediately or directly experienced, and what he calls into question is precisely the claim that any such thing can be a source of meaning. What Jung suggests above, albeit cryptically, is that things may not be so simple. Life might have some say in the matter.

Furthermore, for Derrida, the history that Jung speaks of amounts to a sort of metaphysical heritage, a set of philosophical distinctions, assumptions, and presuppositions bequeathed by tradition that are, more than anything else, in need of deconstruction. Such distinctions and presuppositions are not and have never been based on anything self-evident or conditioned by an implicit logic that precedes them. They are more akin to inherited prejudices. Deconstruction's attitude toward history, which is also the eternal youth's attitude toward the senex and everything senescent, is aptly encapsulated in the following quote by Barbara Johnson, one of deconstruction's better-known advocates, in her introduction to Derrida's *Dissemination*:

> [Deconstruction] reads backwards from what seems natural, obvious, self-evident, or universal, in order to show that these things have their history, their reasons for being the way they are, their effects on what follows from them, and that the starting point is not a (natural) given but a (cultural) construct, usually blind to itself.
>
> *(Johnson, 1981, p. xv)*

For Jung, this sort of either-or approach that would split nature from culture and see history—including the history of language—as merely the opportunity to challenge what had seemed self-evident is a bit foreign. When he looks backward in time, he sees ideas, images, and motifs that have withstood its test, the test of time. History is less an opportunity to undermine conceptions of universality and more an invitation to witness their varied expressions. For this reason, the student of philology—the study of the historical development of languages—is also the student, knowingly or otherwise, of enduring yet evolving human experience, perception, and understanding. The etymologies of words help give us insight into the most fundamental forms of sensemaking that constitute who we are as human beings. Languages contain their own wisdom and studying the root meanings of words can lead to greater insight not only about language but about our own psyches or souls as well. What Derrida considers metaphysical, and the language used to communicate it, is, from Jung's perspective, rooted in experiences so perennial and collective as to be irrevocably sedimented within us. The archetypes, which constitute identical psychic structures common to us all, are "the archaic heritage of humanity, the legacy left behind by all differentiation and development and bestowed upon all men like sunlight and air" (Jung, 1956, p. 178). Jung (1956) describes this heritage as "the mother of humanity" (p. 178), a detail that will be of increasing importance for the present text. The closest equivalent to this in Derrida's thinking is what he calls a metaphysical heritage, the very heritage he seeks to dismantle and that Jung saw as impervious to any such dismantling.

Jung was explicit in his adoption of the philologist's method. In fact, it formed a foundational component of his basic hermeneutic approach, both within the analytic hour and outside of it, insofar as philology applies the logical principle of amplification, the simple seeking of parallels between disparate linguistic forms. Jung's use of amplification, however, was never limited to the strictly linguistic; rather, he sought parallels in the most varied sources: myth, fairy tale, poetry, dreams, symptoms, religions, and philosophies. In all of these areas, the intent was always to find the "tissue that word or image is embedded in" (Jung, 1977, p. 84). This relentless search for parallels was, in part, a means by which Jung collected evidence for his hypothesis of the collective unconscious, but it also had a therapeutic aim: It was a means of broadening a patient's understanding of their own personal neurosis so that they might see it as a more general, perhaps even universal, affliction hardly unique to any given individual. Amplification, for Jung, was a matter of thinking by way of analogy and it followed a certain natural logic, inferring from the similarity of forms a commonality of source or lineage. That is to say, in identifying a formal similarity between words, images, symptoms, and motifs he inferred that they might have a common origin, often one that suggested to him a sort of implicit logic within the human psyche.

Another reason for calling attention to these issues of the derivation and histories of languages at the outset has less to do with the *content* of the present work and more to do with its *form* of argument. One aspect of this form is etymological; I repeatedly draw upon the long-standing associations between words, directing attention to these 'linguistic matrices' so deeply rooted in history. This is a technique of etymological retrieval not unlike Heidegger's, one that recognizes that the meaning of contemporary (synchronic) usage becomes clearer in the light of historical (diachronic) usage. In and of itself, this is a sort of counterargument to some of deconstruction's most fundamental assumptions because, as Derrida was well aware, there is no way of making deconstruction's argument without relying upon the selfsame metaphysical heritage, the linguistic history, that it seeks to dismantle. This fact, and the continued reflection upon history and etymology, also helps explain why changing or co-opting certain words in a manner antagonistic to their historical meaning can prove so futile and amount to such nonsense: Words are rooted in our most primary forms of sensemaking.

The French phenomenologist Merleau-Ponty knew this well. Like Derrida, Husserl, Butler, Jung, Hillman, and von Franz, he plays an important role in the philosophical and psychological drama unfolded in the present pages. His notion of *sedimentation* is relevant as regards the historic aspect of language and his writings serve to counter—or one might even say *heal*—the dissociative tendencies of deconstruction that sever language from the primordial mother and temporal father. Through his work, we attempt the aforementioned therapy of ideas that Hillman (1997) considered so important. Sedimentation, to be explored in greater detail further on, offers a means of thinking about our linguistic inheritance in a way that radically differs from deconstruction and is more kindred in spirit to Jung's approach. Language, for Merleau-Ponty, is of a perceptual order: All of the distinctions, assumptions, and presuppositions bequeathed by our linguistic history—sedimented within us through historic accretion—are also reflections of "the blind and involuntary logic of things perceived" (Merleau-Ponty, 1973, p. 36). Language does not merely cloak the world and prevent our direct perception of it, acting like a sort of cultural bias that thwarts our vision. It is not simply a collection of signs that defer or prevent contact with a world that transcends us. Rather, language is born from the mother of perception. It does not prevent the sort of immediate seeing that is the foundation of Husserl's phenomenology, a seeing that he considered to be the "ultimate legitimizing source of all rational assertions" (Husserl, 2012, p. 36).

Merleau-Ponty's vindication of perception and his insistence on its primacy are not merely simple counterclaims opposing deconstruction, the foundational texts of which he did not live to read, given his untimely death in 1961. Rather, it is an assimilation of many of the insights and trends in continental philosophy that deconstruction would later draw upon. It was an *incorporation* of its insights in the most fundamental sense of this term—a way of bringing them into the body, a way of making them corporeal. Yet by way of this assimilation, he also drew attention to the limitations and blind spots of these insights. With an uncanny prescience, he foresaw the route—one might even say the dead end or cul-de-sac—that a particular way of thinking about language would later lead to. The influence of Saussure, Wittgenstein, and Heidegger is palpable in his writings as it is in the writings of many who have come to be called, for better or worse, postmodernists, including Derrida. But the influence is attenuated, reconfigured, and assimilated by way of a great synthesizing intelligence whose subtle voice is easily lost in the din of those who currently clamor for the deconstruction of every great thinker of ages prior.

In the present volume, I frame Merleau-Ponty's philosophic incorporation as an act of psychological integration, a healing of what could be called a dissociation of ideas. In mythic terms, his assimilation into the body of phenomenology of the insights regarding language—those that latter came to full expression in post-structuralism and deconstruction—represents a rapprochement or reconciliation with the figures of the temporal father and primordial mother. This reconciliation is also, to my mind, evidence of a maturation of desire, a movement from a rather puerile form of eros (known as pothos) toward a more mature eroticism that includes not merely an insatiable desire for what is absent but also a satiable desire for what is present.

The Greek god *Kairos* is an apt deity to represent this more mature, integrated desire, as well as the reconciliation with temporality and primordiality. His appearance in these pages represents an attempt to heal the split between the eternal youth and the temporal father, as well as the ambivalent attachment of this youth to the primordial mother. Kairos epitomizes the moment of this youth's emancipation from Neverland, which is also an acceptance of the present moment. Kairos names in mythic form the very moment that deconstruction attempts to render mute, the moment upon which Husserl's phenomenology rests its claims of veracity, the moment of "the presence of sense to a full and primordial intuition" (Derrida, 1973, p. 5). He represents the selfsame now moment, the moment of lived experience that deconstruction displaces, defers, and delays forever and always.

Invoking ancient deities to critique deconstruction, construing it as myth, and claiming that it is illustrative of a type, much less an archetype, runs counter to its entire ethos. As noted earlier, an archetypal reading of a discourse that is anathema to the archetypal is simultaneously an implicit challenge *to*, and implicitly challenged *by*, the subject matter it addresses. Jung knew nothing of deconstruction, in the strict sense of this word, having died the same year as did Merleau-Ponty. But he did have a great deal to say about repudiation of the archetype, "which in itself is an irrepresentable, unconscious, pre-existent form that seems to be part of the inherited structure of the psyche and can therefore manifest itself spontaneously anywhere, at any time" (Jung, 1964, p. 449). From his perspective, it is when we are most adamant in denying the archetypal that we are most in its grip. This observation is, in fact, fundamental to Jung's entire critique of modernity, which he saw as being a bit too eager to dismiss religious and spiritual traditions through rationalist critiques. It is in denying 'the gods,' although we may no longer name them as such, in failing to pay them appropriate homage or appease them through sufficient sacrifice, that we are most vulnerable to their demands. It is when we most fervently insist on their absence that they are most present. Deconstruction is in many ways just such a fervent insistence, and by Jung's logic, it must be vulnerable to similar demands. It is no surprise then, and even quite expected, that we find the archetype of the puer aeternus, the eternal youth, there, fully present, in the discourse that claims its absence.

## Note

1 The term *lived experience*, which is the English translation of the German *erlebnis*, despite its apparent redundancy given that all experience is in some sense 'lived,' was used by Husserl to make an important distinction in the philosophy of phenomenology. It follows from the same logic that discerns between, on the one hand, a merely physical body (*körper*), which can be rendered as *corpse* in English, the physical body as an anatomical object, and, on the other hand, a lived body (*lieb)*, which is a conscious body, one possessing a sense of 'I can' (Alderman, 2016; Moran & Cohen, 2013). In a similar vein, Husserl distinguished between the merely physical world described by the scientific tradition, a world in the abstract, and our lived experience of this world, which includes the emotional and practical aspects of our existence (Drummond, 2022). The modifier *lived* was intended to emphasize a sense of experience before any appeal to principles, causes, or explanations—what one might call simply *raw* experience.

## References


Alderman, B. (2016). *Symptom, symbol, and the other of language: A Jungian interpretation of the linguistic turn.* Routledge.

Barrie, J. M. (2011). *The annotated Peter Pan: The centennial edition* (M. Tatar, Ed.). W.W. Norton & Company. (Original work published 1911)

Bly, R. (1990 [2004]). *Iron John: A book about men.* Da Capo Press.

Butler, J. (1996 [2011]). *Bodies that matter: On the discursive limits of sex.* Routledge.

Currie, M. (2013). *The invention of deconstruction.* Palgrave Macmillan.

Derrida, J. (1967 [1978]). *Writing and difference* (A. Bass, Trans.). University of Chicago Press.

Derrida, J. (1973). *Speech and phenomena, and other essays on Husserl's theory of signs.* Northwestern University Press.

Derrida, J. (1976). *Of grammatology* (G. C. Spivak, Trans.). Johns Hopkins University Press. (Original work published 1967)

Derrida, J. (1982 [1986]). *Margins of philosophy* (A. Bass, Trans.). University of Chicago Press.

Drummond, J. J. (2022). *Historical dictionary of Husserl's philosophy.* Rowman & Littlefield.

Greene, L., & Sasportas, H. (1987). *The development of the personality.* Seminars in psychological astrology (Vol. 1). Weiser Books.

Hillman, J. (1975a). *Loose ends: Primary papers in archetypal psychology.* Spring Publications.

Hillman, J. (1975b). *Re-visioning psychology* (1st ed.). Harper & Row.

Hillman, J. (1979). *Puer papers.* Spring Publications.

Hillman, J. (1997). *The myth of analysis: Three essays in archetypal psychology.* Northwestern University Press.

Hillman, J., & Slater, G. (2005). *Senex & puer.* Spring Publications.

Husserl, E. (2012). *Ideas pertaining to a pure phenomenology and to a phenomenological philosophy: First book: General introduction to a pure phenomenology.* Springer Netherlands.

Illbruck, H. (2012). *Nostalgia: Origins and ends of an unenlightened disease.* Northwestern University Press.

Johnson, B. (1981). Introduction. In J. Derrida (Ed.), *Dissemination* (pp. vii–xxxiii). University of Chicago Press.

Jung, C. G. (1953). Two essays on analytical psychology. In *The collected works of C. G. Jung* (Vol. 7, R. F. C. Hull, Trans.). Princeton University Press.

Jung, C. G. (1956). Symbols of transformation. In *The collected works of C. G. Jung* (Vol. 5, R. F. C. Hull, Trans.). Princeton University Press.

Jung, C. G. (1959). Aion: Researches into the phenomenology of the self. In *The collected works of C. G. Jung* (Vol. 9.2, R. F. C. Hull, Trans.). Princeton University Press.

Jung, C. G. (1964). Civilization in transition. In *The collected works of C. G. Jung* (Vol. 10, R. F. C. Hull, Trans.). Princeton University Press.

Jung, C. G. (1969). The archetypes and the collective unconscious. In *The collected works of C. G. Jung* (Vol. 9.1, R. F. C. Hull, Trans.). Princeton University Press.

Jung, C. G. (1970). *Mysterium coniunctionis*: An inquiry into the separation and synthesis of psychic opposites in alchemy. In *The collected works of C. G. Jung* (Vol. 14, 2nd ed., R. F. C. Hull, Trans.). Princeton University Press.

Jung, C. G. (1977). The Tavistock lectures, Lecture III. In *The collected works of C. G. Jung: The symbolic life: Miscellaneous writings* (Vol. 18, R. F. C. Hull, Trans.). Princeton University Press.

Jung, C. G. (1983). *The essential Jung* (A. Storr, Ed., R. F. C. Hull, Trans.). Princeton University Press.

Kundera, M. (1976 [1986]). *Life is elsewhere* (P. Kussi, Trans.). Faber & Faber.

Lamont, M. (1987). How to become a dominant French philosopher: The case of Jacques Derrida. *American Journal of Sociology*, *93*(3), 584–622. https://doi.org/10.1086/228790

Merleau-Ponty, M. (1973). *The prose of the world* (C. Lefort, Trans.). Northwestern University Press. (Original work published 1969)

Moran, D., & Cohen, J. (2013). *The Husserl dictionary*. Bloomsbury.

Porterfield, S. F., Polette, K., & Baumlin, T. F. (2009). *Perpetual adolescence: Jungian analyses of American media, literature, and pop culture*. SUNY Press.

Romanyshyn, R. (2007). *The wounded researcher: Research with soul in mind*. Spring Journal Books.

Stevens, A. (2001). *Jung: A very short introduction*. Oxford University Press.

Stewart, A. F. (1993). *Faces of power: Alexander's image and Hellenistic politics*. University of California Press.

Von Franz, M. L. (1970 [1992]). *The golden ass of Apuleius: The liberation of the feminine in man*. Shambhala Publications.

Von Franz, M. L. (1970 [2000]). *The problem of the puer aeternus* (3rd ed.). Inner City Books.

Wood, D., & Bernasconi, R. (Eds.). (1988). *Derrida and différance*. Northwestern University Press.

Yeoman, A. (1998 [1999]). *Now or Neverland: Peter Pan and the myth of eternal youth: A psychological perspective on a cultural icon*. Inner City Books.

# 1

# THE NEVERLAND OF DIFFÉRANCE

## I

J. M. Barrie (1911) tells his reader in the opening lines of his classic novel *Peter and Wendy*, better known to many as *Peter Pan*, the following:

> All children, except one, grow up. They soon know that they will grow up, and the way Wendy knew was this. One day when she was two years old she was playing in a garden, and she plucked another flower and ran with it to her mother. I suppose she must have looked rather delightful, for Mrs. Darling put her hand to her heart and cried, 'Oh, why can't you remain like this for ever!' This was all that passed between them on the subject, but henceforth Wendy knew that she must grow up. You always know after you are two. Two is the beginning of the end.
>
> *(p. 1)*

All children, except one, grow up. All children, except one, are ordinary, mortal children like Wendy. But Peter Pan alone is extraordinary and immortal. By some form of magic, perhaps pixie dust, this motherless child has managed to postpone his entry into time and space and lives forever in a timeless, placeless place known as Neverland. There, all accepted laws of causality are suspended, and memory is fleeting, erased in the very act of its formation. Such is the premise of J. M. Barrie's children's tale. The flying youth is exceptional. He is not like others. He is very, very different.

Jacques Derrida (1973) tells his reader in *Speech and Phenomena* "*Différance* is neither a *word* nor a *concept*" (p. 130). All words, except one, are ordinary, human words. They have not fallen from the sky. They have their history, their reasons for

DOI: 10.4324/b23321-2

being the way they are and meaning what they mean. But one word—différance—is different. It has deferred its entry into time and space. This word that is not a word is timeless and placeless. It exists outside history's grasp. Yet it is primordial: It has always already existed. It is so primordial, in fact, that it *constitutes* both time and space, yet is subject to neither (Derrida, 1973). Différance—ostensibly ten letters forming a single linguistic unit—is, nonetheless, *avant la lettre*, before the letter, that is to say, before a concept was invented or a term created. It is even anterior to time itself (Wood, 2001). How can this be?

Both Peter Pan and différance are exceptional in similar ways. They both *disrupt sequence* as conventionally understood. Put differently, the two seem to cheat time: The former is a boy who does not age. The latter is a word that existed before words, a word that is not a word. Both exceptionalism and cheating time are well-known characteristics of the puer aeternus but perhaps more important is the fact that this figure's exceptionalism resides precisely *in* his cheating of time. He is *sui generis*, or at least believes himself to be, because he never puts his uniqueness to the test, the test of time. In this regard, both Peter and différance are the same. They remain exceptional by residing outside the temporal flux. Both are different because they defer and their deferral is absolute, which makes Peter very different from other children and différance very different from other words.

Yet what if différance, despite appearances, is not a word at all, neither spoken nor written? What is it then? In *Speech and Phenomena* (1973), Derrida tells us that it has neither existence nor essence, that it, in fact, "*is not*, does not exist" (p. 134). Yet he also describes it as a stratagem, the transgressive intent of which is to disrupt presence or, perhaps more precisely, the conceptual order sanctioned under its auspices, the generalized system of schemata he refers to as a metaphysics of presence. It is a stratagem without finality, beyond the collapse of a philosophical edifice erected upon an illusion, a blind tactic intended to bring about the end of an epoch defined by a governing thought: the illusion, the thought of presence. Because its justification is purely strategic, when the tactical ploy has served its purpose or is no longer efficacious, when the non-word and the non-concept is no longer needed, Derrida explains, it will itself be abandoned or replaced. His strategic intent is for différance to erase itself in the very enactment of its purpose. This is an intent that will express itself more overtly in other works (Derrida, 1976) through the typographical convention of *sous rature*—a placing of terms under erasure—which he adopted from the German philosopher Martin Heidegger, who deeply influenced his work.

Despite its dubious linguistic status, Derrida (1973) offers "an approximative semantic analysis" (p. 136) of his stratagem, or what he terms an "assemblage" (p. 131). This is the stratagem that will define, in one form or another, the entirety of his writings, so it is important that we understand it at the outset. What follows, at the risk of needless repetition for those familiar with deconstruction, is a brief delineation of said analysis. The term *différance*, if we can call it this, plays upon dual senses of the French verb *différir*—to defer or delay, but also, to differ or to be non-identical. Fundamental to the production of textual meaning, as deferral it alludes to a temporal lag forever at work within language: The conclusive meaning of a word, a phrase, an utterance can never be truly grasped because it is always dependent upon its relation to other words, or signs, the meaning of which cannot yet be made fully present until other words are present as well. The question of meaning is always subject to postponement. Every time we ask what a word, a sentence, or an entire text means, we can only respond with reference to other words, sentences, and texts, which themselves are subject to similar queries. Différance as deferral signifies the "interposition of a delay, the interval of a *spacing* and *temporalizing* that puts off until 'later' what is presently denied, the possible that is presently impossible" (Derrida, 1973, p. 129). Put differently, the *not yet* of différance vitiates all pretension to the full presence of meaning here and now (Schmidt, 1995).

This is, at first glance, a rather simple idea. If you feel that you have fully understood the preceding paragraph, or if you feel that you have not, the light cast by the paragraphs, pages, and chapters to follow will inevitably throw a different hue upon it. It will come into greater or lesser focus and reveal meanings that are not apparent at present. Words will acquire different connotations as they come to be used in other contexts. You will revise or abandon assumptions. Repeated examinations of the text will reveal different meanings, allusions missed, and metaphors that were not recognized as such. Words that seem odd will grow familiar and what feels familiar will come to feel foreign. Inferences that you could not possibly have made upon first reading will appear obvious in hindsight. Différance as deferral alludes to the fact that the *full* meaning of the paragraph—with every possible connotation and denotation having been recognized and explored—is an impossibility. *That* meaning will never be present.

Such a presence is an impossible possibility. Meaning is always provisional, conditional, and temporary. The decisive moment in which it can be fully adjudicated simply never comes. The gavel never sounds. There is always a step yet to be taken before we arrive at the receding horizon that is the definitive meaning of any written text or verbal utterance. What we attempt to convey is forever absent, forever elsewhere, always desired yet never obtained. The idea of a perpetual absence of something desired, as will become apparent in the chapters to follow, has a long lineage and has been called by many names. Derrida calls it différance: both a detour that aims to return to the *pleasure* of such a presence, and the impossibility of such a return. Meaning, in its fullness, is irreparably lost (Derrida, 1982 [1986]), although our longing for it persists. Returning to it is impossible, and the loss is irreparable because all conclusions are inconclusive. Closure and finality are impermanent and illusory because "every time you try to stabilize the meaning of a thing, try to fix it in its missionary position, the thing itself, if there is anything at all to it, slips away" (Derrida & Caputo, 1997, p. 31).

But the strategic assemblage of différance does not merely allude to deferral, to a semiotic *not yet* forever and always at work within texts. Derrida tells his reader by way of his approximative semantic analysis that the term (that is not a term) also alludes to a *differentiation*. Put another way, he conceives différance both spatially and temporally. Meaning, in its full presence, is both elsewhere and "elsewhen." *Spacing* is the name for this differentiation, which is inseparable from deferral. The two are, in a sense, simply aspects of the same dynamic. Spacing speaks to "time's becoming-spatial or space's becoming temporal (temporalizing)" (Derrida, 1973, p. 143).

What, precisely, is meant by "spacing" is perhaps most easily understood in terms of the iterability of the sign. The iterability of the sign refers to its capacity to be repeated in differing contexts. Although the signifier—the manifest word or linguistic unit, what you see on the page or hear—may appear seemingly identical from one instance to another, its meaning, its signified, cannot. No word, no phrase, no utterance has an identical meaning from one context to another. In this sense, the absolute, unequivocal repetition of a sign, or any meaningful utterance, is an impossibility—because the very act of repetition is transformative. Repetition is transformation. Iteration is alteration. Because the repetition of a sign is always dependent upon a (spatial) gap or (temporal) interval, it is never quite the same sign twice, much like the repetition of a piano chord will never have the same aesthetic effect if it is played within a different measure of a song, or at another tempo, or within another melody. Take any fragment of language, whether it be a single word, an entire phrase, paragraph, or work, then place it in a different context, and its meaning will be altered. Contexts, furthermore, continually change. Read a text, a sentence, or a word at one moment, and then read it at another, and its sense will have shifted. It will have been displaced. Because this is the case, the dual aspects of the sign—the signifier (the manifest word that you see or hear) and the signified (the concept or meaning)—are said to be in disunion: They do not form a coherent, lasting whole, or a single identity. They are fissured, cleaved, and cleft. Because spacing ruptures any possible unity between signifier and signified, words and their meanings are split from one another.

But spacing is more than a fundamental differentiation between signifier and signified. Its import infiltrates more than the space between different iterations of a sign, different instances of a word's usage. There is a far more radical sense to it, one that is of paramount importance to the project of deconstruction and to which we will return in greater detail throughout the present work. For Derrida, spacing is, in fact, "the common root of *all the oppositional concepts* [emphasis added] that mark our language, such as, to take only a few examples, sensible/intelligible, intuition/signification, nature/culture, etc." (Derrida, 1981 [1982], p. 9). Spacing *produces* the differences that make these oppositional pairings possible. It is, figuratively speaking, the forward slash— "/" —used above to delineate such pairings. It alludes to a diacritical dynamic forever reverberating throughout language, one that serves to split one concept from another.

As the source (or root) of oppositional pairings, it is the dehiscence, or the cleaving, that creates seemingly self-evident binaries like hot and cold, light and dark, up and down. Derrida (1981 [1982]) is careful to mention that these binaries are not "inscribed in the heavens, nor in the brain" (p. 9). They are not given by God or biology but are the consequence of the fissuring quality of the temporal, spatial displacement of différance. This distinction is crucial for a few reasons, one of which is that his attribution of these oppositional pairings to différance serves his strategic intent to erode the very foundation of the Western philosophic tradition, with all of its metaphysical assumptions, biases, and baggage, all of which ground themselves in the presumption of presence, that is to say, the presumption that such seemingly self-evident binaries are, in fact, self-evident, given, and *present*. The distinction is also crucial because the contrast with God (the heavens) gives us a sense of what différance is intended to replace. It suggests both a functional equivalence and an analogous placement within a broader structure of ideas; concepts that one might have thought of as God-given are, in fact, the result of this strange word that is not a word called différance.

Derrida (1967 [1978]) describes différance elsewhere as a "non-origin which is originary" (p. 203). Below, he (1982 [1986]) explains that différance is not merely a concept, but the very condition of possibility for all concepts *and* the reason that concepts in their full significance are never quite present:

> The signified concept is never present in and of itself, in a sufficient presence that would refer only to itself. Essentially and lawfully, every concept is inscribed in a chain or in a system with which it refers to the other, to other concepts, by means of the systemic play or differences. Such a play, *différance*, is thus no longer simply a concept, but rather the possibility of conceptuality, of a conceptual process and system in general.
>
> *(p. 11)*

The aspect of différance known as *spacing*, furthermore, refers to not only a gap between signifier and signified, between different iterations of a given sign or word, or between conceptual oppositions. It refers to a gap between language and its other. Put differently, it can be understood in terms of *intra*- and *extra*-linguistic relations, an inside and an outside of language. It is this latter sense of spacing that makes possible the former. The gap between language and its other helps legitimize the contention that oppositional pairings are not self-evident but, rather, have a common root in the temporal, spatial displacement of différance. Because meaning is conveyed and created *within* an infinite matrix of signs, its source cannot reside outside this relational web:

> The meaning of a word is defined differentially, relative to the meaning of other words. What you will never find in the dictionary is a word that detaches itself from these internal relationships and sends you sailing right out of the dictionary into a mythical, mystical thing in itself 'outside' of language, wistfully called the 'transcendental signified'.
>
> *(Derrida & Caputo, 1997, p. 100)*

The meaning that can never be reached, the 'transcendental signified,' is not only yet to come, that is to say, temporally distant; it is spatially distant as well, located in a mythical, mystical 'outside,' a place not here and one that never will be. This sense of spacing renders any contiguity between language and its other impossible because there is always an unbridgeable gap between words and the aforementioned, wistfully termed 'transcendental signified.'

Much of what I have highlighted thus far in the description of Derrida's tactical intervention—his deconstruction of what he calls the metaphysics of presence—is deeply indebted to Saussure's structuralist linguistics, at least insofar as it relies upon, furthers, and radicalizes three prominent traits of Saussure's approach: (1) his emphasis on the diacritical aspect of linguistic signs (i.e., the idea that there are no positive terms—terms that have meaning in and of themselves—but only differences between terms); (2) the division of the sign into signifier and signified (the manifest word, suffix, prefix, or linguistic unit, on the one hand, and what it means, on the other); and (3) the construal of meaning as the effect of intra-linguistic as opposed to extra-linguistic relations.

To gain a clearer understanding of what this gap between words and a transcendental signified might mean, it is worthwhile to consider another of Derrida's primary influences, Edmund Husserl. The German phenomenologist's method, despite inspiring a deep admiration in Derrida, also provoked a perhaps even deeper suspicion in him about "the very notion of presence and the fundamental role it played in all philosophies" (Derrida, as cited in Kearney, 1986, p. 114). Such a suspicion is perhaps most clearly illustrated by contemplating a foundational phrase of phenomenology, the philosophy that Husserl initiated with his work *Logical Investigations* (2001). The phrase is *to the things themselves*. It serves as a guiding notion for all philosophers who work within the phenomenological tradition. *To the things themselves* marks the starting place for all phenomenological reflection. Contrast this with Derrida's insistence that, by virtue of différance, one can never really quite get to the things themselves at all, which, at least insofar as they might be imagined to exist 'outside' of language, would appear to have a somewhat dubious or mythical existence. In other words, they are not quite *present* in the way that one might imagine. The contrast illustrates the fundamental antipathy between Derrida's deconstruction and Husserl's phenomenology (although at the time of his major work on Husserl, Derrida had not yet come to use the term deconstruction). The contrast also illustrates, as I will argue further on, an opposition or philosophical impasse that the phenomenology of Merleau-Ponty is able to overcome. Another contrast worthy of consideration in understanding the aforementioned gap between words or signifiers and a transcendental signified—the thing in itself, an ultimate referent, meaning made fully present—is to focus upon the way that Husserl and Derrida understood the terms *perception*, *phenomena*, and *primordial*. Each term might serve as a stand-in for the mythical, mystical "outside" referred to above and help us make greater sense of what is meant by such an 'outside.'

In *Speech and Phenomena* (1973), Derrida attempted to demonstrate that "the theme or import of 'pure presentation,' pure and primordial perception, full and simple presence" (p. 45n) as developed by Husserl was untenable: It contained metaphysical presuppositions that this same phenomenology intended to contest. Rather than forming a critique of metaphysics, it exemplified it, and in so doing, betrayed itself "as a moment within the history of metaphysical assurance" (p. 5). In contrast to the pure primordial perception and full and simple presence that Husserl affirmed, Derrida contended that "perception does not exist or that what is called perception is not primordial, somehow everything 'begins' by 're-presentation'" (p. 45n). There is no "thing in itself" that presents itself to us, through perception, and is later *re*-presented by us through language. Not only does perception not exist, it never has: "there never was any 'perception'; and 'presentation' is a representation of the representation that yearns for itself therein as for its own birth or its death" (Derrida, 1973, p. 103).

Our perceptions and experiences of the world are always already re-presentations. As Jürgen Habermas (1987) noted, for Derrida, experience "is indebted to an act of representation, perception is indebted to a reproducing recognition" (p. 174). Nothing is quite self-evident because evidence—which is understood as that which is perceptible, obvious, clear, or apparent—is always already vitiated, always already rendered non-evidential by virtue of this indebtedness. Perceptual presentation is a misnomer because everything begins by representation. Derrida called the mistaken belief in such a presentation *logocentrism*, a colossal blunder and delusion from which all of Western thought has suffered and continues to suffer (Johnson, 1981). Yet the supposed blunder, it should be noted, results from what we might call a nested inversion, a reversal of the presentation-representation binary that grants primacy to a term that had previously been considered secondary.

This strategic expropriation of presentation by representation—of perception by language—is a variant of the aforementioned insistence that seemingly self-evident binaries like hot and cold, light and dark, and up and down are not given by God or nature. They neither fall from the heavens nor are inscribed in the brain. In a similar vein, they are not given by our perceptions or the contours and qualities of phenomena. The radicality and importance of Derrida's subversion of the long-held assumption that perception is primordial, that it is somehow fundamental and primary, has several consequences. One immediate and significant consequence is that self-evidence, or perhaps more appropriately, 'self-evidence,' is always the result of a metaphysical heritage, an inherited history of philosophical distinctions, assumptions, and presuppositions. Simply put, it is the result of the past rather than the present.

The key philosophic elements here—oppositional concepts or binaries, metaphysical heritage, perception and its primordiality—have their mythic correlates or parallels, which we will explore in greater detail further on. For the moment, the intent is merely to delineate their outline and give a fair, albeit schematic, account of the deconstructive critique of Husserlian phenomenology. The critique is particularly damning because it undermines phenomenology's principle of principles, namely that "*immediate 'seeing,'* not merely sensuous, experiential seeing, *but seeing in the universal sense as an originally presentive consciousness of any kind whatever*, is the ultimate legitimizing source of all rational assertions" (Husserl, 2012, p. 36). Such an immediate seeing is apparent even in the word *evidence* itself, insofar as it is from the Latin *ex* plus *videntem*: 'out, out of, fully' plus the present participle of *videre* 'to see.' Evidence is what is seen. It is through this seeing, which should be understood to include other forms of perceiving like fantasizing and remembering, as well as bodily sensations, that he attempts to free philosophy of its contestable presuppositions. On his account, this seeing is made possible through what is known as the phenomenological reduction, a setting aside or bracketing of the 'natural attitude,' which is understood as inherited theoretical and philosophical preconceptions. True to the Latin roots of the word *reduction*, this refers to the restoration of, or return to, a former state, in this case, one *preexisting* the self-same philosophical distinctions, assumptions, and presuppositions that deconstruction attempts to dismantle.

To return somewhere implies that there is somewhere to return to—in this instance, a primary perception in all of its immediacy. But for Derrida, there is no such perception, at least not one that precedes the differential, deferential dynamic of différance. Without the reduction, phenomenology's primary imperative—to explain the non-evident by the evident, rather than the evident by the non-evident—is rendered inconceivable. There is no evidence, as previously understood. One does not *see* as Husserl would have it and his belief that all language and all meaning is founded on a prelinguistic strata of sense is completely delegitimized, and with it, the entire phenomenological project. Deconstruction not only disenfranchises the idea that language has its origins in a level of experience that precedes the mediation of language; it inverts this relationship so that experience—and all of the sensing, perceiving, and intuiting that this word implies—has its origins in language.

For Husserl, the medium through which we may access whatever exists for us, or may be considered valid for us, is consciousness, and this consciousness includes a prelinguistic realm of experience (Gurwitsch, 1979). His phenomenology is an attempt to describe primal impressions that are present to the consciousness of the mind or what he called the *transcendental ego*, as well as the workings of consciousness itself, but it is not an attempt to explain *the provenance* of what is present to consciousness or to delineate the unseen causes of what presents itself. It eschews any judgment as to the ultimate nature of reality (which, on Husserl's account, would itself be an incursion into the realm of metaphysics), and instead focuses upon an analysis of experience. Put differently, his phenomenology is committed to *describe* rather than *explain* what is present to consciousness. But because Derrida seeks to "insinuate language into the very functioning of consciousness itself" (Evans, 1991, p. 24), the phenomenological reduction is not possible, and its principle of principles is disqualified. Reference to phenomena or perception can be made, but they are vacuous references, always already emptied of their putative import.

The conceptual undermining of Husserl's phenomenology by Derridean semiotics represents an *acute* case of a general tendency within the linguistic turn: Denying access to any reality, external or internal, that is not linguistically mediated, said tendency undermines the supposed immediacy of sense impressions (Alderman, 2016; Busch & Gallagher, 1992; Habermas & Fultner, 2003). Différance disenfranchises the immediacy of perception by placing a web of signs between the phenomenal world and those who inhabit it. Once conceived of as present and immediate, this world is now far off, rendered distant by the belief that everything begins by representation. Nothing is quite here and quite now in the way that one might have thought. Nothing is quite *present* in the same way.

But what makes Derridean semiotics an *acute* case of this general tendency to focus on the mediating role of language and the way in which it prevents direct perception is this: As strange as it sounds, for Derrida, nothing is quite 'then' and quite 'there' or even quite 'past' in the way one might have thought. This is because the temporal distance that semiotic deferral implies reaches not only forward, but backward as well. It works to suspend both finality and incipiency and it does so preemptively. Put differently, the *not yet* of différance is coupled by an equally important *always already*. There are no true beginnings because, by the logic of this ubiquitous semiological postponement, everything is *always already not yet*. Language has no origin in perception for the same reason that it does not reach its desired destination of the thing perceived. Derrida employs the same logic regarding the origins of language that he applies to its ends: Because words cannot reach the thing itself, the transcendental signified, because they cannot refer to phenomena or perception, neither can they have arisen from a perceived world of phenomena, of things.

For Derrida, just as the conclusive moment never comes, the originary moment never was; the genesis of all meaning resides in an *absolute* past that is never present, never was present, and never could have been present (Bennington, 2010). There never has been a moment when meaning was not subject to deferral, never has been a moment when terms have referred unproblematically to some indubitable presence, some *thing in itself*, a transcendental signified as he has so wistfully termed it. *Yet, this deferral of meaning is, paradoxically, what creates it.*

In fact, it is only by way of semiotic deferral—fundamental to the creation of all significations all the time—that the idea of an origin or a beginning is even possible. This is, in a sense, the logical consequence of affirming that self-evidence is, and always has been, exclusively the result of a metaphysical heritage, the legacy of assumptions and biases bequeathed by a tradition. If this is the case, then this heritage itself cannot have been grounded in self-evidence. It cannot have arisen from something present to perception, phenomena that were immediately apparent. Différance disenfranchises not only the immediacy of perception but the possibility that perception might form a source from which language might arise. In doing so, it undermines the possibility that *pre-conceptions* might be *post-perceptions*, that is to say, it undermines the possibility that the distinctions made by the metaphysical heritage of our language might be the echo of what prior generations perceived. Nothing is self-evident and nothing ever has been.

If the reader is a bit flummoxed at this point, it is no fault of their own. The logic of différance, even on Derrida's own account, is "difficult and uncomfortable" (1973, p. 142). It is a bit like trying to understand movement in a unidirectional universe—quite a bit, in fact. This logic results in what might charitably be called paradoxes, not the least of which is that différance—as the common root of all the oppositional concepts that mark our language—is, by virtue of that fact, an *origin* of said concepts. Yet, to follow a consistent logic, it cannot be an origin in quite the same way as perception or phenomena or things themselves. For this reason, Derrida (1967 [1978]) describes différance as a "non-origin which is originary" (p. 203).

The phrase 'non-origin which is originary' merits further scrutiny. It suggests the idea of différance as a surrogate origin, a substitute for a missing primordiality. The phrase encapsulates many things at once: what deconstruction is at pains to explain in any attempt at its own self-justification; its need to extricate itself from the metaphysical heritage it seeks to dismantle; the difficulty of following its logic; and, yet again, why it represents such a challenge to Husserlian phenomenology, which was intended to be a "philosophy of the Beginning" (Husserl, 2014, p. 18). Yet it also encapsulates deconstruction's attempts to disrupt sequence or to cheat time, an attempt it shares with Peter Pan, the boy who lived in Neverland. With this latter point in mind, now is perhaps a good moment to remember that Derrida's employment of différance is both strategic and tactical. Its purpose is to disrupt a conceptual order, a generalized system of schemata, and it does so by way of a peculiar sequential, temporal logic. It is a means to an end, and the achievement of this end in no way precludes, and may even require, the erasure of différance itself. It is also a good moment to recall that, on Derrida's account, différance has neither existence nor essence; it "*is not*, does not exist" (1973, p. 134). It is not even a word at all, despite appearances.

But then how are we to judge if it is a worthy, coherent, or effective strategy? How can différance, having no essence and no existence, be adjudicated? And by extension, can the project of deconstruction be evaluated and defend itself through the terms, values, distinctions, assumptions, and presuppositions of the metaphysical heritage, the selfsame conceptual order that it seeks to undermine? Rather than attempt to answer these questions, perhaps for the moment it is best to simply ask them and note, in passing, that Derrida (1976) himself claimed that deconstruction was not a refutation of the standards of philosophical rigor, but must in fact "recognize and respect all its classical exigencies" (p. 158). Deconstruction "requires all the instruments of traditional criticism" (p. 158) and should be judged by its norms. Robert Scholes (1991), in his *Protocols of Reading*, notes that Derrida, in fact, makes a great fuss over this question of rigor and further notes that in many ways it functions within Derrida's writing as a guarantor of truth or legitimacy, much as presence or self-evidence does within the texts whose rigor he contests. That is to say, rigor is invoked in lieu of the immediacy of perception that might make certain claims self-evident.

From his earlier texts, such as *Speech and Phenomena* (1973), to somewhat later works, like *Limited Inc.* (1988), in which the term appears over twenty times, *rigor* is the standard to which Derrida holds both himself and others accountable. This is even more so the case as regards Husserl and others of his ilk—those who found their claims upon arguments of consciousness, subjectivity, perception—of whom he expects the strictest adherence to the philosophic virtues of thoroughness, precision, coherence, and non-contradiction.

Yet despite these professed expectations, even among Derrida's admirers, a good deal of disagreement exists as to the specifically *philosophical* merit of his work. Some writers, like Christopher Norris, Irene Harvey, and Rodolphe Gasché, are impressed by the coherency and consistency of his arguments, but others, like Geoffrey Hartman and Richard Rorty, are not, or are only partially so (Evans, 1991). Rorty, in fact, has suggested that Derrida's works be read *not* as philosophy but rather as a form of literary play accessible only to those adequately steeped in the philosophical tradition that he draws upon. Likewise, Paul de Man, a leading proponent of deconstruction within the United States, proposed that Derrida's reading of Rousseau should be taken as parody or fiction (Evans, 1991).

Husserl scholars generally have reacted unfavorably to Derrida's critique of phenomenology, yet his analysis has undoubtedly had a massive impact on that philosophical school (Wood, 2001). It is clear that few thinkers of the twentieth century have inspired greater disagreement, and the question as to what criteria might be used to evaluate his work has birthed schismatic allegiances of critical praise and antipathy, all of which might best be summed up in the following question: Is Derrida a rigorous philosopher or merely an erudite *enfant terrible* playing in philosophy's sandbox? Ultimately, I imagine, he may be a little bit of both.

One thing is for sure, the seemingly oxymoronic syntax of the phrase *non-origin which is originary* is the direct result of a philosophical commitment that is also a strategic requirement. Deconstruction's preemption of presentation by representation, the assertion that what is called perception is not primordial, and that somehow everything begins by re-presentation requires that non-origins be originary. When representation usurps presentation—that is, when the differential, deferential workings of language assume the primacy once granted to perception—then they assume the role of a surrogate origin, a beginning. Thus, différance, on Derrida's account, is primordial (1973). Yet, because the 're' of representation conveys the sense of *back to the original* or *to return once more*, it is difficult to conceive how this might be so, for if representation is itself originary, how can it return to what is originary? If it is an origin, how can it still be representation? The basic disruption of sequence enacted by the claim that somehow everything *begins* by representation elicits a series of questions as regards our most basic sense of temporal unfolding: How can the prior be former, the precedent be subsequent, the pre be post, and the before be after? Such questions draw attention to the nested inversion referred to earlier, a reversal of sequence embedded within deconstruction that has profound consequences.

According to the classical conception of the sign, it takes the place of a thing perceived, and substitutes for an absence. It is "both secondary and provisional: it is second in order after an original and lost presence, a presence from which the sign would be derived" (Derrida, 1973, p. 138). But because deconstruction places perception and presentation in this secondary, provisional position, by way of asserting that they were never quite present as one might have thought, it cannot later claim while maintaining logical consistency, the *presence* of différance as an origin. The grounds for denying both the presence and primordiality of perception must, inevitably, also deny the presence and primordiality of différance. For this reason, Derrida places the descriptor "*primordial*" within quotation marks when it refers to différance: The term cannot trade in the same temporal distinctions of before/after, primary/secondary, and pre/post that it seeks to disrupt. It must be before, take precedence, and be originary—but in not quite the same way as that bequeathed by the metaphysical tradition. It must be a surrogate origin: function as something that ostensibly it is not. To describe it simply as an origin, ground, or source would be to use the very sort of metaphysical terms that Derrida is deconstructing. The notion of primordiality as a beginning must be maintained somehow when it is différance that is primordial. Yet it must be negated when it is presentation, i.e., perception that is primordial. Likewise, différance cannot be a unity, an undifferentiated whole, as origins are often considered to be. This too would imply a similar logic that Derrida is trying to disrupt, one that assumes that unity precedes disunity, and that simplicity precedes differentiation.

In sum, Derrida's (1973) stratagem is an exceptional word that is not a word, one that, in fact, "*is not*, does not exist" (p. 134), yet one that nevertheless helps explain why other words never quite mean what they seem to mean. They never send us to a mythical, mystical thing in itself 'outside' of language, known as the 'transcendental signified.' This word that is not a word is an origin without quite being one. It makes time possible but does not take place in time (Wood, 2001). Thinking by way of its logic is difficult and uncomfortable. It requires that we see through a prism that inverts our most basic sense of temporal unfolding, making the prior be former, the precedent be subsequent, the pre be post, and the before be after. It also requires that we accept that nothing is really self-evident or ever has been.

Is this philosophy, or should it be read as parody, or fiction, or perhaps fairy tale? The latter option is perhaps not as implausible as it may seem. Marie-Louise von Franz, in her book *The Interpretation of Fairy Tales* (1970 [1996]), notes that such tales invoke time and place in a paradoxical way that actually serves to evoke "timelessness and spacelessness—the realm of the collective unconscious" (p. 39). The 'once upon a time' of fairy tales amounts to a forever and always that is also a never, or no time *in particular*, what most mythologists, like Mircea Eliade call "the *illud tempus*, that timeless eternity, now and ever" (p. 39). Is something akin at work in deconstruction? Does not Derrida invoke a sense of time and place—to speak of deferral already makes use of a temporal notion—only to evoke a similar timelessness and spacelessness? The answer to the question will not be given here, though it will not be deferred indefinitely. Rather, it will unfold in the pages to follow.

To understand the strategy of deconstruction and the question of originary non-origins from a perspective that is less overtly philosophical, and somewhat more literary, we will turn to the question of desire. No discussion of deconstruction is complete without it. Différance is a stratagem of many guises. Its definitions are multiple and protean, but desire inevitably shades any credible portrait. This is because, as John Caputo (2011) has so lucidly noted, the passion of deconstruction desires the impossible.

## II

To move this discussion of ideas from the realm of thought to the realm of psyche, as Hillman has entreated, and to begin to discern the myth at work within the theory, first we need a declaration of principle: *Statements about language and semiotics are also statements by and about psyche*. They are statements about soul. The differing and deferring ostensibly at work within sign systems are also, simultaneously, at work within us, at least potentially so. Deconstruction is not merely a doctrine or a technique. It is also an attitude, a disposition, a style of consciousness, and a psychological pattern endemic to human beings. Différance tells a story of frustrated desire. In this respect it is nothing new, or, at least not as new, not as profoundly and radically different and exceptional, as its adherents would have us believe. It fits a pattern and expresses an attitude, a disposition that, in its perennial appearance and reappearance, suggests something intrinsic, innate, and inherent to the human condition.

Since the dawn of the modern era, with Cervantes' great novel *Don Quixote*, knights errant have told of desire's errancy, the travails incurred in the effort to attain the unattainable *doncella*. The heroes and heroines of literature have plodded the often-torturous path of desire and its denouement, through its eventual gratification or obstruction. The perennial theme of desire and its vicissitudes is as old as literature itself. Its form changes with the ages, and yet it remains constant. The changing face of the changeless, the mutations of the immutable, and variations of the invariable all betoken an enduring identity amid difference. Thus, we hear echoes of the risible adventures of Don Quixote in the no less farcical, though far more tragic love of distant, idealized illusion in Flaubert's *Madame Bovary*, and echoes, too, in the legend of *Tristan and Iseult*, Nabokov's *Lolita*, Pasternak's *Doctor Zhivago*, and Musil's *Man Without Qualities* (De Rougemont, 1963). The chivalric romance provoked by a magical intoxicant; the reprobate affair between an aged expatriate and his pubescent stepdaughter; the epic passion made impossible by political revolution; and the incestuous love of brother and sister all suggest a congruence despite their seeming disparity. This is, arguably, the function of great literature and myth, which "makes it possible to become aware at a glance of certain types of constant relations and to disengage these from the welter of everyday appearances" (De Rougemont & Belgion, 1983, p. 18).

In *Love Declared* (1963), Denis de Rougemont, cultural theorist and author of the now classic *Love in the Western World* (De Rougemont & Belgion, 1983), describes a form of romantic desire that is predicated upon distance. He calls this romantic desire *passion*. It is a form of love that is nourished by withdrawals: In order to perpetuate and replenish itself, it must withdraw from the object of affection. The impassioned lover must remain chaste and defer consummation to kindle and rekindle desire's flame. Such a passion is aroused by the wooing of courtship, yet wanes at the blush of its own fulfillment. It eschews carnal knowledge of the other, and if this is, perchance, attained, it then withers on the vine. Insatiate it thrives; satiate it dies. The beloved must forever transcend the grasp of the impassioned lover, who can only desire the far-off prince or princess, or a beloved made inaccessible by circumstance or prohibition. The yearned-for other must be made distant by the duty of conjugal fidelity, must be too old or too young, belong to an unacceptable ethnicity or social class, or be frowned upon by one's peers. Juliet desires Romeo, and Romeo, Juliet, *because*, and not *despite*, of the distance imposed by the mutual enmity of the Montagues and Capulets. The more remote the object of affection, whether due to literal or figurative distance, the greater the love. In this regard, passion is a "desire [that] demands an Elsewhere" (De Rougemont, 1963, p. 232). Because it is predicated upon a lack of literal or perhaps figurative consummation and must remain, in some sense, virginal, such a passionate love is immature and irreal, knowing little of the reciprocal relation that characterizes true love.

The legend of Tristan and Iseult, the most paradigmatic of chivalric romances, is the most exemplary account of such a love. Although the two infatuated youths are the unwitting victims of an elixir that casts an amorous spell upon them, it is physical distance and prohibition that inspire and revive their mutual affection. What their love requires "is not one another's presence, but one another's absence" (De Rougemont & Belgion, 1983, p. 42). Tristan is duty bound to deliver Iseult to King Mark and fulfill the mission with which the king has entrusted him, for it is the king who intends to wed Iseult. Tristan's moral rectitude compels him to renounce his love. It must remain a clandestine affair of the heart, subsisting on subterfuge and guile. Upon discovery of the illicit romance (one that is more of the sentiments and spirit than of the flesh), the King banishes Tristan to a distant town. Later, the exiled youth rescues Iseult and they escape to a forest, where they are discovered by the king, sleeping with a sword separating the two, a symbol, the king surmises, of their enduring chastity.

A vast body of literature in multiple languages tells and retells the tale, and the legend varies in detail from one version to another, but threaded throughout is the sense that Tristan desires Iseult, and Iseult, Tristan, for the very reason that he cannot possess her, nor she him. All romantic heroes on De Rougemont's (1963) account are Tristan separated from Iseult. All heroines are Iseult separated from Tristan. The legend epitomizes the great passion that has informed the entire history of the modern novel and the romantic literature that predates it, reaching back at least as far as the twelfth century. De Rougemont (1963) goes so far as to christen a "Tristan archetype" (p. 43) in reference to this enduring tale of love predicated upon the literal or figurative inaccessibility of the lovers.

Although De Rougemont (1963) remains agnostic on the question of whether "passion derives from distance, or distance from passion" (p. 41), he does not equivocate in his claim that such a passion must *create distance to exalt itself.* This is, in a sense, its strategic intent. The beloved must remain distant for desire to endure. It is in this exaltation that Tristanian love shows its true stripes: *It is a love of love itself.* Like Cupid piercing his flesh with his own quiver, as recounted in *The Golden Ass of Apuleius* (Apuleius, 2013), it is a desire turned back upon itself. In this regard, romantic lovers "love love more than the object of love" (De Rougemont & Belgion, 1983, p. 50). In fact, therein lies the passion:

> Passion means suffering, something undergone, the mastery of fate over a free and responsible person. To love love more than the object of love, to love passion for its own sake, has been to love to suffer and to court suffering all the way from Augustine's *amabam amare* down to modern romanticism. Passionate love, the longing for what sears us and annihilates us in its triumph. . . . Hardly anything could be more tragic.
>
> *(De Rougemont & Belgion, 1983, p. 50)*

Distance serves the purpose of passion's self-exaltation, one that courts suffering and death. But why? Why is it that, in its own self-adoration, it simultaneously seeks life's negation? Because the love of "profound woe and despair" (De Rougemont & Belgion, 1983, p. 311), exemplified in Tristan's very name, which is itself a cognate of the Latin word for *sorrow*, is a limitless aspiration. Its destructiveness lies in its boundlessness. Because it precludes its own fulfillment, it is an impossible love, at odds with itself. As in the deeper levels of hell depicted by the Buddhist *Bardo Thodol*, in which those with insatiable appetites are tortured by having long throats and tiny mouths, the unequal equation of desire and its fulfillment leads to suffering (Van Scott, 1999). Appetites repeatedly provoked but never satisfied that on principle must remain insatiate cause suffering and sickness, even unto death, as Kierkegaard would have it. Love as passion, on this account, glorifies destruction and even idealizes it. Unchecked, it is love in its most demonic aspect, its most malignant form. It is what the object relations theorists Ronald Fairbairn and Harry Guntrip would have called "love made hungry" (Guntrip, 1992, p. 24), a love caught between a drive toward the beloved and a drive away.

In *Beyond Romance*, the philosopher M. C. Dillon (2001) describes a similar love, invoking the same chivalric tradition of Tristan and Iseult, Lancelot and Guinevere, Abelard and Heloise: This is a love that by way of distance and prohibition also beckons tragedy to itself. It "loves the prohibited object because it is prohibited" (p. 20) and thrives on dissatisfaction, swelling within the "immanent fantasy of the lover rather than the transcendent reality of the beloved" (p. 17). This type of love is not, however, merely an artifact from a far-off, or even recent past, nor is it a relic of troubadour lore, nor the tired trope of great works of a modernity now bygone. Rather, it is fully contemporary, perhaps even quintessentially so. On his account, it is endemic to a "postmodern erotic pessimism [that] offers another variant of the same structure: the satisfaction of desire is the death of desire" (p. 60). Despite this fact, or perhaps in support of it, the romantic love of distance and obstruction also appears "in times and places far removed from the court of the Countess of Champagne. The rape or abduction of Helen by Paris recounted in Homer in the Iliad has romantic tendrils that reach back into the murk of prehistory" (p. 50).

Into this murk we will now descend, tethered to a term that perhaps will make this descent less vertiginous. It is the Greek word *pothos*—the "longing towards the unattainable, the ungraspable, the incomprehensible, that idealization which is attendant upon all love and which is always beyond capture" (Hillman, 1975, p. 53). Pothos, one of many possible manifestations of eros, personifies a particular form of desire: a desire for what is absent. (Illbruck, 2012; Stewart, 1993). The absence can be temporal or spatial and the desired object can exist in the past or future. It is the Tristanian love identified by Rougement, although it predates Tristan by many centuries (Hillman, 1997). Plato speaks of it in his *Cratylus*, and it can also be found in Homer's *Odyssey* (Whitmarsh, 2011). In fact, all odysseys are imbued with it. As a persistent feature of the Greek tradition, present in the *Iliad*, the Dionysian trek through Hades in search of Euripides, and Alexander's dream of the conquest of distant lands, it is the relationship between pothos and its satisfaction that forms "one of the most fundamental models for Greek narrative" (Whitmarsh, 2011, p. 142). It is also the insatiable yearning that characterizes the *puer aeternus* and *puella aeterna* (Hillman, 1975; Hillman & Slater, 2005): You can hear it in the echoes of little orphan Annie's bellowing ode to the ever-longed-for tomorrow, always a day away. The aspects of pothos most relevant here, for the present discussion, are those of the *absence of an object* and the *impossibility of attainment*.

As a desire for something past, pothos forms the basis of nostalgia and was thus understood to be antithetical to happiness. Ancient Greeks associated it with destruction, both for the desirer and for that which is desired. Nostalgia, which combines the Greek words for return, *nostos*, and suffering, *algos*, is the suffering provoked by an unappeased yearning to return (Kundera & Asher, 2003). A destabilizing and disconcerting emotion, pothos often foretells tragedy for those possessed of it (Whitmarsh, 2011).

Imagined through the mythic figure of the eternal youth, différance is a manifestation of this figure's voracious yet unrequited yearning; within the confines of the logic of semiotic deferral, the term *transcendental signified* can only allude to what is both absent and unattainable. Therein lies the aforementioned wistfulness with which Derrida imbued the term—to be wistful is to be filled with nostalgia, filled with a pensive and melancholic longing. If, according to the logic of semiotic deferral, "the thing itself always escapes" (Derrida, 1973, p. 104), this implies that it is, nevertheless, always pursued, always desired. Consequently, there is an insatiate hunger and unquenchable thirst in différance. The stratagem of the deferral of meaning in its plenitude is both an expression of the homelessness of the inquiring intellect and its desire for home. Despite its pretense to the contrary—as a means of undermining the very idea of an origin—it reflects a nostalgia for origins. The seemingly oxymoronic syntax of the phrase *non-origin which is originary* is not only the direct result of a philosophical commitment and a strategic requirement, one that admits to a certain contradiction; it is also a phrase that admits to a certain affliction—that of an unappeased yearning to return. Every time that it is invoked, one can hear both desire at a distance and the impossibility of that desire's fulfillment.

The case that I am making here is that the claim that the transcendental signified will always and forever remain transcendent is not merely a statement regarding semiotics. It is also a claim regarding the human heart, and a veiled, perennial story in a clever disguise. So is the belief that the living present is "*in fact*, really, effectively, etc., deferred *ad infinitum*" (Derrida, 1973, p. 99). Such claims and beliefs are not grounded, or are only grounded tangentially, in the logical consequence or the inevitable conclusion of an argument. The assertion of the signified's absolute difference and distance from the signifier, the assertion that the two—word and meaning—are cleft by an unbridgeable abyss, is the consequence of a psychological pattern, as is the attempt to usurp the idea of primordiality. Literature and myth the world over, time and again, have made this pattern evident. As De Rougemont (1983) has pointed out, this is their function: To make us aware of certain types of constant relations and disengage them from the welter of everyday appearances. Through such a disengagement, a pattern of relations becomes clear: The temporal and spatial distance separating signifier and signified, word and meaning, language and its origins is the same distance that separated Tristan from Iseult. The characters in the story of an insuperable distance have changed their names, but the outlines of the drama remain relative constants. They still tell the tale of the same impossible love.

With these reflections in mind, the argument against the phenomenological reduction as conceived by Husserl, that is to say, the argument against a return to an original, primordial perception, is not a foregone conclusion. Or, put differently, it is foregone for reasons other than those that are claimed. The seemingly inevitable and absolute dissociation of signifier and signified is not warranted by rigorous argument, nor is the ostensible inaccessibility of a realm of prelinguistic experience. References to phenomena and perception are not vacuous or voided of their putative import, at least not for the reasons given. Deconstruction does, as Caputo (2011) claimed, desire the impossible. But the consequences of this fact are formidable and inevitably call into question the validity of deconstructive logic itself, with its pretense to recognize and respect all the classical demands of philosophic reason and traditional criticism.

By way of the postulates of semiotics, différance articulates a wanderlust and proclaims, perhaps tragically, the very impossibility of its fulfillment, because the boon of meaning in its plenitude is, on principle, always to be had elsewhere and at another time, be it past or future, but certainly not now. The promise of a living present will be forever deferred. Seen through the prism that reveals myth even within the realm of philosophic, semiotic theory or stratagem, the signifier's failure to reach the transcendental signified reflects not only nostalgia but also a subtle duplicity. Différance is the repeated invocation of something that can never be possessed, can never be made present, because it "suspends the accomplishment or fulfillment of 'desire' or 'will'" (Derrida, 1973, p. 136) and by definition "carries desire or will out in a way that annuls or tempers their effect" (p. 136). A double bind doubly bound, différance summons what it denies and conjures what it negates. It "produces what it forbids, making possible the very thing that it makes impossible" (Derrida, 1976, p. 143). As a desire that defers its own consummation, it is a want that is at odds with itself (Dillon, 1995, 2001). Like the yearning to be elsewhere, it cannot be satisfied, even momentarily, because one's very presence makes the *elsewhere* into a *here*, and the future *then* into a present *now*.

If the eternal youth, by way of the pining that is pothos, is driven "to inquire, quest, travel, chase, search, to transgress all limits" (Hillman & Slater, 2005, p. 187), then Derridean deferral is a conceptual correlate of this drive, at least insofar as it speaks to a forever renascent pursuit of meaning that is as imperative as it is unappeasable. Such is the duplicitous desire of the eternal youth, which also must suspend its fulfillment, and temper or annul its effect. Tristan desires Iseult—whom he cannot have—as language desires the signified that forever eludes it. This elusion is the imperative of a love that is at odds with itself. *It is its strategic intent:* When one's pleasure lies in the pursuit rather than the capture, prolonging pleasure requires postponing the apprehension of what is ostensibly pursued. The signified *must* remain utterly transcendent, distant, absent; the referent, the thing itself, the living present *must*, by design, exceed the grasp of the language that would hope to attain it. All of these things must remain there, in the realm of the transcendent, just beyond our grasp, out of a psychological necessity.

Understood as pothos, différance as a "non-origin which is originary" (Derrida, 1967 [1978], p. 203) reflects a duplicitous desire that both yearns to return to origins and also prohibits the return. Like a Freudian parapraxis, it suggests a dual intention. Such an originary non-origin reflects the dueling imperatives of an impossible want, one that must move toward its object and must, simultaneously, remain distant from it. Deconstruction's preemption of presentation by representation—the assertion that what is called perception is not primordial, and that somehow everything begins by re-presentation—requires that non-origins be originary. It reflects a desire that is nostalgic and ambivalent, one that yearns to return home, yet prevents the return. The desire is the strategy, and the strategy is the desire. The name of this strategic desire is multiple: For the Greeks it was pothos. Others have called it passion. One of its more recent incarnations goes by the name of différance.

These dueling imperatives find their expression in numerous typological strategies that deconstruction employs to simultaneously evoke and deny, suggest and refute the ideas of both origin and presence. Quotation marks, italics, parenthesis, and an erasure of terms (*sous rature*) all reflect a form of eros that longs for what it cannot, or will not, have. Derrida does not merely deny origins, but also pursues them and even, in the words of philosopher Edward Casey (1984, p. 602), "clandestinely commemorates them—so long as they are placed under the suspension of double marks (quotation marks, parentheses, and those crossings-out which are a legacy from Heidegger)." The suspension of double marks, as is often required in reference to "primordiality," to give but one example, not only allows the clandestine commemoration, it is, in a sense, the commemorative act; it reflects both the longing for origins, for home, for beginnings, and the futility of this longing.

The trifecta of nostalgia, destructiveness, and a dual imperative that characterize both pothos and différance is perhaps best brought into relief by way of this fragment from *Margins of Philosophy*:

> We must not hasten to decide. How are we to think simultaneously, on the one hand, différance as the economic detour which, in the element of the same, always aims at coming back to the pleasure or the presence that have been deferred by (conscious or unconscious) calculation, and, on the other hand, *différance* as the relation to an impossible presence, as expenditure without reserve, as the irreparable loss of presence, the irreversible usage of energy, that is, as the death instinct, and as the entirely other relationship that apparently interrupts every economy?
>
> *(Derrida, 1982 [1986], p. 19)*

In response to Derrida's query '*How are we to think . . .*', I would like to offer that we think by way of a figure of archetypal provenance—that of the eternal youth with his unique form of desire. With him in mind, the aforementioned economic detour, the conscious or unconscious calculation, and the sense of impossibility all bespeak a strategic desire that is at odds with itself and dissimulates itself. It is the strategic desire of a dual and dueling imperative, one that seeks what it cannot or will not have, one that defers the attainment of what is ostensibly desired. This desire, known by many names and chronicled through the ages, aims to return, yet purposely defers the return. The reference to the impossibility of presence and irreparable loss echoes nostalgia and the suffering provoked by an unappeased yearning to return. Completing the trifecta, there is the destructiveness of the death instinct that, on this account, involves an irreversible use of energy, the utter depletion and expenditure of forces, the result, apparently, of a desire that requires endless detours and is ultimately doomed to fail.

## References


Alderman, B. (2016). *Symptom, symbol, and the other of language: A Jungian interpretation of the linguistic turn*. Routledge.

Apuleius. (2013). *The golden ass* (S. Ruden, Trans.). Yale University Press. (Original work published c. late 200 AD)

Barrie, J. M. (1911). *Peter and Wendy*. Charles Scribner's Sons.

Bennington, G. (2010). *Not half no end: Militantly melancholic essays in memory of Jacques Derrida*. Edinburgh University Press.

Busch, T., & Gallagher, S. (Eds.). (1992). *Merleau-Ponty, hermeneutics, and postmodernism*. State University of New York Press.

Caputo, J. D. (2011). The return of anti-religion: From radical atheism to radical theology. *Journal for Cultural and Religious Theory*, *11*(2), 32–125.

Casey, E. S. (1984). Origin(s) in (of) Heidegger/Derrida. *The Journal of Philosophy*, *81*(10), 601–610. https://doi.org/10.2307/2026262

De Rougemont, D. (1963). *Love declared: Essays on the myths of love*. Pantheon Books.

De Rougemont, D., & Belgion, M. (1983). *Love in the western world*. Princeton University Press.

Derrida, J. (1967 [1978]). *Writing and difference* (A. Bass, Trans.). University of Chicago Press.

Derrida, J. (1973). *Speech and phenomena, and other essays on Husserl's theory of signs*. Northwestern University Press.

Derrida, J. (1976). *Of grammatology* (G. C. Spivak, Trans.). Johns Hopkins University Press. (Original work published 1967)

Derrida, J. (1981 [1982]). *Positions* (A. Bass, Trans.). University of Chicago Press.

Derrida, J. (1982 [1986]). *Margins of philosophy* (A. Bass, Trans.). University of Chicago Press.

Derrida, J. (1988). *Limited Inc* (A. Bass & S. Weber, Trans.). Northwestern University Press.

Derrida, J., & Caputo, J. D. (1997). *Deconstruction in a nutshell: A conversation with Jacques Derrida*. Fordham University Press.

Dillon, M. C. (1995). *Semiological reductionism: A critique of the deconstructionist movement in postmodern thought*. State University of New York Press.

Dillon, M. C. (2001). *Beyond romance*. State University of New York Press.

Evans, J. C. (1991). *Strategies of deconstruction: Derrida and the myth of the voice*. University of Minnesota Press.

Guntrip, H. (1992). *Schizoid phenomena, object relations and the self*. Karnac Books.

Gurwitsch, A. (1979). *Phenomenology and theory of science*. Northwestern University Press.

Habermas, J. (1987). *The philosophical discourse of modernity: Twelve lectures*. MIT Press.

Habermas, J., & Fultner, B. (2003). *Truth and justification*. MIT Press.

Hillman, J. (1975). *Loose ends: Primary papers in archetypal psychology*. Spring Publications.

Hillman, J. (1997). *The myth of analysis: Three essays in archetypal psychology*. Northwestern University Press.

Hillman, J., & Slater, G. (2005). *Senex & puer*. Spring Publications.

Husserl, E. (2001). *Logical investigations* (Vol. 1, D. Moran, Ed.). Routledge.

Husserl, E. (2012). *Ideas pertaining to a pure phenomenology and to a phenomenological philosophy: First book: General introduction to a pure phenomenology*. Springer Netherlands.

Husserl, E. (2014). *Ideas: General introduction to pure phenomenology*. Routledge.

Illbruck, H. (2012). *Nostalgia: Origins and ends of an unenlightened disease*. Northwestern University Press.

Johnson, B. (1981). Introduction. In J. Derrida (Ed.), *Dissemination* (pp. vii–xxxiii). University of Chicago Press.

Kearney, R. (1986). *Modern movements in European philosophy*. Manchester University Press.

Kundera, M., & Asher, L. (2003). *Ignorance*. HarperCollins Publishers.

Schmidt, L. K. (1995). *The specter of relativism: Truth, dialogue, and phronesis in philosophical hermeneutics*. Northwestern University Press.

Scholes, R. (1991). *Protocols of reading*. Yale University Press.

Stewart, A. F. (1993). *Faces of power: Alexander's image and Hellenistic politics*. University of California Press.

Van Scott, M. (1999). *The encyclopedia of Hell: A comprehensive survey of the underworld*. St. Martin's Press.

Von Franz, M. L. (1970 [1996]). *Interpretation of fairy tales*. Shambhala Publications.

Whitmarsh, T. (2011). *Narrative and identity in the ancient Greek novel: Returning romance*. Cambridge University Press.

Wood, D. (2001). *The deconstruction of time*. Northwestern University Press.

# 2

# TRACES OF THE HOLLOWED NOW

## I

One can argue that différance as doomed desire does not equate to deconstruction as failed philosophy. If, in fact, the desire to reach the transcendental signified is fated to fail and if, in fact, to reach the things themselves is truly an impossibility, is this not evidence of deconstruction's lucidity? There is a good deal of merit, and much of it undeniable, in the logic of semiotic deferral and differentiation, the temporal and spatial workings of signifiers and signifieds: Conclusions *are* inconclusive. Words never quite mean what we want them to, or they mean quite more, and this meaning is protean: Like Proteus himself, that old man of the sea from Greek lore shape-shifting to avoid capture who was as slippery as the seals that he tended, meaning morphs in myriad ways. There is some truth to the idea that no word, no phrase, no utterance has an *absolutely* identical significance from one context to another. The repetition of a sign is always dependent upon a (spatial) gap or (temporal) interval, and in this sense, it is never quite the same sign twice. Context changes the significance of words, and contexts are far more fluid than our desire for certainty and fixity would have us imagine. Interpretations *are* provisional, conditional, temporary, and makeshift shelters from doubt falter from even the feeblest breeze of ever-changing circumstance. Concepts creep, albeit slowly, and signifiers slide, albeit in due course. The paradox of arriving anywhere is that it also marks a place of departure. This is true not only of literal, geographic space, but also of the metaphoric space of interpretation: Arriving at one interpretation eventually leads to yet others. There is something to be said for the undeniable validity of the 'not yet' of différance and the way that it undermines all pretension to the full presence of meaning and certainty. Words convey so little. They satisfy our desire for communication so poorly.

DOI: 10.4324/b23321-3

One might also argue another point, no less relevant, by way of corollary questions arising from our current account: Are the resemblances described thus far valid, those between the form of desire attributed to the figure of the eternal youth, on the one hand, and deconstruction, on the other? Or are they just convenient likenesses twisted into the service of an argument, superficial similarities drawn between essentially disparate forms? Jung's technique of amplification, which seeks to draw parallels between seemingly dissimilar materials, unlike the Freudian technique of free association, requires one to return time and again to the object of interpretation. It is not entirely free. This doubling back was essential, from Jung's point of view, so that interpretation did not simply amount to a purely subjective flight of fancy, unmoored from any objective element whatsoever. Perhaps then it is best that we turn once more to the object of the present amplification, the original texts to which we are drawing parallels. It is only fair that we restore Derrida's strategy to its intended context and purpose, and only fair to move it from the realm of psyche back to the realm of ideas from which it came. After all, although statements about language and semiotics may also be statements by and about psyche, they are also what they say they are, and should be treated as such.

With that in mind, certain elements of Derrida's thought need to be explained in greater detail. How can it be that perception does not exist or that what is called perception is not primordial? How can it be that somehow everything begins by re-presentation? How is it that there is no 'thing in itself' that presents itself to us, through perception, and is later *re*-presented by us through language? Is nothing ever self-evident because language itself renders it non-evidential? Derrida's answers to such questions, from my perspective, are counterintuitive and result in seemingly incongruous affirmations that create a certain cognitive dissonance. So, we need to go beneath the surface, beneath the strata of deconstructive thought that goes by the name of representation, down to a layer that would account for that which makes representation possible. A great weight rests upon the 'somehow' of the claim that perception is not primordial and that somehow everything begins by re-presentation. Exactly how is this possible? As before, Derrida's response will involve an argument as regards sequence, that is to say, temporal unfolding. The undermining of primordiality and perception is carried out through a critique of time, which is always an undermining of the idea of *presence* as traditionally understood.

He attempts to lighten the weight of this *somehow*—which places representation at the beginning—by the introduction of *the trace*, a concept that, again, results from his engagement with Husserl's phenomenology. As with his indebtedness to Saussure's structuralist linguistics, Derrida's debt to Husserl furthers, radicalizes, and yet in many ways undermines the philosophical project of the latter. In this regard, the trace shares many parallels, both formal and functional, with what Husserl called *protention* and *retention*, two terms by which he attempted to explain our sense of temporal unfolding, that is to say, how it is that we perceive time. Yet the similarities at the level of form and function belie profound dissimilarities at the level of content. This, parenthetically, can be said of much regarding Derrida and Husserl: Often in reading the former, it is difficult to discern where the latter's thought begins or ends. Derrida at times appears to be engaged in "high-grade mimicry of transcendental arguments" (Wood, 2001, p. 274) like those of Husserl: What might be called his linguistic transcendentalism shadowboxes against the backdrop of phenomenology with such alacrity that the two are not always easily discernible.

On Husserl's account, the living present—the milieu within which perception takes place—has a tripartite structure consisting of retentions, primal impressions, and protentions: Perception happens within a temporal horizon of recollection and anticipation, immediate memory and expectation. Echoes of moments past and future reverberate throughout the here and now. What happened a moment ago and what may happen a moment from now, moments that are no longer and that are not yet, gather within the present and coalesce in the here and now. Past experience is always present in its absence, as is the expectation of future experience, which acts like "a shadow projected ahead, an inverted memory" (Husserl, 2001, p. 424). Life itself is a stream of lived experiences and they are strung together by way of this tripartite structure.

This same gathering, furthermore, takes place within moments other than the living present: The immediate past likewise retained the past that preceded it, past moments compounded by other past moments, *ad infinitum*. Likewise, pending future moments exist within a horizon of expectation no less infinite. Furthermore, within past moments congregate pending future moments, and these moments, yet to come, retain within themselves their own pasts, so that the present is perceived as the future of those past moments. Moreover, as each moment arrives, preceding moments are modified by present moments, which are themselves pregnant with expectations fulfilled and unfulfilled.

For Husserl, the living present, with its originary (or primal) impressions, involved an *unceasing synthesis* and gathering of retentional vestiges and protentional openings that enrichen it, giving context and significance to perception in the here and now. Without this synthesis, perception would hardly be possible or meaningful. Protention and retention help form an indissoluble unity of the living present, providing it with a certain cohesiveness and perceptual continuity. The retentional horizon of the past and the protentional horizon of the future grant the impressional present a thickness and extension it would not otherwise have. The present is not an isolated and therefore meaningless point, not a discrete, clearly delineated unit, separated from other moments, but a unitary and unifying stream, a transitional synthesis of past and future in which perception takes place.

The thickness of the living present allows for a sense of temporal and perceptual unfolding without which, for example, the perception of a melody would not be possible, for it requires that we hold within our awareness both vestiges of the notes that have sounded and anticipations of notes to come. The apprehension of tonal sequence requires that perceptual presence contain within itself memory and expectation as it segues from past to future. As Derrida (1973) notes, for Husserl, "it belongs to the essence of lived experiences that they must be extended in this fashion, that a punctual phase cannot be [simply] for itself" (Derrida quoting Husserl, p. 61).

This temporal extension granted to the present through protention and retention is also, in a sense, spatial. The transitional synthesis of moments is a synthesis of perspectives, allowing for one perspective to pass seamlessly into another, as seamlessly as a ball flies through the air: When we witness such an occurrence, we do not see a collection of images passing one after another in quick succession, but a flow, a flux, a smooth movement without fault lines. Nor do we see a series of snapshots, each of a different ball, appearing in different locations and moments, because the protentional, retentional structure of consciousness provides perceptual continuity and thereby allows for the constitution of temporal objects or object permanence: The perception of the enduring presence of an object through different temporal phases, its perceived identity over time. Protention and retention act like threads of continuity that allow us to confer an *enduring identity* over manifold moments and infer the abiding phenomenal and perceptual presence of persons and things, although they appear at different times and places.

This includes a person's own self-identity: Without protention and retention there could be no continuity of self, no awareness of a person's own abiding individuality. Husserl's theory was not merely a way of describing the temporal givenness of objects, that is to say, a way of explaining the awareness of objects with temporal extension, but also a description of the temporal self-givenness of consciousness itself (Zahavi, 2005). Merleau-Ponty (1964), in describing this perspectival synthesis notes that it "constitutes the unity of perceived objects" and that it is not "an intellectual synthesis" (p. 15) requiring mediation by way of signifiers or representation. It is perceptual. Signifiers are not a condition of possibility for the identification of an object from one moment to another, just as they are not the condition of possibility for identifying one's own consciousness.

Put differently, the 're' of retention should not be confused with the 're' of representation. Signifiers do not provide a sense of perceptual continuity or the enduring identity of objects over time. My perception of a single ball flying through the air—as opposed to a series of fragmented perceptions with no relation one to another—does not depend upon the articulation that "the ball is flying through the air." It requires no linguistically mediated mentation whatsoever. Rather, it is a bodily, perceptual form of synthesis, a seamless layering of moments absent the need of any intellectual act, intercession by language, or reliance upon a conceptual order. In fact, Husserl's term 'lived experiences,' as cited by Derrida earlier, was intended to speak to precisely this. All experience is, of course, lived. But Husserl intended the term to refer specifically to *pre-reflective* experience, experience in its immediacy before it has been reflected upon. In his words, lived experience is "pregiven to the I" (Zahavi, citing Husserl, 2005, p. 51). In a similar vein, he used the term 'life world' or *Lebenswelt* to refer to the world as immediately or directly experienced in everyday life, as opposed to the 'objective' world as conceived by the sciences.

For Derrida, as admirable as Husserl's analysis of time-consciousness may have been, it contained within itself conclusions that the latter failed to ascertain. His critique of Husserlian phenomenology proceeds by way of simply making manifest what is already there in latent form, teasing out its inherent implications. The thickness of the present moment that, for Husserl, provides a form of temporal and spatial continuity also implies a dependence of the living present upon moments other than itself: The now can only appear insofar as it is compounded with past and future. The present moment is an amalgam of moments, a composite of memory and anticipation. For Derrida, this implies that the present is not so much informed or enriched by moments past and future, but that it is always already haunted by those moments. As such, it is not simple and pristine but differentiated and corrupted. Husserl's protention and retention amount to an inclusion of the just-past and the just-future within the immediacy of the living present. The consequence of this inclusion is that there is no unspoiled present that is not *always already* contaminated by moments other than itself. By virtue of this, the identity of the present as present, as that which is taking place in the here and now, is subverted by an alien element, undermined by alterity. It is not what it appeared to be.

On Derrida's reading, this fundamental otherness at the heart of the now precludes any possibility of it serving as source or origin as Husserl had envisioned. Because its own self-identity as presence has been undermined and its purported primacy and primordiality has been disqualified, the living present can no longer serve as a source of certitude. The moment that, for Husserl, is pregnant with past and future is, for Derrida, and by virtue of this same logic, hollowed out by past and future. The dynamics of protention and retention serve the former to envision the now in its synthesizing, unifying aspect as a moment that provides continuity, while the latter envisions the now as dispersed, dissipated, dissociated from within. It is radically deficient, emptied of its pretense and privilege as a source of sense and meaning. On his account, although we can continue to use the language of perception and phenomena, with its presumption to immediacy, such language has been *de facto* emptied of its time-honored illusion of presence and thereby deprived of its previous role as origin. Presence is an illusion. What appears to be here and now is not so much enriched but rather corrupted by the elsewhere and the elsewhen. In a similar vein, experience of oneself or what Derrida (1973) would call auto-affection is likewise contaminated by an element of otherness and, as such, is a hetero-affection. It is not what it appears to be.

Husserl provides the opportunity for such a reading, one that sees difference within the living present—a fundamental otherness at the heart of the now—by way of an unresolved tension within his description of temporal continuity on the one hand and his vocabulary of temporal atomism on the other. Derrida exploits this opportunity that, on his reading, is decisive in undermining Husserl's project. There is a cleft that separates Husserl's understanding of time as continuity and his description of the present moment as point of origin, precisely because it is a *point*, it is an instant. The former perspective portrays the present moment as permeable and diffuse, without definitive beginning or end, while the latter portrays it as impermeable and encapsulated, as succinct and distinct as a *point* in time or the period at the end of this sentence. And, by his own account, it is the latter, more 'punctual' portrayal of the perceptual moment, that must prevail. Thus, for example, he speaks of "the individuality of the time-points as they sink back into the past" (Husserl, 1999, p. 208) and, more importantly, claims that "the actual *now* is necessarily something punctual and remains so, *a form that persists through continuous change of matter*" (Derrida, 1973, p. 63 quoting Husserl).

The continuity of the present moment that the concepts of retention and protention provide is at odds with the discontinuity of its punctuality. The present moment has no unambiguously discernible beginning or end, so to clearly differentiate it from moments other than itself is not, in principle, possible. This is, for Derrida, not something of secondary or tertiary importance, a mere oversight as regards careful descriptive language. Nor is it indicative of an inevitable paradox that is, nevertheless, inconsequential as regards Husserl's project. It is more akin to a linchpin without which the entire unity and cohesiveness of the project fall apart.

Such observations provide Derrida an opportunity to see a differing and deferring movement of discrete, individual moments within the seamless temporal stream. He applies the same analytical wedge that splits signifier from signified, and even signs from different iterations of themselves, to the question of temporal continuity. He transfers his differential, deferential logic from signs to moments: Just as no sign is identical to itself, no moment is. Just as the full meaning of a word or text never arrives, no moment does. But even to say that he has 'transferred a logic' is a bit misleading because the strategy of différance is as temporal as it is semiotic. It is a ploy utilized to disrupt both a particular understanding of time and a particular understanding of language. If time is a language, each moment is non-identical to itself. Furthermore, the present moment is not the present moment in the same way that the bipartite sign is not the sign it purports to be: Signifiers are not identical with signifieds.

No less troubling than the observation that one can see a differing and deferring movement of discrete moments within an ostensibly seamless temporal stream is the observation that there also appears to be a stream within each moment: The punctuality of the now, its pointedness, on Derrida's reading, requires that it be as instantaneous as the blink of an eye. But there is duration even to the blink, and within that duration there is memory and anticipation, clouding the vision and calling its perception into question:

> As soon as we admit this continuity of the now and the not-now, perception and nonperception, in the zone of primordiality common to primordial impression and primordial retention, we admit the other into the self-identity of the Augenblick; nonpresence and nonevidence are admitted into the blink of an instant.
>
> *(Derrida, 1973, p. 65)*

In calling attention to the issue of temporal continuity vis-à-vis divisibility, Derrida points to a conundrum that is infinitely exploitable. This is the conundrum to which he will return time and again: Dueling conceptions of the present that make time itself an impossible possibility because it "is continuous according to the now and divided according to the now" (Derrida, 1982 [1986], p. 54). These dueling conceptions will also form the basis of his critique of Aristotle, for whom "time is divisible into parts" (Derrida, 1982 [1986], p. 40), yet also for whom the inverse hypothesis is true: Time is not divisible into parts, or 'now moments.' Every claim that there is duration within the blink of an eye provides an opportunity for the counterclaim that there are blinks of an eye within any duration, and this tit-for-tat would seem to undermine the purported primacy and primordiality of presence upon which Husserl's entire project depends.

Derrida exploits this conundrum in a way that warrants particular attention. He does not content himself by merely highlighting a logical inconsistency in Husserl's thought or a potentially dizzying cul-de-sac of cognition implicit in such issues. Rather, he uses it as leverage to make an assertion with profound implications. The other within the identity of the blink, the alterity or non-presence introduced by implication of Husserl's logic of protention and retention, not only infiltrates and undermines presence, it is, on Derrida's account, its necessary *precondition*. Presence is not only infiltrated by its other, it is parasitic to it, even *derived from it*, as is perception from nonperception. The present moment is not only not a source, not an origin, it is a by-product, an after-effect. Such a claim corresponds to a general strategy of deconstruction that, in making what is secondary primary, also makes what is derivative constitutive. The alterity at the heart of the now "not only must inhabit the pure actuality of the now but must constitute it through the very movement of differance it introduces" (Derrida, 1973, p. 67).

But why *must* it? Why must différance not only inhabit but actually *constitute* presence? And by invoking the theme of constitution, is Derrida not, a bit surreptitiously, also invoking the same transcendental arguments that he has set out to critique? These questions, veiled in a more temporal vocabulary, merely give fresh clothing to a familiar query put forth previously: How can non-origins be originary? Now, as then, we may ask what warrants such assertions. What rationale might justify such constitutional claims? How can absolute deferral and differentiation create presence or at least the illusion of presence? How can différance act as a surrogate origin without being one? Also, is it not possible to accept Derrida's critique of Husserl's conception of presence without accepting his own constitutional claims?

Such questions—and even more so Derrida's ripostes—require an almost vertiginous level of abstraction, a disorienting degree of intellection that can leave one light-headed in the thinning ether of ideas, and one might wonder whether this is not the intention—to leave the reader without nary a foothold on the firm ground of any certainty. The means by which Derrida puts forth his argument throughout his career, at times, offer little to grab hold of, not even a meager crevice to grip: His perplexing syntax, filled with parenthetical phrases and qualifications, themselves qualified; subordinate clauses rendered superordinate by subsequent clauses; self-reflective asides indicative of a persistent philosophic vigilance; erudite, seemingly superfluous allusions that later prove substantive; literary puns, double entendres, and general lexiphanic fun, much of which constitute subtle tactical ploys; innumerable graphic and lexical innovations as well as a formidable vocabulary drawing upon a deep reserve of semantic and etymological associations, all of these do a great deal to both impress and confuse the reader, but do little, in my view, to warrant philosophical claims. One is, having traversed the perilous trek of Derrida's argument, left breathless and vulnerable to the sheer force of his assertion: Différance *must* constitute presence. Bald assertions aside, and mindful that deconstruction does not refute the standards of philosophical rigor, the reader can only resume the perilous trek.

Derrida claims that différance constitutes presence by way of something called the *trace*. This trace shares a marked similarity with Husserl's protentional, retentional logic as regards its form and function, but it is belied by a profound dissimilarity as regards its content. What Derrida calls the trace allows for a sense of temporal continuity or identification through time, and in this regard it is functionally similar to Husserl's protention and retention, yet it works in a remarkably different way. In understanding this semblance that is also a dissemblance, it is perhaps best to recall the previous Husserl quote italicized by Derrida: *a form that persists through continuous changes of matter*.

Functionally, the trace opens the present to past and future in a way that formally parallels Husserl's description, yet it attempts to do this in a way that is consequent with the claim that perception is not primary but derivative. Whereas protention and retention explain the *temporalization* of perception—that is to say, the location of a perception in time—within a conceptual framework in which perception is primary, the trace does so within a framework in which perception is not primary. It accounts for the temporalization of perception and experience on the plain of signification, that is, at the level of the signifier, or perhaps, in a sense, just beneath it. The trace is an attempt to explain the "temporalization of a lived experience" (Derrida, 1976, p. 65) when perception is no longer granted primordiality, primacy, or firstness, when experience cannot be an experience of the present, when what is called 'the present' is merely a simulacrum, when it is merely *a form that persists through continuous changes of matter*, and nothing else.

Yet when perception is no longer primordial, experience is no longer lived. As ironic or nonsensical as that might sound, this is certainly the case if we grant the term *lived* experience the meaning that Husserl did, alluding to something pre-reflective and perceptual that, as Merleau-Ponty stressed, was *not* an intellectual synthesis requiring mediation by way of signifiers or representation. The trace denies this fundamental aspect of Husserl's sense of the term *lived*. Its logic suggests, in a way perhaps not intended by Derrida, that experience is *unlived*. We will return to this idea of *unlived experience* later on to explore some of the more psychological interpretations that one might read into such a phrase. But for now, let us simply note that the logic of the trace, or what I call *the logic of the hollowed now*, is a way of thinking that allows for the present moment to exist as an abstraction or a placeholder of sorts, but nothing more. In some sense it allows experience to be, but not be lived. It allows experience to exist as a term in a discourse, but the term, in a sense, is drained of its blood, robbed of its *élan vital*. This is because for Derrida (1982 [1986]), the present becomes the sign of a sign, and the trace of a trace, it is reduced to "a function in a structure of generalized reference" (p. 24).

The dissimilarity as regards content between protention and retention on the one hand, and the trace on the other, is that the former *has* content while the latter does not. Through one hand sieves the sands of an hourglass while the other hand remains empty. Comparing Husserl and Derrida, respectively, David Wood (2001) writes in *Deconstructing Time*:

> The present is from the very beginning permeated with past and future, as retention and protention. But the past and future are here each grasped as presents, albeit potential presents. That is, they are experiences that we once were having, or may soon be having. In this expanded living present, the value of experiential evidence, of "presence," remains and is indeed shored up. And it is this very value that the trace denies. There can be no phenomenology of the trace.
>
> *(p. 271)*

The logic of the hollowed now that drains the present of its vital impulse amounts to a denial of the experiential evidence that phenomenology stakes its claims upon. The present persists as form, but what any present moment ever contained as regards content is vacated, so that moments no longer *matter* in quite the way as they once did.

Unlike Husserl's protention and retention, the trace does not merely complicate the present moment by imbuing it with past and future, nor does it relegate the present to one side of a dialectic—two approaches that admit, at least superficially, to a certain commonsense plausibility. On the contrary, just as was the case with the logic of ubiquitous semiological postponement described in the opening chapter of the present work, according to the logic of the hollowed now, everything is *always already not yet*. . . even the present! Presence is *pre-emptively* deferred. Just as the genesis of all meaning resides in an *absolute* past, so does the genesis of presence itself. There never has been a moment when meaning was not subject to deferral.

Likewise, according to the logic of the trace, *there never has been any presence to complicate by way of protention and retention*. The present cannot be an "unceasing synthesis—a synthesis constantly directed back on itself, gathered in on itself and gathering—of retentional traces and protentional openings" (Derrida, 1982 [1986], p. 21). Because of this, the logic of the trace is not concerned with "horizons of modified—past or future—presents, but with a 'past' that has never been present, and which never will be, whose future to come will never be a *production* or a reproduction in the form of presence" (Derrida, 1982 [1986], p. 21). The trace is incompatible with the concepts of both retention and protention, despite formal similarities, because that would imply "the becoming-past of what has been present. [But] one cannot think the trace—and therefore, *différance*—on the basis of the present, or of the presence of the present (Derrida, 1982 [1986], p. 21).

Nicholas Royle (2003) has understandably called such a line of thought "mind-boggling" (p. 71) and in confronting Derridean texts many readers are probably struck by the odd amalgamation of rigorous argument coupled with seemingly non-sensical conclusions. It is as if an expert mathematician had set out for himself the challenge of carefully, systematically, and in a way completely in accordance with all known laws of mathematics, to solve a complex equation under the assumption that $2 + 2 = 5$. The end result would undoubtedly be faulty, but the origin of the fault would not be found anywhere in the procedural advance of the mathematical solution. It would only be found in the initial assumption. Derrida's initial assumption, which could be stated in multiple ways, always amounts to some variation of the insistence that representation precedes and accounts for presentation (i.e., perception, phenomena). Following through on the implications of such an insistence is difficult and uncomfortable, as Derrida himself acknowledged.

The difficulty, to my mind, only increases as we proceed. According to deconstruction, it is by way of *repetition* that the trace constitutes presence. Repetition is what makes *the form that persists* persist. The hollowed now endures because it can be repeated: "The ideality of the form (*Form*) of presence itself implies that it be infinitely re-peatable, that its re-turn, as a return of the same, is necessary *ad infinitum* and is inscribed in presence itself" (Derrida, 1973, p. 67). According to the logic of the trace, the very idea of the now moment implies a uniformity, a sort of minimal repeatability. Although every now moment is finite and fleeting, the fact that we can recall or anticipate other moments of its kind suggests that it is repeatable. There is a form called 'the present' that persists through the continuous changes of matter. The trace is the name of the inscription that makes possible this general sense of 'nowness,' this repeatability of the idea, or the form of the present. The now presents itself again and again. It re-presents and repeats itself, but what appears time and again is only that—an appearance, an apparition, a vacuous form, a hollowed now.

Mimicking the functional attributes of Husserl's protention and retention, the trace makes possible this formal sense of presence by carrying forth the past into the (empty) present while opening it toward the future. Derrida (1973) often describes this 'carrying forth' and 'opening' in terms of 'the movement' of différance, which allows what appears to be present, to be "related to something other than itself, thereby keeping within itself the mark of a past element and already letting itself be hollowed out by the mark of its relation to a future element" (p. 142). This movement does not imply the retention or protention of anything perceived. Rather, it "presupposes a retention and protention of differences, a spacing and temporalizing, a play of traces" (Derrida, 1973, p. 146). The trace, like Saussure's portrayal of an entirely diacritical sign system with no positive terms but only differences between terms, functions without the retention and protention of any perception or presence but only differences between them. Putting it somewhat differently, yet alluding to what I believe to be this same fundamental emptiness, David Wood (2001) describes both différance and the trace as terms that "make meaning possible without themselves having meaning" (p. 114).

The trace, understood as the possibility of repetition, is not only a means to account for presence as *constituted*, it is also a means by which Derrida opens a conceptual domain. This domain, if it can be called as such, is not only more fundamental, more primordial, and prior to experience, as one might expect given deconstruction's strategic intent. It is more fundamental, more primordial, and *prior to representation as well*, insofar as the trace, understood as the possibility of repetition, is the common root that makes *both* retention and representation possible:

> Without reducing the abyss which may indeed separate retention from representation, without hiding the fact that the problem of their relationship is none other than that of the history of "life" and of life's becoming conscious, we should be able to say *a priori* that their common root—the possibility of re-petition in its most universal sense—is a possibility which not only must inhabit the pure actuality of the now but must constitute it through the very movement of differance it introduces. Such a trace is—if we can employ this language without immediately contradicting it or crossing it out as we proceed—more "primordial" than what is phenomenologically primordial.
>
> *(Derrida, 1973, p. 67)*

But is the abyss so easily dismissed, this abyss so cryptically alluded to as 'life,' but a life enclosed within quotations and founded upon a primordiality similarly enclosed? And is this enclosure not, precisely, the issue? And can the chasm between perceptual retention, on the one hand, and representation, on the other, as well as the problem of the relationship between the two, the problem of "life's becoming conscious" be discharged so summarily with an *a priori*? And might this problem of life's becoming conscious be in some way related to the aforementioned and tentatively suggested idea of *unlived experience*? Lastly, do the 're' of retention and the 're' of representation merit the two ideas being corralled within the all-encompassing category of repetition?

If we do not allow, as Derrida requests, the employment of (a previously deconstructed) primordiality to underwrite the trace—the 'movement' of différance—we are left with a contradiction and a very familiar problematic within the history of philosophy: How can one attribute to a condition of possibility the very thing that makes it possible? In other words, how can we attribute primordiality to the trace and différance if they are what makes any sense of primordiality possible? Derrida is obviously aware of such quandaries; otherwise, he would not suggest the need to cross out or erase the language that he has just employed. This, it should be noted, is a strategy he often uses. He employs terms that are crossed out, permitting him to rely upon their meaning while simultaneously disavowing them.

Husserl's portrayal of retention is that of a sensation that lingers within immediacy and slowly subsides from it, granting the present a certain thickness that is also an openness, a duration to the blink of an eye, whereas the 're' of repetition relies upon a more staccato, or punctual disappearance and reappearance of moments. Repetition, by way of the trace, seems to presuppose a sort of temporal atomism, a reliance on the idea of time's infinite divisibility (Dillon, 1992). Such an atomism or divisibility is congruent with the idea of representation, insofar as representation is a re-presenting of another, temporally discrete moment, a presenting again of something now past. Husserl's thick, continuous moment does not require that retention be a form of representation, as Merleau-Ponty pointed out. Nothing needs to be 'presented again' because there is continuity. If I *retain* an object in my hand, I have not let go of it and then grabbed it again. It has never left my hand to begin with, and retention is a bit like that. It differs from the trace: The former *keeps* present what the latter *re*-presents. One suggests seamlessness, like an extended note fading slowly out of perception. The other suggests something more akin to a series of separate sounds like a beat, like a rhythm.

Time's divisibility into discrete moments is conducive, at least on its surface, to a privileging of representation over presentation. Yet it creates other issues to be resolved because it raises, in a slightly altered form, the same issue of divisibility versus continuity that Derrida understandably objects to in Husserl's account of the present moment. Having identified the cleft between the present as continuous and the present as punctual, then using it as the basis for a critical reading, Derrida privileges the latter (punctuality) through the dubious subsumption of both representation *and* retention under the rubric of repetition. He accounts for the sense of uninterrupted duration by way of repetition, which itself implies an interruption or an interval. Derrida's strategy of thinking, so attuned and adept at spotting incongruent elements and exploiting discernible difficulties in a philosophy like Husserl's, seems ill-equipped, from my perspective, at overcoming similar incongruities.

But is this even the point? Does Derrida's deconstruction of presence, or the metaphysics that is its namesake, depend upon a sense of logical congruency? If its transgressive intent is to disrupt presence or, perhaps more precisely, the conceptual order sanctioned under its auspices, if it is a stratagem without finality, beyond the collapse of a philosophical edifice erected upon an illusion, does it need to appeal to a sense of coherency? Derrida's claim that deconstruction must recognize and respect all the traditional demands of philosophical rigor would seem to suggest that the answer is yes, it does require such an appeal. Yet his claim that différance is simply a tactical ploy that is not intended to survive its own efficacy would suggest that the answer is no.

Paradoxically, the upshot of this attempt to explain both the temporalization of lived experience and representation by way of the trace *qua* repetition amounts to a collapse of the logic of representation itself: If the trace is a repetition, it must be the repetition *of* something by virtue of the same logic that claims representation must be *of* something. In the detritus of this collapse, what is left is a sort of protolinguisticality, a "writing before the letter" (Derrida, 1976, p. 1). The opening of this new domain underlying, or prior to, both representation and retention serves the same strategic purpose of disenfranchising both presence and perception, though it does so, as it were, on a different conceptual plane: If *différance* usurps perception by way of representation, the trace does this by way of proto-representation:

> The use of language or the employment of any code which implies a play of forms—with no determined or invariable substratum—also presupposes a retention and protention of differences, a spacing and temporalizing, a play of traces. This play must be a sort of inscription prior to writing, a protowriting without a present origin, without an *archē*.
>
> *(Derrida, 1973, p. 146)*

But why *must* the play of traces be an inscription, or a protowriting? Why is it that what precedes representation is yet another form of representation, another form of writing? The answer is that both the prefix *proto* and the phrase *without an archē* serve the strategic intent of disrupting sequence. In effect, they up the ante in a poker game in which Derrida has wagered that representation must, at all costs, take precedence and priority over that which had previously been understood to precede it. What has changed is that now the apriority of language is explained through the apriority of proto language, a writing 'before the letter.' The simple addition of the prefix *proto* amounts to yet another insistence on priority, primacy, and primordiality. Yet the phrase *without an archē* suggests a contradiction, given that *proto* and *arche* are at least similar if not synonymous in meaning, just as are *prototype* and *archetype*. *Arche* is a word that means *something that was in the beginning*. It is a first principle, a substance or primal element.

Derrida's attempt to overthrow Husserl's phenomenology, and with it an entire metaphysic known as presence, always amount to allusions to other linguistic forms, other forms of markings made upon a tablet: protowriting, inscriptions, traces, even *arche*-writing. Somehow, these forms of writing can *be archai* but they cannot *have archai*. Regardless the form, they must always exist without an origin, yet serve as origins themselves. They must be without an *archē*, even though the very sense of *proto* that they attempt to communicate would seem to require it. The problem lies in the fact that this requirement forms part of the very system of thought from which Derrida attempts to escape. According to this system, there is a subject, or an object, a *something* that language is derived from and returns to. Language has both origin and end. To disrupt the system, which is, in fact, his strategic intent, concepts like trace, protowriting, différance, etc. must undermine both. In Derrida's (1973) words:

> Since language (which Saussure says is a classification) has not fallen from the sky, it is clear that the differences have been produced; they are the effects

> produced, but effects that do not have as their cause a subject or substance, a thing in general, or a being that is somewhere present and itself escapes the play of difference. . . . I have tried to indicate a way out of the closure imposed by this system, namely by means of the "trace."
>
> *(p. 141)*

Yet Derrida's attempted escape from such an enclosure raises difficult philosophical problems that cannot be hidden for long behind a passive grammatical construction: If the differences communicated by language 'have been produced,' then it would seem that some subject, substance, thing in general, or being has done this producing. We can deny the risible claim of such differences falling from the sky without denying that they must have some origin somewhere.

The insistence on the absence of an origin grounded in perception or presence continues to raise difficult philosophical problems that the trace is ill-equipped to resolve. With all of its formal and functional similarities to perceptual retention and protention, which themselves serve to explain perceptual continuity and the existence of temporal objects, the trace *should* offer some account of this same perceptual continuity, a sense of how objects are identified through different temporal manifestations. Because Derrida claims the apriority rather than the aposteriority of signifiers in one form or another—whether they are understood as traces, inscriptions, protolanguage, or by some other name—it has led some critics to discern at least an implicit model of cognition in which something must be cognized in language *first* for it to be perceived. Such cognition of an object cannot take place *after* its perception. Rather, it is the condition *for* its perception. Because *everything* begins by representation, the perceptual continuity that allows for the identification or recognition of temporal objects must take place on the plain of signifiers.

M. C. Dillon (1995) is one such critic, and a trenchant, divisive one at that. He expresses this implied model of cognition, and its difficulties, succinctly when he writes, "No recognition without signifiers, no signifiers without recognition" (p. 203). But if there is no recognition without signifiers, how can signifiers function at all? Put differently, when words confer identity, when they are the means by which the existence of an enduring *something* is established, it raises the question as to how this conferral might take place:

> Empiricism maintains that we see natural groupings, things that resemble one another in some respect at the perceptual level, then induce a signifier to name that grouping or property, and finally identify things bearing the property by calling them by the name that signifies the property: My perception of the black cat as a cat and as black allows me to refer to it as a black cat. Transcendentalism maintains that I could not see the cat as a cat or as black were it not for the a priori operation of the signifiers "cat" and "black."
>
> *(Dillon, 1998, p. 81)*

The logic of the trace, on Dillon's reading, makes it difficult to understand how anything might be recognized or identified without a signifier (a word, a name) being associated with it in some way: I could not recognize a person without the use of their name, or in lieu of their name, some other set of signifiers like "unnamed person." But how would I even be able to use these signifiers if I had not *previously perceived* unnamed persons? All of this raises questions regarding what philosophers call *natural kinds*, that is to say, groupings that are not arbitrarily or artificially imposed by human beings but exist as part of the natural world.

Regardless of the answers to these questions or even the way in which they have been framed, the conflict with empiricism would seem to be inevitable. The irrelevance of the empirical dimension and empirical research runs throughout Derrida's (1989) writings and appears in his first major published work in 1962, an *Introduction* to Husserl's "The Origin of Geometry." The conflict holds for phenomenology as well which, on Husserl's (2014) account, was actually the truest and purist form of empiricism. Both schools of thought hold firm to a sense of experiential evidence and the etymological roots of empiricism point to precisely this: It is a form of knowing that grounds itself in experience and therefore, it would seem, all that the logic of the trace denies.

The reader of Derrida's texts, as well as the reader of the present work, having reviewed multiple descriptions of the trace, may perhaps be left with little more than the scantest sense of what the term refers to. In this regard, it is appropriately named: traces are so scant, so sketchy, so gossamer, thinner even than Ariadne's thread. Yet it appears to be Derrida's hope that they might lead us, like Theseus on his heroic journey, outside the labyrinthine enclosure imposed by a metaphysical system.

But perhaps traces are more akin to the breadcrumbs left by Hansel and Gretel, abandoned in a maze of trees. Hungry birds consume the hope that the meager morsels might show a path back out of the forest the children find themselves in, and they are left lost. Crumbs, then, are perhaps better metaphors than threads when it comes to defining the trace. Traces are, like such crumbs, similarly consumed and equally transitory, even more so. They must be. They cannot be an enduring presence because this would implicate them in the same metaphysical logic of origins that deconstruction seeks to overcome. For this reason, the trace must *erase* itself. Derrida (1982 [1986]) writes

> Since the trace is not a presence but the simulacrum of a presence that dislocates itself, displaces itself, refers itself, it properly has no site—erasure belongs to its structure. And not only the erasure which must always be able to overtake it (without which it would not be a trace but an indestructible and monumental substance), but also the erasure which constitutes it from the outset as a trace, which situates it as the change of site, and makes it disappear in its appearance, makes it emerge from itself in its production.
>
> *(p. 24)*

Erasure must characterize the trace from the outset so that it vanishes in its very advent, otherwise it would be merely another of the enduring origins that Derrida disavows. Put simply, the trace requires its own erasure so as not to be present. It must be self-effacing, even preemptively so, or self-effacing in the very process of its inscription for the same reason that originary différance must be a *non*-origin. Erasure must belong to the structure of the trace by virtue of the same logic that inverts the sequential order of presentation and representation, yet this is also why the logic of the trace appears incongruous. It raises the same questions. How can a trace be effaced at all without ever having been present? It cannot. How can it disappear in its appearance if the very idea of simultaneity that this implies is denied by the logic of différance? Then again, if the strategic intent of différance is to erase itself in the very enactment of its purpose, do any of these questions even matter? Logic and rigor suggest they do, but the strategic intent suggests they might not.

The word *obliterate* is a useful one when thinking about the concept of erasure. It means to blot out and is derived from the Latin *ob*, meaning *against*, plus *littera*, meaning letter or script. To obliterate, in its root sense, means to blot out letters or to erase. Yet the connotations of the word suggest a sense of oblivion, that is to say, a pleasant forgetfulness, a blessed incognizance, a desirable amnesia or ignorance. This sense of erasure as the desirable oblivion of forgetting will be of particular importance further on in Chapter 4, in which Peter Pan's Neverland is portrayed as a form of eternal amnesia, much like Wonderland and other imaginary realms typical of children's fiction. This land of oblivion, it should be noted, is also a realm unhindered by the empirical and pragmatic concerns that come with time and space, a realm in which the mundane matters of living and the usual laws of causality do not apply, a world in which experience and the lessons learned from it are rendered mute. Oblivion too will be addressed in the chapter immediately following the present one, though it is oblivion of a different sort, one that, in a sense, renders experience unlived.

## II

In an effort to move the discussion of deconstruction from the realm of thought to the realm of psyche once more, I want to offer an alternative semantic analysis to the one put forth by Derrida. It is also an attempt to further illustrate the previously stated principle that *statements about language and semiotics are also statements by and about psyche*. The strategy of différance is an attempt to disrupt a conceptual order that Derrida calls a *metaphysics of presence*. This disruption is its *raison d'être*. Yet, if we simply omit the words 'metaphysics of,' we can easily turn a philosophical statement into a psychological one. We are then left with something quite different, something perhaps less daunting in its intellectual sophistry, yet, in a sense, more daunting in its implications: Différance is an attempt to disrupt presence, but of what?

There is a particular strategy of the psyche, well known to all forms of depth psychology, that could also rightly be described as an attempt to disrupt presence. Its parallels with différance, from a purely semantic perspective, are striking, so much so that any attempt to place deconstruction within the realm of psyche would be remiss not to address them. It has been conceptualized in countless psychological texts of numerous schools of thought, from the foundational works of Janet—who systematically elaborated the workings of this strategy—as well as Bleuler, Charcot, Binet, James, Freud, Jung, and innumerable others (Ellenberger, 1970) to the works of Winnicott, Bion, Bowlby, Guntrip, Klein, Fairbairn and those who carry on their legacy into the present (Kalsched, 2013). It is a strategy of the psyche to protect itself from an unbearable affect and is a key concept in trauma theory. When a person experiences something so painful or injurious that it overwhelms their ability to consciously cope, it serves as a psychological defense that preserves the individual, although at a cost. It allows for survival, although at the price of psychological integrity, or even more precisely, psychological integration, for this strategic defense is in fact a form of disintegration, one that splits affect from image, body from mind, memory from identity, sensation from thought, and thought from meaning.

This strategy is implicated in an armory of defenses and dynamics, an inclusive, though not exhaustive list of which contains *projection, introjection, projective identification, repression, displacement, regression, reaction formation, transference, doubling, conversion,* and *compartmentalization.* It is also implicated in almost innumerable pathological conditions from schizophrenia to multiple forms of affective, obsessive-compulsive, schizoid, and bipolar personality disorders. The idea of archetypal possession, to be addressed further on, would make little sense without it, nor would individuation, which for Jung is the never fully realized goal of psychological development. You can hear echoes of it in Jung's pithy, memorable definition of neurosis as a state of being in disagreement with oneself, as well as in Bion's (2013) no less memorable phrase, 'attacks on linking.' Without it, arguably, modern psychology in its myriad and far-reaching forms would look little like it does today, the concept has been so foundational. This attempt to disrupt presence is known as *dissociation.*

My semantic, or perhaps psychosemantic, analysis of différance will begin with the prefix *dis* and with the observation that *dif*, as in the French verb *différir* and the English verb differ, is one of its assimilated forms. Etymologically speaking, the *dif* of différance is simply a variation of the *dis* of dissociation. This Latin prefix of Proto-Indo-European origin made its way into both French and English and evolved into forms like *des*, *de*, *di*, *dif*, and even, by way of semantic confusion, *def*, as in defer. In classical Latin, *dis* had much the same meaning as the prefix *de*. Both denoted lack, opposition, and a sense of being apart, away, or asunder. Through the Proto-Indo-European *dwis, dis* is related to the Latin *bis* (originally *dvis*) as well as *duo*, both of which carry the notion of being split in two.

*Dis*, to be found in words like *disarm*, *disorient*, *distrust*, *discourage*, and *disown* reverses what it is affixed to, in effect, turning a word's meaning into its opposite or communicating a deficiency. Such is the case as well for the variant *de*, in words like *destabilize*, *depersonalize* and even *deconstruction*, all of which convey a reversal of a given sense offered by their root words. Yet, along with its other variants *des*, *di*, and *dif*, *dis* also speaks to a splitting or divisive action, as in *discrimination*, which is the careful differentiation or discernment of two or more things from one another. In this sense, *dis* cleaves, cuts, splays. As with its Greek correlate *di*, it expresses the meaning of making twofold, taking apart or away. These three senses of *dis,* that of reversal, lack, and taking apart or making twofold are best epitomized, perhaps more than anywhere else in the English language, in the word *dissociation* itself, by virtue of its root word *associate*. From the Latin *ad*, meaning *to*, and *sociare*, meaning to join, to associate is to bring together in a relationship. Dissociation, in turn, is a reversal and deficiency of relationship, but it is also a taking apart specifically that which bonds, that which associates.

With these etymological reflections in mind, Derrida could not have chosen a better neologism than différance to affect his strategic dismantling of a metaphysics of presence. Although new, a linguistic innovation, this word (that is not a word) draws from a bottomless well of semantic associations that reaches down into the obscure depths and the abyssal darkness of prehistory. His attempt to dismantle a tradition draws power from these associations even as it attempts to disrupt them.

Différance is a form of dissociation: The latter of the two terms refers to an attempt to disrupt presence, while the former is an attempt to disrupt the metaphysics operating under its auspices. Dissociation is the core psychological truth of deconstruction as well as the reason for the failings of its argument: Such a stratagem offers a temporary respite from an unbearable presence but is ultimately one that is doomed to fail or at least provide a somewhat diminished version of the fullness of psychological being.

Such claims rest on much more than the filial ties of *dif* and *dis*. Deconstruction operates by way of an incessant splitting, a repeated emphasis on the fissuring quality of the temporal, spatial displacement. It cleaves, clefts, and fractures, speaking the language of endemic divergence and abyssal rupture, a dialect of pure division founded upon an absolute belief in the diacritical. It disengages the dual aspects of the sign, signifier and signified. It severs presentation from representation, perception from language. It places an unbridgeable gap between words and a realm—mystical and mythical on Caputo's account—that transcends them. Deconstruction is nothing if it is not, to use Bion's phrase, an attack on linking, the linking between word, meaning, and perception. Framing deconstruction in terms of dissociative dynamics may shed light on many of its conceptual difficulties—aspects that seem philosophically untenable or incongruent—but do so from an angle slightly adjacent to the conceptual, *stricto sensu*. It may also help answer the question posed earlier as to whether the failure of différance is the failure of deconstruction, or, on the contrary, evidence of its lucidity.

Faced with Husserl's description of the present as a synthesis of past and future, retention and protention, the dissociative logic of différance disrupts the synthesis by construing it as dispersed and dissipated, vacuous and vacant. Somehow, by way of repetition, or some evanescent trace, it construes an abyss into which 'life' disappears, like a gaping maw that consumes experience and renders life unlived. It tears presence asunder, rendering it incoherent. Identifying a contradiction between Husserl's account of presence as both continuous and divisible, it does not attempt to reconcile the contradiction, or accept it as an inevitable paradox, but doubles down on the side of infinite divisibility. No less dissociative is the disruption of sequence that différance introduces in its attempt to make the primary be secondary and the before come after. The sum consequence of such a temporal, or perhaps *dis*temporal logic is a hollowed now, a presence made absent. Is this not exactly what dissociation does, make the present absent, alienating one from his or her experiential depths?

It is only with the slightest change of vocabulary and syntax that one can move, almost seamlessly, from speaking of the dissociative impact of trauma to the disintegrative impact of différance. If one describes an attack upon the link between sensation and thought, then moves to describe a severance of thought from meaning, is one describing différance in the former and dissociation in the latter, or vice versa? It makes little difference. At heart, they are one and the same. *Différance is to the metaphysics of presence what dissociation is to psychological presence*: a strategy of disruption, a means of evasion, a defensive maneuvering, one that is undoubtedly necessary at times when being more fully present is simply unbearable. It may form part of a necessary process. But it can no more serve as the guiding principle or lodestar of a coherent philosophy than dissociation can serve a similar role in psychological well-being. Dissociation is a defense against presence, the presence of an unbearable affect, an overwhelming experience the likes of which requires that the psyche be fragmented, divided into compartments. The elements of unified experience must be held separate, severed, so that between words and their meaning there is always an impassible chasm, so that the immediacy of perception be held at a safe distance, so that moments past, present, and future appear discontinuous. In deconstructive terms, it disrupts being *as* presence.

The effect of dissociation is, in a sense, to 'hollow the now.' It leaves a vacuous form in lieu of a moment pregnant with meaning. Once existing within a temporal flux uniting past and future into a coherent whole, the present moment stands bereft, isolated, tethered to other moments only by the faintest of traces, the vaguest sense of a moment compulsively repeated ad infinitum. In its stead lies an eviscerated, or perhaps bloodless body, once sensate, feeling, perceptive, responsive to the phenomenal world like the skin's pores to the slightest breeze.

In furtherance of this alternative psychosemantic analysis of différance by way of the prefix *dis*, and to add a mythic dimension to it, we will turn to the seminal work of Donald Kalsched. In *Trauma and the Soul*, Kalsched (2013) offers an account of *dis* not merely in its etymological aspect, but first and foremost in its mythological aspect through a detailed reading of Dante's *Divine Comedy*. This epic poem of the fourteenth century, with its tripartite vision of life after death—Inferno, Purgatorio, and Paradiso—begins with an imagined descent into hell in search of the source of the poet's suffering and is followed by a sojourn in purgatory, both of which are guided by the ancient Roman poet Virgil. During the last portion of the journey, into the heavenly realms, Dante is guided by his beloved Beatrice, a woman who, in the life of the Italian poet, was the object of his courtly love, his chaste passion in the chivalric tradition of Tristan and Iseult. With this in mind, we might imagine Dante's trek through the inferno, when he is furthest from his beloved, as a trek through the tortures of pothos or what Denis de Rougemont called romantic love. Kalsched's reading focuses on the first of the three books, that of the journey into the underworld in which Beatrice is nowhere to be found, the hellscape in which she is most *dis*tant, the depths of Hades ruled by the dark lord known, in Dante's poem, as none other than *Dis*. This is the name given to the governing spirit of the underworld, the fallen angel Lucifer, that presides over hell and resides in its deepest layer, and the name, in the hands of the great poet, is no mere happenstance.

On Kalsched's reading, the descent into the netherworld offers a powerful portrayal of the inner world of trauma and the psychological defenses marshaled to survive its overwhelming effect. Through its medieval Christian imagery, the poet's journey into the depths of hell parallels the trauma survivor's descent into his or her own private hell of paranoia and persecution. Trauma is by definition an unbearable pain, and in response to this unbearable pain, a person's psyche or soul marshals its own defenses to ensure survival, although, as was mentioned earlier, at the price of his or her own psychological integrity. Survival comes at the cost of a nightmare, an inner landscape riddled by defenses that never allow a person to fully enjoy life. Dante's hell, marked by its successive 'rings' or levels, serves as a model description of the successive layers of psychological defenses against intolerable suffering and, paradoxically, the suffering that these defenses perpetuate. In the deepest layer, the dark crypt of the trauma survivor's torment and the poet's theological vision stands the devil himself, the dark lord Dis.

Such an epithet is only fitting, for each step in the descent toward increasingly torturous levels of the poet's hellscape represents a greater state of psychological rending and tearing apart, and the role of Dis is that of an agent of dissociation. He is a personification of the psyche's divisive defenses and the poet's redemptive journey into hell is to "confront the dark Lord of Dissociation otherwise known in Latin as 'Dis'" (Kalsched, 2013, p. 20). These three simple letters name the violent effects of all the forms of psychological rupture and the persecutory powers of a defensive system erected in response to an unbearable experience. They name the hell of a soul's disintegration, the suffering of a strategic dissociation that through tearing affect from image, body from mind, memory from identity, sensation from thought, and thought from meaning, satisfies a need. Such a tearing apart is simply what the psyche does in response to trauma: To protect us from the unbearable, "different aspects of the traumatic experience (sensation, affect, image) are fragmented, divided into compartments" (Kalsched, 2013, p. 23). The elements of unified experience are severed so as to prevent the integration of feeling, sensation, image, and word. Jung, says Kalsched (2013), "probably would have seen Dis as personifying that *disintegrative effect* of what he called the autonomous fragmentary systems that appear from the collective layer of the unconscious, possessing the ego in mental disturbances" (p. 93). Following such a line of thought and translating Kalsched for the purposes of the present text, we might say that deconstruction is the philosophic expression of the dissociative tendency of archetypal possession.

Dis, the lord of the flies, Lucifer within the Christian tradition, is the angel who led the revolt against god's intention to incarnate as Christ. For this reason, the fallen angel offers a "mytho-poetic description of how a splitting defense comes into being—as a prideful refusal to embody" (Kalsched, 2013, p. 89). The Luciferian defense within the trauma survivor prevents him or her from being 'made flesh,' as it were, but the acute suffering that this might entail, a living or re-living of the original injury, is exchanged for the chronic, repetitive torment of the damned, which is without respite and without hope of redemption.

Such a distinction between acute and chronic suffering may be familiar to readers of both Freud and Jung. The former made a similar distinction, contrasting hysterical misery with common unhappiness, while the latter spoke of illegitimate versus legitimate suffering (Freud, 1953; Jung, 1973). The binary oppositions of acute and chronic, common and hysterical, legitimate and illegitimate, incarnate and disincarnate all allude to fundamentally the same dilemma, and it is the devil of dissociation that holds people prisoner within the crypt that the latter halves of these pairings represent. This is the Beelzebub that perpetuates a disembodied existence in the phantasmal realm of the underworld.

The machinations of Dis that prevent a person from becoming flesh, on Kalsched's reading, amount to what is known as a *schizoid* compromise or a schizoid withdrawal. The term and its relation to Dis is only appropriate, for this diabolic spirit is schismatic and the word *schizoid* derives from the Greek *skhizein*, meaning to split. But what exactly is this compromise and how might it serve as a way of furthering this psychosemantic analysis? How might it shed light on the parallels between deconstruction and the figure of the eternal youth?

In response to the first question, the schizoid withdrawal, to revisit Fairbairn's phrase, is based on a 'love made hungry,' one that can only gravitate toward a "desirable deserter" (Guntrip, 1992, p. 24), can only love someone or something that eludes it. Thus, a person with such a hunger:

> . . . wants what he has not got, and begins to lose interest and wants to get away from it when he has it. This particularly undermines friendships and love relationships but can become a general discontent with most things. '*Absence makes the heart grow fonder*' is true of schizoid people unless too much fear is roused,

> and then it turns love to hate. The schizoid individual can often feel strong longings for another person *so long as he or she is not there, but the actual presence of the other person causes an emotional withdrawal* which may range from coldness, loss of interest and inability to find anything to say, to hostility and revulsion: '*presence makes the heart grow less fond*' [emphasis added].
>
> *(Guntrip, 1992, p. 59)*

Because absence makes the heart grow fonder and presence makes the heart grow less fond, schizoid love is made hungry by its own demands. To sustain itself it must remain insatiate. It must either choose an 'object,' a beloved that will always thwart its intent to possess, or choose a circumstance that will likewise thwart possession. Like pothos, it must create a metaphorical or literal distance to exalt itself. Because it is nourished by withdrawals, like Rougemont's romantic love, it requires not another's presence but another's absence.

But why? On Guntrip's account, heavily influenced by the works of Ronald Fairbairn, Melanie Klein, and Michael Balint, love is made hungry during the primary experiences of early infancy, specifically those of the parental attachments that will set a precedent for later relationships. The dissociative dynamic of the schizoid defense at the most fundamental level involves a withdrawal from the external world where love was frustrated or inadequate and a struggle for possession of that lost love via the internal world. Put in yet simpler terms, it is a turn "into oneself and out of the body" (p. 78) as R. D. Laing (1960 [2010]) has described it in his own account of the schizoid condition. The turn into oneself is a response to an unmet dependency on love objects. One turns inward to possess what one cannot find elsewhere. The less satisfactory an infant's relationships are with parental figures, especially with the mother in the preoedipal phase of infancy, the more he or she remains entrenched in those relationships through a complex dynamic of passive identification and active incorporation.

*Passive identification* is related to an ambivalent fear of engulfment and overwhelm, a sense of being flooded, coupled with a regressive desire to return to the womb, to the undifferentiated state of symbiotic union. Clinically, the dynamics of passive identification take many forms as the dissociative splits carry forth into young adulthood and later life. Passive identification insinuates itself into any close relationship and with it comes the fear of a loss of self. Even the experience of being understood, seen, cared for by another person can provoke the panic of being swallowed, smothered, lost in the other (Guntrip, 1992; Laing, 1960 [2010]). Love threatens annihilation. Being in love means being *in* the beloved, or even *being* the beloved, becoming the other, being subsumed within someone else and losing any sense of one's own independent identity. The slightest trickle of love can portend a flood. Relationship *with* another person means relationship *within* another person, and the imagery brought forth by such a fate is that of being absorbed, drowned, devoured.

These dynamics of passive identification extend beyond relationships with individuals to relationships with the entire objective world. The individual is "perpetually uncommitted 'to the objective element'" (Laing, 1960 [2010], p. 88) because contact with external reality itself threatens the person with implosion, as if the barricades of an inner bastion might collapse upon him or her. A primary maneuver to avoid such a catastrophic engulfment is isolation. In lieu of a relationship based on the polarities of separateness and relatedness, schizoid splits impose a dynamic of absorption and aloneness.

*Active incorporation* is a means to avoid being incorporated and, in this regard, it is the counter dynamic to passive identification. So as not to be engulfed, yet faced with the failure to outgrow a dependency on love objects, the person establishes an inner world that in many regards duplicates the original relationship with 'bad objects,' or original caregivers. Active incorporation is more closely related to the post-natal oral stage of the infant at the mother's breast and a desire to not merely take from it but, rather, due to unmet needs, to devour the breast entirely. When the child depends upon an undependable mother, when 'the breast' (both literally and metaphorically) cannot be relied upon, when love relationships with external objects (i.e., persons) in general are precarious or bad, the child tends to retain his or her love inside himself or herself, turning it toward internal (i.e., imagined) objects. Put differently, the person incorporates the external, objective world within an internal world of representations.

To the extent that a person's infantile needs were not met, the child, and later the adult, will remain unconsciously embedded in those relationships. He or she remains attached, but not to the caretakers *per se*, not the people themselves, not to the 'objects themselves.' The schizoid person, in response to frustrated attachments, feels overwhelmed by the external world and takes flight from it. Yet, in a sense, his or her attachments take the flight as well. Through the dynamic of active incorporation, they simply transfer to internal objects that both excite and deny satisfaction (Guntrip, 1992). The external world is rendered internal, and the desire for attachment is satisfied surreptitiously, although not in a way that will prove satisfactory:

> It is bad objects which are internalized, because we cannot accept their badness; we seek to withdraw from them in outer reality and yet cannot give them up, cannot leave them alone; we cannot master and control them in outer reality and so keep on struggling to possess them, alter them and compel them to change into good objects, in our inner psychic world.
>
> *(Guntrip, 1992, p. 22)*

The dissociative dynamic of the schizoid defense involves a withdrawal from the external world and a struggle for possession of love via the internal world. It works by way of introversion and the abolition of external relationships, or perhaps more precisely, the establishment of pseudo relationships with others through introversion. The halfway-in-halfway-out compromise seeks to satisfy two contrary needs "the need to withdraw from intolerable reality and the need to remain in touch with it" (Guntrip, 1992, p. 82).

Like many psychological defenses, such a dissociative/incorporative strategy offers a means of survival but is not ultimately satisfactory. Suckling upon an imaginary breast may offer the illusion of nourishment but it does not nourish. With his or her love made hungry, a person "at bottom feels overwhelmed by the external world and is in flight from it both inwards, and, as it were, backwards, to the safety of the womb" (Guntrip, 1992, p. 44). But, of course, this cannot be the actual womb made of living human flesh. It must be a womb made of dream and fantasy, imagination and idea. This may be a refuge of astonishing wealth, like a citadel furbished and provisioned, seemingly, with all the requisites of a prolonged sequester, which is, in a sense, exactly what it is intended to be. The flight to the safety of an inner world is a protracted sojourn that becomes a habitus, a way of being. But, like the imagined breast that cannot truly nourish, the inner womb of imagination can offer only an illusory respite.

When a pronounced schizoid state intervenes, it may appear as a patient who dispassionately reports a vivid inner world of dream and fantasy as if he or she were a detached third-party observer. There is a similar attitude of non-involvement and clinical detachment toward the external world. Affect and action, in both cases, are notably absent as if the person had no personal investment, nothing at stake in his or her own life and therefore feels no compulsion to act (Guntrip, 1992). Suspended in an emotional and impulsive stasis, such a person seeks an equipoise between two worlds. A bit like Goldilocks who needs her porridge neither too hot nor too cold but just right, such a person requires just the right distance, neither too close, for fear of a loss of identity, nor too far, for fear of a sense of isolation. Passive identification and active incorporation form the dueling imperatives of the schizoid's compromise which, in the simplest of terms, is an attempt to *always be halfway in and halfway out* of relationships with others, as if suspended "in between two worlds, internal and external, and having no real relationships with either of them" (Guntrip, 1992, p. 18).

Ronald Fairbairn (1952) described three primary consequences of the schizoid withdrawal and subsequent compromise. First, there is an attitude of omnipotence. Within the sphere of internal objects, a realm of image and idea only tenuously referential to a world from which the person has withdrawn, anything is possible. One can be or do anything because, untethered to external demands, there are no limitations. A person can be anyone, anywhere, anyhow. Second, there is a deep feeling of isolation and detachment, albeit at times disguised by a façade of sociability. Because contact with the external world is so slight, like an umbilical cord thin as a thread, it can offer only the most meager of emotional sustenance. Yet such "shut in personalities" (Fairbairn, 1952, p. 15) must remain shut in and withdrawn as a defense against engulfment and overwhelm: the specter of love arouses the specter of annihilation. Guntrip (1992) described this common schizoid symptom as "the feeling of a plateglass wall between the patient and the world" (p. 63). Third, and most importantly, there is a preoccupation with an inner realm which may be "substituted for outer reality, identified with outer reality, or superimposed upon outer reality" (Fairbairn, 1952, p. 7). The more a person withdraws from the external 'real' world, the more their libido turns toward an inner mental world: *into oneself and out of the body*, as Laing so pithily summarized.

Schizoid love is a love made hungry. It can only desire that which eludes it. This is what the child has been taught through the repeated frustration of his or her legitimate dependency needs, and this experience sets a precedent. As a consequence of the frustration, the child is forced to withdraw love—let us call it eros—from his or her environment, where it is unrequited, and turn it inward:

> He becomes afraid to love: and therefore he erects barriers between his objects and himself. He tends to both keep his objects at a distance and to make himself remote from them. He rejects his objects: and at the same time he withdraws libido from them. This withdrawal of libido may be carried to all lengths. It may be carried to a point at which all emotional and physical contacts with other persons are renounced; and it may even go so far that all libidinal links with outer reality are surrendered, all interest in the world around fades and everything becomes meaningless. In proportion as libido is withdrawn from outer objects it is directed toward internalized objects: and in proportion as this happens the person becomes introverted.
>
> *(Fairbairn, 1952, p. 50)*

Such is, in its most schematic form, the schizoid's strategy of dis-incarnation, his or her enthrallment to the dark lord Dis, that mythic personification of the refusal to embody that resides in the depths of the inferno. The goal of the schizoid defense requires that the subject be:

> disembodied, encapsulated, or otherwise driven out of the body/mind unity—foreclosed from entering time and space reality. Instead of slowly and painfully incarnating in a cohesive self, the volcanic opposing dynamisms of the inner world become organized around defensive purposes, constituting a 'self-care system' for the individual. Instead of individuation and the integration of mental life, the archaic defense engineers dis-incarnation (dis-embodiment) and dis-integration in order to help a weakened anxiety-ridden ego to survive, albeit as a partially 'false' self.
>
> *(Kalsched, 1996, p. 38)*

*Foreclosed from entering time and space* is a resonant phrase, one that helps unite seemingly disparate themes, both within Kalsched's work and within the one at hand: For Kalsched, the schizoid dilemma is also that of the eternal youth. Both have a problem with entering time and space completely, and opt to withdraw to a place beyond the realm of circumstance and consequence. Neither, in a sense, incarnates. Both lead provisional lives. Kalsched (2013) makes explicit the equivalence of this schizoid dynamic and the psychology of the eternal youth when he writes that "the experience of not yet being fully 'in life' describes a typical feature of what Jungian theory describes as 'Puer' psychology, based upon the writings of M.L. von Franz" (p. 318), adding that the deeper meaning of this *not yet* at the threshold of life is "captured by Guntrip's description of the schizoid compromise" (p. 318). The limbo of the provisional life is the limbo of this compromise.

Because this limbo allows for no transformative, redemptive, or legitimate suffering, it leads to what Kalsched terms *malignant innocence*. Driven out of the body/mind unity, dis-incarnated and dis-integrated, normal childhood omnipotence and innocence are not allowed to be transformed by experience. They remain forever in the halfway house of the compromise. Innocence is not relativized and constantly evolving but remains absolute and static. Omnipotence, held within the dissociative crypt, never confronts face to face its own limitations. The fact that Dis reigns over a realm of innocents in Dante's poem is an expression of this sort of innocence that is malignant because it is *absolute*: It is not alterable by further experience.

The present work adds yet another element to the unity of these seemingly disparate themes: différance. Its dissociative dynamics that split language from meaning and hollow presence, are another variation upon the schizoid strategy, which is itself a form of the eternal youth's *not yet*. Seen by way of schizoid dissociative dynamics, the transcendental signified, "the thing itself [that] always escapes" (Derrida, 1973, p. 104) is something like a 'bad object' for deconstruction, as are phenomena, perception, and primordiality. Its philosophical strategy is to withdraw from the signified by claiming its utter transcendence, yet it cannot truly give up the transcendental signified. The same can be said as regards phenomena, perception, and primordiality, without which there would be nothing to deconstruct.

In effect, deconstruction is stuck in a form of schizoid compromise: It renders what might be considered 'outside' language as inside and, in so doing, satisfies its attachment surreptitiously, although not in a way that proves satisfactory or philosophically coherent. Deconstruction enacts its own introversion and abolition of external relationships and its own establishment of pseudo relationships through introversion every time it places the word *primordial* within quotation marks, which allows it to act like a pseudo presence. The quotation marks satisfy the dueling imperatives of the schizoid compromise: "the need to withdraw from intolerable reality and the need to remain in touch with it" (Guntrip, 1992, p. 82). The quotation marks allow for deconstruction to relinquish yet surreptitiously satisfy its attachment needs. Despite appearances, it is a form of thought that is deeply attached to a sense of primordiality, much like the phenomenology that it mimics. Yet it must simultaneously withdraw from this primordiality because it is anathema to its project of disrupting the metaphysics of presence.

The need to withdraw yet remain in touch runs throughout deconstruction. We can find it in the reliance upon the very system of metaphysical distinctions that it seeks to dismantle. It withdraws yet remains in touch in the peculiar fashion by which it seems to vacate the meaningful content of words yet retain their functional equivalence, use them yet erase them. It is there in the tendency to justify itself by way of the very ideas of primacy and firstness that it also refutes. It is there in the functioning of the trace, which hollows the now, allowing presence to endure, yet merely as an empty form. It is there in *sous rature*, a typographical innovation that allows Derrida to plant an idea in the reader's mind while simultaneously disavowing its consequences. Such a planting then disavowing is typical of Derrida's form of argument. He remains in touch even in the very act of his withdrawal. The stratagem of différance works by way of a similar dissociative/incorporative ploy as that of the schizoid's compromise, which attempts to be halfway in and halfway out of relationships. In a similar vein, Derrida's references to primordiality or a transcendental signified are halfway references that always seem equivocal or paradoxical. Somehow, to use Laing's phrase, such references remain perpetually uncommitted to the objective element.

## References


Bion, W. R. (2013). Attacks on linking. *The Psychoanalytic Quarterly*, *82*(2), 285–300. https://doi.org/10.1002/j.2167-4086.2013.00029.x

Derrida, J. (1973). *Speech and phenomena, and other essays on Husserl's theory of signs*. Northwestern University Press.

Derrida, J. (1976). *Of grammatology* (G. C. Spivak, Trans.). Johns Hopkins University Press. (Original work published 1967)

Derrida, J. (1982 [1986]). *Margins of philosophy* (A. Bass, Trans.). University of Chicago Press.

Derrida, J. (1989). *Edmund Husserl's origin of geometry: An introduction*. University of Nebraska Press.

Dillon, M. C. (1992). Temporality: Merleau-Ponty and Derrida. In T. W. Busch & S. Gallagher (Eds.), *Merleau-Ponty, hermeneutics, and postmodernism* (pp. 189–212). State University of New York Press.

Dillon, M. C. (1995). *Semiological reductionism: A critique of the deconstructionist movement in postmodern thought*. State University of New York Press.

Dillon, M. C. (1998). Beyond semiological reductionism. In A. Tymieniecka (Ed.), *The reincarnating mind, or the ontopoietic outburst in creative virtualities*. Analecta Husserliana (The year book of phenomenological research) (Vol. 53, pp. 75–88). Springer.

Ellenberger, H. F. (1970). *The discovery of the unconscious: The history and evolution of dynamic psychiatry*. Basic Books.

Fairbairn, W. R. D. (1952). *Psychoanalytic studies of the personality*. Routledge.

Freud, S. (1953). *The standard edition of the complete psychological works of Sigmund Freud: Studies on hysteria*. W.W. Norton & Company.

Guntrip, H. (1992). *Schizoid phenomena, object relations and the self*. Karnac Books.

Husserl, E. (1999). *The essential Husserl: Basic writings in transcendental phenomenology*. Indiana University Press.

Husserl, E. (2001). *Analyses concerning passive and active synthesis: Lectures on transcendental logic*. Springer Netherlands.

Husserl, E. (2014). *Ideas: General introduction to pure phenomenology*. Routledge.

Jung, C. G. (1973). Psychology and religion, west and east. In *The collected works of C. G. Jung* (Vol. 11, R. F. C. Hull, Trans.). Princeton University Press.

Kalsched, D. (1996). *The inner world of trauma: Archetypal defenses of the personal spirit*. Routledge.

Kalsched, D. (2013). *Trauma and the soul: A psycho-spiritual approach to human development and its interruption*. Routledge.

Laing, R. D. (1960 [2010]). *The divided self: An existential study in sanity and madness*. Penguin Books.

Merleau-Ponty, M. (1964). *The primacy of perception: And other essays on phenomenological psychology, the philosophy of art, history, and politics* (J. M. Edie, Trans.). Northwestern University Press.

Royle, N. (2003). *Jacques Derrida*. Routledge.

Wood, D. (2001). *The deconstruction of time*. Northwestern University Press.

Zahavi, D. (2005). *Subjectivity and selfhood: Investigating the first-person perspective*. MIT Press.

# 3

# THE IMPERATIVE OF ARCHETYPAL POSSESSION

## I

One can, in principle, extend the logic of the hollowed now indefinitely: Perhaps there is a proto-protowriting, and preceding this a proto-proto-protowriting, as well as a trace of the trace and a trace of that trace. But the insistence upon priority veils the paucity of the argument and suggests the need to place it within another context, the context of psyche, and more specifically, the archetypal psyche as conceived by Jung and those influenced by his work. There, we can at least ask whether what appear to be systemic flaws in the premises of deconstruction have a correlate in psychological and archetypal terms. There, perhaps the argument will gain greater clarity.

Theoretically, one can defer ad infinitum the conclusive refutation of the deconstructive approach through a never-ending appeal to priority, adding prefixes to prior arguments thereby refurbishing them with ever-renewed assertions as to what *must* come first, themselves bolstered by an ever-renewed appeal to inconclusiveness. One side of the argument is bookended by the appeal to absolute priority, while the other side is bookended by the appeal to an equally absolute inconclusiveness. Perhaps they are one and the same bookend, both alpha and omega. *Theoretically* one can defer in such a manner, although the arguments made by human beings are subject to the limits of the human; Mortality, whether we like it or not, limits even our ability to defer.

A purely philosophic critique of deconstruction might content itself with pointing out that différance is, despite arguments to the contrary, the very sort of presence that it attempts to undermine. Deconstruction is vulnerable to this type of critique whenever it affirms that différance is in any way constitutional, in any way an origin. This is, in effect, what an astute observer like Wood (2001) is pointing

DOI: 10.4324/b23321-4

out in his description of Derrida's mimicry of Husserl's transcendental phenomenology. To substitute différance for presence as an origin, or to center a principle of de-centering, does not so much undermine the thought of a metaphysics of presence as much as revamp its façade.

Yet for a critique that attempts to move from the realm of thought to the realm of psyche, pointing out such seeming contradictions is merely a stepping stone. The path through the realm of psyche is paved with opportunities to discern projective dynamics, dissociative tendencies, and even 'gods' at work within ideas—archaic emissaries alive in even the most abstruse of abstractions—as well as constellations of themes that cluster around such emissaries, like time and eternity, love at a distance, nostalgia, and others yet to be explored.

The effectiveness of the deconstructive argument depends upon the primordiality, the firstness of différance, yet this dependence betrays the project's implicit agreement with the metaphysics it seeks to dismantle. Both share the assumption that what comes first is what matters most. Primacy is both determinative and constitutive. Despite his opposition to transcendental arguments, Derrida "retains the value of privilege and priority that only such arguments bestow" (Wood, 2001, p. 274). Therein lies his insistence that différance is originary and that the alterity at the heart of the now "not only must inhabit the pure actuality of the now but must constitute it through the very movement of differance it introduces" (Derrida, 1973, p. 67). Such observations are what lead Wood (2001) to describe Derrida's argument as a form of mimicry of the selfsame transcendental positions that he takes issue with. They evoke the image of a shadow boxer stealthily squaring off against a wall, sparring with an ever-elusive specter.

The metaphor, I think, is *à propos*, but it may appear exceptionally so to the reader familiar with Jungian terminology and metapsychology, for the term *shadow* inevitably implies a degree of self-deception and lack of self-awareness as well as dissociative and projective dynamics. The shadow, which often takes on the guise of a nemesis or antagonist, also implies a "moral problem that challenges the whole ego-personality, for no one can become conscious of the shadow without considerable moral effort. To become conscious of it involves recognizing the dark aspects of the personality as present and real" (Jung, 1959, p. 8).

It is tempting to say that the moral challenge that the shadow presents is always one of identification; it asks of us that we say to ourselves, *I am what I claim I am not. I may even be what I most vociferously insist that I am not*. This is, inevitably, a bitter pill to swallow, for it confronts a person with the sort of inner cleavage that, for Jung, is definitive of neurosis, a state of being at war with oneself and "what drives people to war with themselves is the intuition or the knowledge that they consist of two persons in opposition to one another" (Jung, 1933, pp. 236–237). But *tempting* is an important qualifier here, for what Jung recommends is not mere identification but, rather, integration. The moral challenge of the shadow, ever-present and never fully met, requires that one understand oneself to be neither identical to nor absolutely different from it: The shadow is merely an aspect of the greater whole that one is.

The challenge the shadow presents is not merely intellectual. Jung characterizes as *moral* both the challenge the shadow presents and the effort the challenge requires. In part, this is because resistance to the shadow's assimilation often involves the recognition of the most recalcitrant projections. Its content, the qualities that must be acknowledged as one's own, inevitably appear to lie entirely outside oneself. One's own shadow is seen in the *other person*. "Projections change the world into the replica of one's own unknown face" (Jung, 1959, p. 9), as Jung so pithily remarked. When left unacknowledged, they isolate the individual, leading to what he described as an autoerotic or autistic state. These projections are, furthermore and most importantly, emotionally toned: They are imbued with often disagreeable affects that one is, understandably, reluctant to fully feel and make conscious. Put differently, the shadow's assimilation requires a great deal of affect tolerance, the ability to unflinchingly accept embodied emotional experience, albeit difficult.

The story of Peter Pan offers a beautiful depiction of the unintegrated shadow: Peter, famously, loses his shadow from time to time. He tries to stick it on with soap, to no avail, but later allows his companion Wendy to sow it onto his feet, so that he might not lose it again. The shadow, detached from the body (and its affect), appears as *other*. It seems to have its own volition. The challenge of the eternal youth is to keep it close, to not let it act in a way that is utterly independent (i.e., dissociated) from the rest of one's personality. Peter's detached shadow succinctly depicts in graphic form the surprising autonomy that split-off aspects of the psyche can possess, as well as the particular challenge that they offer for the eternal youth.

The determinative, constitutive aspect of différance—its role as privileged non-origin that is, nevertheless, originary—raises the issue of Husserl's phenomenology as deconstruction's shadow. This is an important means of framing the issue because it helps us move beyond merely pointing out evidence, perhaps circumstantial and contested, of a philosophical contradiction. It helps us to move beyond simply noting somewhat egregious examples of mutually untenable claims or the unconscious committal of a sin so incisively reproached in others. The idea of a philosophical shadow places philosophical claims within a psychological context and is an implicit acknowledgment that these ideas are emotionally charged and are subject to the sorts of psychological dynamics that depth psychology has elucidated throughout its history. It also helps us see beyond the limitations of argument and raises the question of how contrary claims might be integrated into a coherent, that is, less dissociated whole.

Furthermore, raising the issue of Husserl's phenomenology as deconstruction's shadow helps us detect an *archetypal imperative*. From a viewpoint informed by Jungian and post-Jungian psychology, the shadow dynamics at play within deconstruction suggest the machinations of an archetypal possession—the domination of consciousness by an intrusive, irrational, autonomous fragment of the psyche, one that is both archaic and typical. On Jung's account, "the domain of the 'gods' begins where consciousness leaves off, for at that point man is already at the mercy of the natural order, whether he thrive or perish" (Jung, 1973, p. 156). Such shadow dynamics suggest an interference from this domain. Under the influence of an archetypal imperative, possessed of an *idée fixe*, one bends logic to fit a preordained conclusion, twists syntax to hide the agency, and places the reasoning mind at the service of an unreasoned compulsion. Enthralled by the archetype and following its edict, one often does and says exactly what one so vociferously denounces in what others do and say.

According to Jung, when no longer personified as gods, the archetypes, with their readiness to produce over and over again the same or similar mythical ideas, merely take on new forms. They manifest themselves despite the fact that the secular intellect imagines itself to be beyond such superstitious, anachronistic beliefs. He warns that "what we have left behind are only verbal specters, not the psychic facts that were responsible for the birth of the gods. We are still as much possessed by autonomous psychic contents as if they were Olympians" (Jung & De Laszlo, 1991, p. 366). One might say that, on his account, the verbal specters that we refer to as 'gods' can be deconstructed: One can apply any variety of literary-philosophic techniques to deny their *presence*, but what these specters allude to remains ever potent, more so in fact. The power wrested from yesterday's deities somehow endures and, in actuality, may even grow stronger in direct proportion to the perceived abrogation of divine authority. We may believe that we have vanquished the powers beyond our ken, but this is an impossibility. These powers, which, for Jung, emanate from the unconscious psyche, not only persist, but are even strengthened by the belief that they have been defeated. There can be no ultimate conquest, no final overcoming of the psychic facts that gave birth to them (Jung, 1953), just as the conscious ego can never do away with the unconscious psyche. We can explain away the existence of the ancient Greek god Pan, but the *panic* that this god is a proxy for or an expression of will be left untouched. Human beings are still vulnerable to what in other ages would be described as possession by Pan because we are still vulnerable to being possessed by panic.

It is precisely at the moment when we believe that we have dominated the unconscious that we find ourselves most possessed, most at the mercy of powers that exceed our comprehension. Jung's word for this type of phenomena is *enantiodromia*—the process by which something turns into its opposite—the moment, in this case, when our imperious consciousness, convinced of its ultimate conquest, experiences its own abject, inevitable defeat. And, for Jung (1953), the defeat *is* inevitable, for it is "a delusion to think that by some kind of magical theory or method the unconscious can be finally emptied of libido and thus, as it were eliminated" (p. 285). It is precisely when we believe ourselves to be subject to no force, no truth, no dynamic, no divinity, no *presence*, to nothing greater than ourselves that we are most vulnerable to possession by the very forces we believe we have vanquished.

The new forms that the gods take, are often "phobias, obsessions, and so forth; in a word, neurotic symptoms. The gods have become diseases; Zeus no longer rules Olympus but rather the solar plexus, and produces curious specimens for the doctor's consulting room" (Jung & De Laszlo, 1991, p. 366). Like the gods of old, these gods in new form can compel certain behaviors, manifest by way of obsessions, and grab hold of our thinking (Jung, 2011). They still bewitch, enthrall, and place people under a spell. But they take other forms as well. Not only can they manifest as disease, they can also manifest as ideologies, what Jung referred to as *isms*, sacrosanct belief systems beyond refute. He writes,

> The old religions with their sublime and ridiculous, their friendly and fiendish symbols did not drop from the blue, but were born of this human soul that dwells within us at this moment. All those things, their primal forms, live on in us and may at any time burst in upon us with annihilating force, in the guise of mass-suggestions against which the individual is defenceless. Our fearsome gods have only changed their names: they now rhyme with *ism*.
>
> *(Jung, 1953, p. 204)*

More than anyone, it was undoubtedly Nietzsche who influenced Jung on this issue, both in his prophetic discernment and in his tragic folly. For Jung, the philologist's well-known proclamation that 'God is dead' was both a profound truth and a profound delusion. Nietzsche's mental illness toward the end of his life served as a perfect exemplar of what Jung meant by possession and the inflation that accompanies it. It served to illustrate the dangers of attempting to abolish god or gods and the grotesque, inflationary, megalomaniacal dynamics that accompany the attempt.

> Modern iconoclasts are unconscious of the one in whose name they are destroying old values. Nietzsche thought himself quite conscious and responsible when he smashed the old tablets, yet he felt a peculiar need to back himself up with a revivified Zarathustra, a sort of alter ego, with whom he often identifies himself in his great tragedy *Thus Spake Zarathustra*. Nietzsche was no atheist, but his God was dead. The result of this demise was a split in himself, and he felt compelled to call the other self "Zarathustra" or, at times, "Dionysus." In his fatal illness he signed his letters "Zagreus," the dismembered god of the Thracians. The tragedy of Zarathustra is that, because his god died, Nietzsche himself became a god.
>
> *(Jung, 1983, p. 245)*

Jung's entire psychology, in one form or another, grapples with Nietzsche's dilemma, which was also the dilemma of a growing number of Jung's contemporaries as well as his own. The passage above illustrates with unusual clarity what he saw as the need to express religious thought in a more modern idiom amenable to the scientific rationalism of modernity, an endeavor that, in his view, might save us from the very dynamic that Nietzsche so lucidly described and so tragically suffered. He believed we needed to find a new way of speaking of 'gods' lest we become their victims, a new way of acknowledging that we are subject to psychological forces outside of consciousness.

He knew too well that the death of God was profoundly true: Traditional religious forms simply did not mean for moderns what they had meant for their ancestors. To increasingly many, they appeared to be little more than antiquated absurdities and superstitious beliefs worthy of ridicule. Yet he also knew too well that the death of God was profoundly false: God had merely taken on a new form, and our failure to recognize this left us woefully vulnerable to possession by him, although in another guise. Increasingly, he believed that what in other ages had been known as gods or spirits, fairies, or demons, with all of their supernatural power, took the form of unquestioned ideologies and dogmatic beliefs that seized moderns with no less ferocity than their more religious forebearers. Such possession, on his account, was not only a personal occurrence, but a collective one as well, and this collective aspect was particularly worrisome for him. Entire populations, as he saw in his own lifetime, could be swept up in such a dynamic. As he observed, "in so far as psychiatrists are concerned with the psychic treatment of such [archetypal] complexes, they have to do every day with 'demons,' i.e., with psychic factors that display demonic features when they appear as a mass phenomenon" (Jung, 1977, pp. 600–601).

Jung often referred to the aforementioned ideologies and dogmatic beliefs as 'isms,' with the clear intent of evoking the dueling specters of Nazism and Marxism, two ideologies that he witnessed grab hold of a massive swath of the world and cause undeniable devastation. The death of God had as its consequence a "fog of -isms, [and] the catastrophe" (Jung, 1973, p. 88) of World War II. He wrote:

> Perhaps, we could say with Nietzsche, "God is dead." Yet it would be truer to say, "He has put off our image, and where shall we find him again?" The interregnum is full of danger, for the natural facts will raise their claim in the form of various -isms, which are productive of nothing but anarchy and destruction because inflation and man's hybris between them have elected to make the ego, in all its ridiculous paltriness, lord of the universe. That was the case with Nietzsche, the uncomprehended portent of a whole epoch.
>
> *(Jung, 1983, p. 247)*

The lesson learned from Nietzsche is not so much that God has died as much as that he has changed his form. Or, put differently, although God may have died, whatever it is that inspired this term, it still persists and may even have grown in its power by virtue of its apparent disappearance.

Derrida, it would seem, learned very different lessons from Nietzsche. If for Jung, Nietzsche, with hubristic zeal, went a bit too far in his dismissal of the deity, for Derrida, he did not go quite far enough. Despite, like Jung, having a deep admiration for his prophetic genius, he believed that Nietzsche (and Heidegger as well) fell short in his attempt to overcome the metaphysical legacy of the West. Jung, on the other hand, was less intent on overcoming that legacy and more intent on translating it into a more modern idiom, as well as drawing parallels with the traditions of other cultures. From a Jungian perspective, Derrida's attempt to dismantle the tradition *more* thoroughly is an invitation to the same possessive and inflationary tendencies found in Nietzsche, perhaps an even more explicit and insistent invitation. If, as he claimed, because Nietzsche's god had died, he himself 'became' a god, one might similarly claim that, because Derrida deconstructs gods, he 'becomes' one as well. He invites possession.

Because Nietzsche was Jung's mentor in this regard, he understood that the death of the Christian deity and the twilight of prior idols were accompanied by a trend toward Dionysian thought among intellectuals, one that often favored the irrational and particular over the rational and universal. The result was a fierce, even fundamentalist belief in ideologies, in *isms* that strangely mirrored archaic forms of belief despite their modernist pretense of having overcome the prima facie absurd narratives of the religious imagination.

Comparing the paragraph from Jung cited earlier with another from Derrida that we have already considered is instructive for understanding their differing beliefs as regards our metaphysical heritage, that is to say, the historical categories and linguistic matrices we use to assign meaning. It is also instructive for understanding the idea of archetypal possession with all of its annihilating force:

> Since language (which Saussure says is a classification) has not fallen from the sky, it is clear that the differences have been produced; they are the effects produced, but effects that do not have as their cause a subject or substance, a thing in general, or a being that is somewhere present and itself escapes the play of difference. . . . I have tried to indicate a way out of the closure imposed by this system, namely by means of the "trace."
>
> *(Derrida, 1973, p. 141)*

Note, first, the use of the passive voice—differences 'have been produced'—and the insistence that the differences produced through language have no subject or substance, no thing or being that is involved in said production. The producer of language is absent. Indeed, for Derrida (1973), the "movement of *différance* is not something that happens to a transcendental subject; it produces a subject" (p. 82). Somehow, by means that are never made clear, humans have inherited an entire metaphysics, a conceptual order, a generalized system of schemata that Derrida refers to as a *metaphysics of presence*, but the entire process is clouded in obscurity.

Jung sees things differently: The forms we use for assigning meaning, our 'linguistic matrices,' or what Derrida would call our 'metaphysical heritage,' are derived from the same primordial ground of experience as that of myth and religion, with all of its sublime and ridiculous, friendly and fiendish symbols. They did not drop from the sky but were born of the human soul, or psyche.

Thinking in this way is important because it allows us to return ideas to their psychic, archetypal ground. Then, their symptomatic and symbolic content can be engaged because their more fully human provenance has been acknowledged. Abstract ideas are no longer seen merely as abstract ideas. In the *aporia* of ideas one finds the pathos of psyche, with all the splits, fissures, and doublings, with all the rage, sadness, and anxiety that can cleave a person from himself or herself, or make one cling with irrational zeal to one claim or another. One finds trauma, with all of its unbearable affects. Returning ideas to this psychic ground was Jung's, Hillman's, and von Franz's approach. As the vast body of Jung's work testifies, these traumatic dissociations run along archetypal lines (Jung, 1969, 1970, 1973; Kalsched, 1996, 2013). They manifest through figures that are archaic and typical. The failure to return ideas to this archetypal context obscures psyche and the foci of sickness remain opaque. We are left with the brilliant opining of savants, but the archetypal syndrome that possesses them remains shrouded, and behind a façade of theoretical plausibility hides pathology.

Deconstruction invites possession in another way. As mentioned earlier, Marie-Louise von Franz and others have noted that fairy tales invoke time and place in paradoxical ways that evoke timelessness and spacelessness, on her account, the realm of the collective unconscious. Deconstruction evokes a similar timelessness and spacelessness in its basic disruption of sequence and the associated reconfiguration of the meaning of words like *past*, *present*, and *future*. All of this functions as its own *once upon a time* that encourages the reader to suspend belief and enter an *illud tempus*, a timeless eternity. There, in that realm, where one is not reminded of one's own finitude and mortality, where one is embodied, time-bound and, as Nietzsche might say, human all too human, one is left vulnerable to possession by what were once called gods. The invocation *once upon a time* is a pact of sorts, an agreement, a voucher or ticket to another realm, perhaps no less real, but a realm from which one must return. It is like a magic portal of sorts that leads to a timeless realm but does not necessarily lead back.

Just as a poker player exhibits certain *tells*—idiosyncratic mannerisms and reflexes that reveal hidden intent—the machinations of the archetype make themselves evident covertly but are nevertheless decipherable to the perceptive observer. One such tell discloses itself in the insistence that the trace not only must inhabit the now, but must *constitute* it (Derrida, 1973). To claim that the present is inhabited by moments other than itself is a reasonable claim, one that Husserl would not contest and one that, nevertheless, might serve to undermine his particular conception of presence as originary. Yet the claim that the trace *constitutes* the present is something quite different. Not only does it mimic the phenomenological presumptions that it seeks to undermine, it also grants to the trace an almost demiurgic status, a god-like quality, as do claims that différance is the origin of the experience of time and space. One can, in complete agreement with deconstruction, incant in tones evocative of the Torah, the words *in the beginning there was différance*.

A similar tell involves the closely related claim that the trace is not concerned with "horizons of modified—past or future—presents, but with a 'past' that has never been present" (Derrida, 1982 [1986], p. 21). A past that has never been present implies again a demiurge, a deity beyond the vicissitudes of temporality that is, nevertheless, responsible for them. Pasts that have never once been present are not pasts at all, and the repeated insistence that they are—particularly when it involves the governing principle and *spiritus rector* of an entire philosophical project—is indicative of an imperative that lies outside the reasoning mind in that place where consciousness leaves off.

Derrida (1973) is quick to assure his reader that although the phrases and syntax that he resorts to in his description of *différance* "will sometimes be practically indiscernible from—those of negative theology" (p. 134) they are not what they appear to be. Negative theology is an attempt to describe a supreme being that is beyond human categories. If it claims that god does not exist, it does so only "to recognize him as a superior, inconceivable, and ineffable mode of being" (Derrida, 1973, p. 134). But *différance*, he (1973) assures us, is irreducible "to every ontological or theological—onto-theological—reappropriation" (p. 134). He is right to use such a preemptive defense because this is where he is most vulnerable.

*Différance is Derrida's god.* This is evidenced by its omnitemporal ubiquity: The temporal distance that semiotic deferral implies reaches not only forward but backward as well. It suspends both finality *and* inception. Everything is *always already not yet*. Everything is preemptively deferred. According to its logic, the genesis of all meaning resides in an *absolute* past (Bennington, 2010) and it is this absoluteness that hints at its archetypal constitution. To claim that meaning is subject to deferral is a fairly straightforward and reasonable claim, but to found a philosophical project upon the principle that this has *always already* been the case is to ratify a unidimensional and unidirectional understanding of both time and language. To claim that meaning is subject to deferral is to point to an aspect of its temporal unfolding. But deferral, when infinite, amounts to never, just as distance, when infinite, leads nowhere. To acknowledge *différance* as an aspect of a more complex, rich, varied understanding of both time/space and language is analogous to a humble acknowledgment that the eternal youth is but one deity in a broader pantheon, but one force among many. But to claim that it plays the role of an origin, to ally it with the absolute, to provide no substantial countervailing principle to it, and to grant it the power of the infinite, is to succumb to possession by this same eternal youth. Such an attitude fetishizes the *not yet*, making it an object of exclusive, undue reverence.

To claim that différance is Derrida's god and that he is, in a sense, possessed by this god is a bold claim that warrants unpacking, or perhaps translating. For Jung (1973), "that psychological fact which is the greatest in your system is the god, since it is always the overwhelming psychic factor which is called god" (p. 81). From his point of view, 'gods' are akin to supraordinate ideas or reigning principles, often ones that carry with them an unusually strong emotional charge. They express themselves in what Jung, borrowing from anthropology, referred to as *représentations collectives*. He writes:

> Now religious ideas, as history shows, are charged with an extremely suggestive, emotional power. Among them I naturally reckon all *représentations collectives*, everything that we learn from the history of religion, and anything that has an "-ism" attached to it. The latter is only a modern variant of the denominational religions. A man may be convinced in all good faith that he has no religious ideas, but no one can fall so far away from humanity that he no longer has any dominating *représentation collective*. His very materialism, atheism, communism, socialism, liberalism, intellectualism, existentialism, or what not, testifies against his innocence. Somewhere or other, overtly or covertly, he is possessed by a supraordinate idea.
>
> *(Jung, 1969, pp. 61–62)*

Jung is unequivocal in this regard: A person may be convinced that he or she has no religious ideas, just as Derrida can be convinced that différance is irreducible to every 'onto-theological reappropriation,' but this is simply not the case. If Jung's reading is correct, then it would seem that deconstruction(ism) is something like a religious denomination that worships at the altar of *différance*.

Another 'tell' that Derrida is, uncritically, under the influence of a supraordinate idea, resides in deconstruction's understanding of the disjuncture between signifiers and signifieds: To acknowledge the protean quality of a given word as it slides from one context to another is fairly incontrovertible. Recognizing that signifiers slide, that words change their meaning, serves as a healthy reminder to check the hubris of any interpretation enthralled by its own certainty and the pompous belief in its own authority. But the deconstructive project recognizes no other dynamic, no other master: It is a thinking by way of disunion and disruption. Countervailing principles like identity, presence, continuity, and synthesis, although acknowledged, are themselves understood as arising from, and being secondary to, the non-identity, absence, discontinuity, and divisiveness of différance, given that it is the common root of *all* oppositional concepts (Derrida, 1981 [1982]).

Such one-sidedness, such a lack of any truly counterbalancing force, on Jung's (1964) reading, is symptomatic of the gravitational pull of the archetype, which renders even the best of us, at times, "liable to possession by an infatuation, a vice, or a one-sided conviction" (p. 139). Under the sway of an archetypal imperative, certain things simply *must* be so. In lieu of an argument to provide sufficient warrant, and despite repeated logical incongruities requiring that terms be either oxymoronic or enclosed within qualifying quotations, the repeated insistence that presence *must* be constituted by différance and that representation *must* precede presentation suggests a demand that lies outside consciousness. Similarly, the assertion that différance is neither a word nor a concept, despite evidence to the contrary, suggests an equally imperious need. This is the one word that must be exceptional, that must not, under any circumstances, be subjected to the provisions that other words are subjected to. The bulwark of its absoluteness, its privileged status of being always already in play, must remain unquestioned.

Von Franz (1980), in *Projection and Re-collection in Jungian Psychology*, writes of the possessive states of autonomous complexes that they

> upset the total equilibrium of the personality by compelling one-sidedness. One among other easily recognizable symptoms is the way in which the thoughts and deeds of the possessed person tend to circle, in incredible monomania, around the one complex-theme, to the damage of the whole personality.
>
> *(p. 100)*

In such a state, one is like Polyphemus or other one-eyed creatures like those that often appear in Grimms' fairy tales; that is to say, a person becomes not only monomaniacal but *monocular*. Seeing with one eye focused on one object and lacking binocular vision, a person fails to perceive the depth of a third dimension. Then, one is *ver-rückt*, a German word that means crazy or insane, but also carries the meaning of being *displaced* (Von Franz, 1980). Such a double meaning is also conveyed by the English expression that a person is 'not all there.'

Another name for this one-sidedness is reductionism, or the tyranny of the *nothing but*. Deconstruction is reductive to the extent that it construes meaning as something produced exclusively by the differential, deferential play of signs. Insofar as it contends that "from the moment that there is meaning, there are *nothing but* signs [emphasis added]" (Derrida, 1976, p. 50), insofar as it insists that the use of language or the employment of any code implies a play of forms with "no determined or invariable substratum" (p. 146), it is one-sided. Within this *nothing but* its reductionism resides. Jung describes the *nothing but* temperament as "the insistent leitmotiv of all one-sidedness" (Jung, 1981, p. 83). An equally insistent leitmotiv goes by the name of ad infinitum. By its very nature, the one-sidedness of archetypal possession knows no limitation. Childlike in its sense of omnipotence, it lacks epistemic humility. In this regard, it is not the mere acknowledgment of semiotic deferral that is indicative of such a one-sidedness, but the belief that presence is "*in fact*, really, effectively, etc., deferred *ad infinitum*" (Derrida, 1973, p. 99). Presence is not merely put off until later. Later, when infinite, amounts to never.

Let us, for a moment, consider Derrida's (1973) description of the trace, the play of différance, as a kind of protowriting "without an *archē*" (p. 146). As acknowledged in the introduction, *archē* and all that is synonymous with such a term, is a favorite target that deconstruction takes aim at. Construing deconstruction itself in terms of the archetypal, therefore, implies starting from premises that are antithetical to its fundamental critical thrust. *Archē* implies such invariable presences as essences, substances, consciousness, gods, or universals, which are the very ideas that deconstruction attempts to dismantle. An archetypal reading of a discourse that is anathema to the archetypal is simultaneously an implicit challenge *to*, and implicitly challenged *by*, the subject matter it addresses.

One way of tackling this challenge is to point out that, for Jung, it is when we are most adamant in denying the archetypal that we are most in its grips. It is in denying 'the gods'—although we may not name them as such—in failing to pay them appropriate homage or appease them through sufficient sacrifice, that we are most vulnerable to their demands. This observation is, in fact, fundamental to Jung's entire critique of modernity and a guiding impulse behind his psychology, which is, to a great extent, an attempt to put into a more contemporary language the past insights of fairy tale, myth, and religion. For Jung (1964), it was

> . . . just when people were congratulating themselves on having abolished all spooks, [that] it turned out that instead of haunting the attic or old ruins the spooks were flitting about in the heads of apparently normal Europeans. Tyrannical, obsessive, intoxicating ideas and delusions were abroad everywhere, and people began to believe the most absurd things, just as the possessed do.
>
> *(p. 212)*

If Jung is correct, then the words *without an archē* are indicative of not merely a philosophical claim but a psychological attitude fraught with peril. The aforementioned critical thrust of deconstruction, which seeks to dismantle any such presence, surreptitiously invites the very presences, gods, or archaic and typical psychological dynamics that it attempts to dismantle. Like a person who denies the reality of gravity, it invites a fall. Jung (1964) writes:

> No one will deny the important role which the powers of the human psyche, personified as "gods," played in the past. The mere act of enlightenment may have destroyed the spirits of nature, but not the psychic factors that correspond to them, such as suggestibility, lack of criticism, fearfulness, propensity to superstition and prejudice—in short, all those qualities which make possession possible. Even though nature is depsychized, the psychic conditions which breed demons are as actively at work as ever. The demons have not really disappeared but have merely taken on another form: they have become unconscious psychic forces.
>
> *(p. 211)*

For Jung, the undeniable enlightenment of our present era, with its scientific and technological progress, leaves us vulnerable. Despite our pretenses, despite the feeling that we are beyond the silly beliefs of our ancestors, we are not. In fact, "mankind, *because* [emphasis added] of its scientific and technological development, has in increasing measure delivered itself over to the danger of possession" (Jung, 1969, p. 253). It is as if there is an inverse or compensatory relationship between the belief that we possess knowledge and our vulnerability to possession.

The demon, the spirit, the god, the archetype, the tyrannical, obsessive, idea that intoxicates the advocates of deconstruction is différance, a principle of absolute, infinite deferral, ostensibly responsible for the experience of time and space yet existing beyond it. Let us call it the god of the *not yet*, the god of temporal displacement whose desire, as pothos, must be a desire for something so transcendent, so beyond grasp that he will never attain it, something as transcendent as, we are told, is the transcendental signified.

Seen in this light, the strategy that attempts to dismantle a metaphysics of presence, and the *archai* that are characteristic of it, is itself symptomatic of an *archē*. It is archetypal. It is when we are most convinced of the non-existence of the archetypes that we are most in their grip. It is when we most fervently insist on their absence that they are most present. As Erasmus knew, and as Jung carved above the entrance to his home, *Vocatus atque non vocatus deus aderit*: Called or not called, God is there.

It cannot be overstated the degree to which deconstruction is an attempt to undermine the archetypal, in the broadest sense of the word. Its critique of origins is just such an attempt. Its endeavor to disrupt a metaphysics of presence is an endeavor to disrupt a metaphysics of presences:

> It could be shown that all the names related to fundamentals, to principles, or to the center have always designated an invariable presence—eidos, arche, telos, energeia, ousia (essence, existence, substance, subject) aletheia, transcendentality, consciousness, God, man, and so forth.
>
> *(Derrida, 1967 [1978], pp. 279–280)*

Deconstruction is a strategy to undermine appeals to such originary principles and generative centers as those listed earlier, but also those that go by the names of *truth, reality, self, center, unity*, and *nature* (Alderman, 2016). It is an attempt to steal something of their *élan vital*. They are, to borrow Jung's language, the spooks it wishes to abolish, or, to borrow Derrida's language, the *god-terms* it desires to destabilize.

From Jung's perspective, " 'principalities and powers' are always with us; we have no need to create them even if we could" (Jung, 1983, p. 246). We cannot do away with them, and to think otherwise is hubris. The challenge is not to abolish the archetypal powers or undermine our belief in the presence of things like consciousness, or substance, or transcendentality, but to find the right relationship to them. On his account, "the chief danger is that of succumbing to the fascinating influence of the archetypes, and this is most likely to happen when the archetypal images are not made conscious" (Jung, 1969, p. 39). Awareness is essential. Jung (1969) writes:

> The constellation of archetypal images and fantasies is not in itself pathological. The pathological element only reveals itself in the way the individual reacts to

> them and how he interprets them. The characteristic feature of a pathological reaction is, above all, *identification with the archetype*. This produces a sort of inflation and possession by the emergent contents, so that they pour out in a torrent which no therapy can stop. Identification can, in favourable cases, sometimes pass off as a more or less harmless inflation. But in all cases identification with the unconscious brings a weakening of consciousness, and herein lies the danger. You do not 'make' an identification, you do not 'identify yourself,' but you experience your identity with the archetype in an unconscious way and so are possessed by it.
>
> *(pp. 351–352)*

What he means by identification is perhaps better understood as *becoming identical with*. In order not to become identical with a god, one must discern its form and find the right relationship to it, rather than being swallowed up by it.

A right relationship is becoming neither absolutely identical nor absolutely different from a deity, a split off fragment of a greater psychic whole. This fact brings us to the potential dangers of the present diagnostic argument. It risks the same sort of shadowboxing that I attribute to deconstruction: Critics are always well advised to suspect themselves of the foibles they so lucidly detect in others and remain mindful of their own complicity in the phenomena critiqued. It risks reducing the complex genius of deconstruction to nothing more than a set of intellectual defenses dressed up as theory. Such a reading flirts with the same one-sidedness or reductionism, the same tyranny of the *nothing but* that characterizes the psychological state under discussion. The present text is not exempt from risking its own form of reductionism. And substituting one reductionism (the linguistic) for that of another (the psychological or archetypal) is hardly progress if a greater integration is the goal.

With these thoughts in mind, it should be noted that other readings from within the Jungian community cast a far more sympathetic light on Derrida's work. Stanton Marlan (2005, 2020, 2022), whose writings on Jungian and post-Jungian approaches to alchemy offer detailed, nuanced, masterful readings, has portrayed in numerous works not only deconstruction but post-structuralism more broadly as being far more kindred to Jung's work than the present text would suggest. A superficial reading of Marlan's work and the present text might lead to the conclusion that his account and my own could not be more antithetical to one another. This is understandable but perhaps only partially true.

For Marlan, it was in particular Jung's alchemical studies that moved him toward a more fluid, self-reflective, and contextual thinking akin to Derrida's. In addressing Jung's approach, he notes, "there has been a tendency to understand his use of archetypal material as an essentialist paradigm, insofar as he places an emphasis on a universal, fixed, and unchanging (essential) meaning" (Marlan, 2020, p. 60). This is, to an extent at least, an unfortunate tendency that does not grant Jung the sophisticated reading that he merits; Marlan sees Jung as less essentialist than some give him credit for and notes that "since meaning is never completely known (a position that Jung also takes)" he cannot be characterized as the rigid thinker that some might see him as. In fact, since he takes meaning to never be completely known, his similarity to Derrida is all the more apparent.

Furthermore, Derrida's similarities to James Hillman's re-visioning of Jung's work are even more conducive to a perceived alliance between post-Jungian studies and deconstruction. Marlan's writings are indicative of a general shift in Jungian and post-Jungian thinking toward a more postmodern and relativistic sensibility, one that Hillman was certainly an integral part of. Yet Marlan notes that Hillman could be likewise critical, seeing deconstruction as "playing with the ambiguity of the 'trace,' troping, displacing, and insisting upon difference and, as well, the absenting of all certitudes from positive propositions [which] becomes one more habitual concretism of Western thought" (Marlan quoting Hillman, 2020, p. 127). In terms of the interpretation to be given in a later chapter of the present work, this might be thought of as the secret alliance of the eternal youth with his polar opposite, the senex, whose tendency is toward the concrete and immutable, but more of this later.

For Marlan, deconstructing presence into absence is what makes cultural evolution possible. If ideas, words, and cultural forms cannot be dismantled then there is stasis. On his account, then, Derrida is an integral part of a cultural evolution that sees beyond the tendency of the West to privilege its own set of biases and assumptions, its own version of reason, as if it were a universal form. In particular, it is Enlightenment reason that is at issue, insofar as said 'enlightenment' is an expression of the West's privileging of light over dark. Derrida's work, on this account, points to the shadow of the West's own power dynamics (Marlan, 2020). His undermining of the logic of representation, Marlan rightly notes, is in many ways conducive to Jung's own thinking as regards symbols as infinitely generative sources of meaning that resist any totalizing, final interpretation. It likewise has an affinity to Jung's proclivity to use ideas only as provisional structures that could never adequately grasp the full complexity of the subject at hand. Marlan emphasizes that, in freeing the mind of literalism, deconstruction senses fluidity in language, one that is open to paradox, contradiction, and ambiguity, and is attuned to the historically contingent nature of truth. These are all valid observations.

More importantly, and perhaps more pertinent to the present work, Marlan (2005, 2020) places deconstruction within the context of Jung's thinking on alchemy, associating it with such alchemical stages as the *nigredo*, *putrefactio*, and *mortifactio*. The latter stage is one in which "the primitive King is tortured, beaten, humiliated, poisoned, drowned, dissolved, calcined, and killed" (Marlan, 2020, p. 156). Likewise, Derrida's "idea of erasure lends itself to comparison with certain operations of alchemy that have to do with the processes of mortification, calcination, and dissolution and entering into the blacker-than-black aspect of the nigredo" (Marlan, 2005, p. 188). Such descriptions are conducive to an understanding of deconstruction as a dissociation, a dissolving, a process of de-integration, as construed in the previous chapter, and I have no desire to take issue with any of them. Rather, I want to simply place deconstruction with its dissociative tendencies within a broader alchemical process. This broader process will be more fully articulated in the final chapter by way of the image of the uroboros, the self-consuming and self-generating serpent that, on Jung's account, was a symbol of psychological wholeness.

## II

Derrida tells his reader that *différance* involves the pleasure of an impossible presence, one irreparably lost that, nevertheless, cannot fail to provoke an unappeasable desire to return. Like schizoid love, it suffers from dueling imperatives. The reading of a love made hungry offered by Guntrip, Fairbairn, Klein, Balint, Laing, Kalsched, and others, so briefly sketched previously, suggests that the source of this insatiable hunger lies in infancy.

In keeping with our psychosemantic analysis, and in the attempt to move the discussion of deconstruction from the realm of thought to the realm of psyche, it should be noted that infancy—as the etymology of the word *infant* attests—is the age before speech. Deriving from the Latin *in*, meaning *not* or *opposite*, and *fans*, meaning *to speak*, infancy is a time preceding the use of language. If there is—to co-opt Derrida's words and place them in a context that he did not intend—an age of *pure and primordial perception, full and simple presence* that *precedes representation*, then infancy is that age. It is before speech, before writing and, as différance itself is said to be, it is *avant la lettre* in all senses of the phrase. If there is a time in psychological development that might refute, confirm, or merely shed light on the claim that perception does not exist or is not primordial, and that somehow everything begins by re-presentation then infancy would be that time.

And if there is another name for the primordial presence irreparably lost, perhaps that name is *mother*. Is she not such a presence? After all, what is primordiality? To what does that word, often invoked by both Jung and Derrida, refer? It is inseparable from a sense of sequence. From the Latin *primus* "first" and *ordiri* "to begin," it denotes a first beginning and alludes to that which is primal and primeval, primary and precedent. To speak of it is to summon the idea of an origin, and for each of us individually, this origin is our own mother. She is our first beginning. There is something primordial in the very idea of *mother*: She enwombs us, enwraps us within her flesh, enspheres us within her universe. She births us and later, with luck, she will nourish us at her bosom, cradle us within her embrace, and enswathe us within her affection. She is always already there as an ever-present surround, a ubiquitous feminine presence as we progress from zygote to embryo, from fetus to the nascent being that we all once were. In the age before speech, she enfolds us, for:

> Mother is a separate object only from the standpoint of an adult observer: for the infant, Mother is a global presence whose being is not yet distinct from

> the infant's own being. *Différance* has not come into play; it is only a portent existing in the demand of the transcendent world to have its articulations acknowledged.
>
> *(Dillon, 2003, p. 133)*

A time when différance has not yet come into play—this is exactly what deconstruction fails to account for, because its 'count' or sense of sequence is amiss. Mother is, as it were, the gap that creates deconstruction's peculiar temporal discontinuity: She is the primordiality forever denied and commemorated, the experience, to borrow Husserl's phrase, pregiven to the I.

Antepartum, and to varying degrees postpartum, she is that which envelops us. She is ambience, from the Latin *ambiens* "a going around." She is an *environ*, an encircling, as the Latin roots of the word tell us: en=in and viron=circle or circuit. Mother is a phenomenal and perceptual field inhabited before we, swaddled infants, can clearly sense self and other. She is an original symbiosis, a 'living together.' She is our primal love object, though only subsequently perceived as such, well after she has been lived as milieu and medium, well after an original fusion preceding the diffusion of our world into an 'I' or 'you' or 'she.' Within that fusion, we are shrouded by a sonorous field of echoing cries and placating coos, entwined within a tactile reciprocity of the sentient and sensible before we even know that we are persons as such. She is "the totality of life of which we are a small and helpless part" (Jung, 1969, p. 92), even before we know that we are a 'part.' She is the totality because during the first months of life, infants cannot distinguish between subject and object, self and other, self and mother (Guntrip, 1992). Prior to these distinctions, there is only one seamless flesh.

Each mother is also a Pandora, in the sense given that name before the time of Hesiod, before she became the epithet of a disaster bequeathed in the guise of a gift, a box containing calamity: Each mother is the giver of all for her infant, and this is, indeed, the root meaning of the goddess' name, as its Greek etymology attests: *pan* is all and *doron* is gift, from the root *do*, meaning to give (Dougherty, 2006). Each mother is the giver of all because without her, the infant's world would not exist. Each mother is the given, in the sense that she is immediately present in experience. She is given and we are derivative. She is the other out of which we all individuate—in the most literal and material sense at the moment of physical birth and the cutting of the umbilical cord—yet also in the most metaphorical sense as we cut, over and again, invisible umbilical ties that persist long after. Through developmental stages, we recognize her as other and recognize our own consequent difference from her. Within months, mother is not an environ, but a figure within it, one among others, albeit a special one. She becomes a means to an end and a reflective presence as we begin to recognize ourselves as recognizable by others. Slowly our world differentiates itself and mother, once a global presence, becomes circumscribed and singular. Mother—the great container, the great surround, whose continuity with ourselves felt seamless—is now contained, surrounded by the same world that contains and surrounds us. Yet who better to symbolize the sense of a primordial, enveloping presence, even once she has ceased to be so?

Let us imagine that the metaphoric, associative matrix of 'mother' is not arbitrary, nor the exclusive result of a metaphysical heritage or cultural bias. Rather, the full meaning of 'mother' is rooted in experiences so perennial and collective as to be sedimented within us. 'Mother,' although a term that may imply a system of oppositional concepts like mother/father or mother/child, has not acquired its meaning *solely* through the interplay of such oppositions. 'Mother' has a meaning that—although not inscribed in the heavens or in the brain as Derrida would remind us—forms part of an inheritance grounded in such universal experiences as those described earlier.

Much of the resonance of mother metaphors, as well as the connotations of the word itself, can appear self-evident if one takes a moment to reflect. *Mother*, in a greater, figurative sense, is simply everything that functions as she does, so that anything with an "enveloping, embracing, and devouring element points unmistakably to the mother" (Jung, 1959, p. 11). Because of this encircling or containing quality, the resonance of the mother archetype reaches all things that might serve as containers, from ovens and cups to bowls and baskets, reservoirs and lakes, and, of course, the uterus and vagina (Jung, 1959). Because of our personal, individual experiences of our own mothers, the archetype—the greater, metaphoric, figurative sense of the mother motif—is often expressed through her image:

> The carrier of the archetype is in the first place the personal mother, because the child lives at first in complete participation with her, in a state of unconscious identity. She is the psychic well as the physical precondition of the child.
>
> *(Jung, 1969, p. 102)*

Yet she is still but one carrier, one idiosyncratic expression peculiar to our own experience. The less idiosyncratic expressions take the form of myth and metaphor. We speak of *mother nature* for example, because *nature*, insofar as the idea is inseparable from the *natal* and *native*, that is to say, from birth and place of birth, is related to mother. We speak of *mother earth* because the earth insofar as it is our place of origin, the creative, living environ from which each of us has been born shares the qualities of a mother.

Perhaps less apparent is the idea of mother as matter, yet both terms, the former and the latter, derive from the Latin *mater*. The inheritance is not merely a Western one. The linking of mother and matter is evident in the Mesopotamian lore of Ereshkigal, queen of the underworld and representative of the "seeming stasis and the coalesced, unitive solidity of matter as a cosmic principle" (Perera, 1981, p. 25). Moving farther east, to the Sankhya philosophy of India, mother is matter by way of the concept of *prakrti* (Jung, 1969). Within alchemy, the protoscience practiced throughout Africa, Asia, and Europe that originated in Egypt in the first centuries of the Christian Era, Mother was often the name of the *prima materia*, the first matter from which alchemists attempted to conjure gold (Jung, 1969). Mother in other ages was termed "anima mundi, . . . the soul in cosmic matter" (Von Franz, 1970 [1992], p. 209).

In the East, she is Maya (Jung, 1969) the creator of illusion. She is Ishtar, Astarte, Atargatis, Aphrodite, Venus, and Cybele. For Jung, she is, in a sense, psychic structure itself, that which is given, what might be called its Pandoric quality, "the precondition that is found to be present in every case . . . this is the *mother*, the matrix—the form into which all experience is poured" (Jung, 1969, pp. 101–102). She is also a "homecoming, shelter, and the long silence from which everything begins and in which everything ends" (Jung, 1969, p. 92). She is both origin and end, birth and death, womb and tomb: "the first world of the child and the last world of the adult. We are all wrapped as her children in the mantle of this great Isis" (Jung, 1969, p. 94). Because mother is our first beginning, our origin, our first presence, she is an apt image or symbol of primordiality itself. If, as Derrida (1981 [1982]) acknowledged, metaphysics is the mythos of an idiom, then the mythic figure of mother has a correlate in the idiom of our metaphysics. If, as Jung (1969) once phrased it, "linguistic matrices . . . are themselves derived from primordial images" (pp. 32–33), then the term *primordial* has in some sense been derived from the mother image or has an enduring relationship to it.

In light of such an observation, it is, symbolically speaking, the mother that deconstruction attempts to usurp with its insistence that the primordial and perceptual are secondary and derivative. The trace, which allows the present to be a form, yet void of matter, voids the present of mother. Yet mother is also what deconstruction returns to, again and again, in its repeated invocation of traces that are "more 'primordial' than what is phenomenologically primordial" (Derrida, 1973, p. 67). She is gone, then there again: *fort-da*, as Derrida plays a game of peekaboo, or hide-and-go-seek with a primordiality that must be denied at the very moment of its invocation, must be reputed and then surreptitiously serve to underwrite the argument that reputes it. Although deconstruction encloses her safely within quotations, it nevertheless needs her to bolster its own arguments, its own privileging. Remember, despite his opposition to Husserl's claims founded on the present as origin, Derrida, nevertheless "retains the value of privilege and priority that only such arguments bestow" (Wood, 2001, p. 274). Although he is opposed to the primordial mother, he attempts to retain the privilege that her firstness confers. He grants this firstness to a surrogate primordiality, the surrogate mother that is différance.

For Marie-Louise Von Franz (1970 [1992]), whose writings on the topic remain authoritative classics within Jungian studies, the *puer aeternus* is the eternal lover of the eternal mother, the Attis of Cybele, Ba'al of Astarte, Oedipus of Jocasta. Unconsciously embedded in the relationship, he is surreptitiously attached to her far beyond due time. Entangled within Maya, men and women who remain puerile well into middle age suffer a " 'longing for the mother,' the nostalgia for the source from which we came" (Jung, 1953, p. 169). One might say they suffer from the irreparable loss of her presence. Peter Pan certainly did; his suffering was so great that he denied even having had a mother. Individuals enthralled by this mythic character, those who see through the eyes of this eternal youth, suffer from a mother complex, one that takes a predictable form that is evidenced the world over in mythological patterns that do not fail to repeat themselves. Von Franz' reading is informed by the observation made by her mentor and others before him that,

> [a]s mythology shows, one of the peculiarities of the Great Mother is that she frequently appears paired with her male counterpart. Accordingly the man identifies with the son-lover on whom the grace of Sophia has descended, with a *puer aeternus* or a *filius sapientiae.*
>
> *(Jung, 1969, p. 106)*

One iteration of this figure upon which von Franz writes extensively is the protagonist of *The Golden Ass*, Lucius—the doppelgänger, or ideal ego of Apuleius, the author of this celebrated Greek novel of antiquity, which, like many such novels, centers upon the relationship between pothos and its satisfaction (Whitmarsh, 2011). In her reading, the problem of Lucius-Apuleius is that he suffers from a mother complex, the fundamental problem of the puer type. He is "threatened by an overwhelming power, namely the archetypal feminine principle" (Von Franz, 1970 [1992], p. 22).

The story of this struggle and its eventual resolution takes the form of an initiation into the cult of Isis, which, in more modern and classically Jungian terms, refers to a maturation of his relation to the feminine. This maturation manifests in the form of an odyssey, a return to his mother's native land, a place that represents her but is not her, a place that serves as her surrogate or proxy. The journey itself is riddled with tragically comic mishaps, not the least of which gives the novel its name: Lucius, the neophyte magician, who dabbles in the occult sciences without ever quite committing to them fully, mistakenly turns himself into an ass, a beast of burden, lowly and laughable. Such are the emasculating tricks that the overwhelming power of the mother complex plays upon him. His odyssey and eventual healing—in the form of a final deliverance from his inept magical spell—result in a renewed sense of relatedness, communion, and spiritual nourishment. But this is achieved only after multiple humiliations, including that of being purchased, when still in the form of an ass, by a band of travelers who are worshipers of the Syrian goddess Cybele, whose priests, called *galli*, in imitation of her son-lover Attis, castrate, whip, and mutilate themselves as an act of devotion to this goddess.

Much of the genius of Jungian and post-Jungian studies lies in the recognition of similarities between the pathos of individuals and the pathos of mythic and literary figures. The similarities are so perennial and typical as to appear intrinsic to the human condition. They suggest fundamental psychological patterns that are not as uniquely individual as they may appear. In fact, the greater the pathology, the greater the typicality. The more we convince ourselves that our suffering is uniquely ours, the more it reveals its collective hue. It is when we most deeply believe in the *sui generis* nature of our affliction that we are most suffering from an archetypal possession, that we are most trapped within a pattern of behavior, thought, and feeling that is endemic to the species.

This possession is a form of identification, a becoming identical to. Therefore, a *puer* personality is deemed as such because he "is merely the archetype of the eternal youth god, and therefore he has all the features of the god: he has a nostalgic longing for death, [and] he thinks of himself as being something special" (Von Franz, 1970 [2000], p. 121), although, in fact, this is what he has failed to become. By succumbing to the archetype, he has become a stereotype. He is a semblance of Attis, Adonis, Osiris, Adam, Corybas, Pan, or Bacchus (Jung, 1969)—though he may not have heard of any of these figures—but he is not a semblance of himself, curious as this formulation may sound. The eternal lover of the eternal mother is merely another iteration of Lucius, the little prince, or Peter Pan.

The god manifests in multiple ways within the lives of those possessed by him. According to von Franz, pueri aeterni—those enthralled by the deity—often consider themselves exceptionally talented, and may even be so, yet they too often avoid putting this talent to the test or developing it through years of discipline and practice, therefore, they remain maladapted and often have megalomaniacal pretensions. An emphatic belief in their own difference from others hides a fear of their own fundamental similarity. They never test the difference because they never quite enter the realm of adults, with its troublesome practicalities, material necessity, and pragmatic demands.

> The one thing dreaded by such a type of man is to be bound to anything whatever. There is a terrific fear of being pinned down, of entering space and time completely, and of being the singular human being that one is. There is always the fear of being caught in a situation from which it may be impossible to slip out again. Every just-so situation is hell. At the same time, there is a highly symbolic fascination for dangerous sports—particularly flying and mountaineering—so as to get as high as possible, the symbolism being to get away from reality, from earth, from ordinary life.
>
> *(Von Franz, 1970 [2000], p. 8)*

One recurrent approach to forestalling entrance into space and time for such a person is through simple inaction. Eternal youths do not seize the opportune moment or act when circumstance calls for it. They fail in decisive moments by simply not deciding. Puer gods are gods of possibility without limitation, mutability without final form, and decisions inevitably suggest finality, which is anathema to this archetypal disposition that insists on having all options open all the time.

It is in the most decisive moments that things become most undecidable for eternal youths. They are "always inwardly toying with a thousand possibilities of life and cannot choose just one" (Von Franz, 1970 [2000], p. 91). They never wholly situate themselves in the here and now, in the immediacy of circumstance that would demand action. Hesitant and indecisive, they would rather fly off into the realm of the intellect or imagination than act unequivocally. To act is to become actual, and this is what such types cannot do. When called to act, they are filled with panic because to act means to become real in the sense of making potential manifest in the here and now. Richard Carstone, the protagonist of Dickens' *Bleak House*, is such a person for whom indecision seems almost innate although it may also be, according to his guardian Mr. Jarndyce, a product of the uncertainty of circumstances he was born into. Perhaps it is this that "engendered or confirmed in him a habit of putting off" and "dismissing everything as unsettled, uncertain, and confused" (Dickens, 1853 [2003], p. 197).

The eternal youth, in Aristotelian terms, is pure *potentiality*, and those enthralled by this deity fail in the struggle to manifest the contrary pole, that of *actuality*. To better understand this fear and its relation to the puer problematic, consider the English word *actually* and its cognates in other languages: The French *actuellement* and the Spanish *actualmente*. Both, like their English counterpart, are derived from the Latin *actus*, yet they have come to mean *currently* or *of the present moment*. The nexus of meaning derived from the original Latin suggests that there is a relation between the real, the now, and action—three terms that highlight stumbling blocks for the eternal youth. To better understand the relevance of these etymological observations, keep in mind that what deconstruction takes issue with is precisely this—both what is present and what is actual, or more precisely, the way presence has been used to underwrite actuality, the way it has been used to claim what is real.

To act implies limitation. Once we have decided to act in one way, we have foreclosed the possibility of acting in certain other ways. But because the eternal youth does not want to narrow his horizons or be limited in any manner, and may feel that such limitations are oppressive, he opts to do nothing, which grants the illusion of infinite possibility yet to come. As long as he does nothing, he could be anyone, and his potential remains intact, although at the price of him being no one in the here and now. Decisions take place in finite moments, and he demands infinity. Such is the oft-mentioned neurosis of his provisional life—the chronic attitude of the not yet. The words *not yet* epitomize an attitude that is in many ways fully appropriate to youth because youth is a provisional age: There is so much life yet to live and the future is a distant horizon of infinite and indeterminate possibility. The *not yet* attitude has its place, but when held onto for too long as a means to avoid acting in the present, it serves as a defense against entering space and time completely.

On von Franz' reading, in addition to sheer indecision, another such defense, which also represents an ambivalent avoidance/attachment to mother matter, is to scurry off into the realm of idea and fantasy. The person replaces impulse with reflection and forestalls action in the present with endless subterfuge, so that acts become fantasies about acts or theories about action (Von Franz, 1970 [2000]). In his desperate attempt to flee mother, "he escapes into the intellect where generally she cannot follow him" (Von Franz, 1970 [1992], p. 22). He flies into the stratosphere of ideas and imagination, but at the cost of his relationship with a more earthly plane:

> It is a trick which many pueri aeterni perform; the realization that they should adapt to reality is an intellectual idea to them which they fulfill in fantasy but not in reality. The idea is executed only in reflection and on a philosophical level, but not on the level of action.
>
> *(Von Franz, 1970 [2000], p. 46)*

In the case of Apuleius, an "intellectual who cuts himself off from the immediacy of life experience through his intellectual theories" (Von Franz, 1970 [1992], p. 21), his scholarly training is of great benefit. It allows him to establish a certain ironic, rational distance from what he might otherwise experience more directly, not unlike Guntrip's description of the schizoid defense strategy of "non-involvement and observation at a distance without any feeling" (Von Franz, 1970 [1992], p. 18). His is a "pseudo-philosophy, the wrong kind of intellectualism induced by the mother complex" (Von Franz, 1970 [2000], p. 167). He addresses the threat of the archetypal feminine by attempting to de-potentiate her through abstract thought and fantasy.

Although the eternal youth may be touched by the world, emotionally moved, he quickly pulls away and hovers ironically above the emotion, gazing at it from a distance. In his escape into intellectualism, he refuses to suffer life. Although he is driven by the hunch that there is a knowledge that can only be attained through being suffered or lived rather than through intellectual studies, he only flirts with such a knowledge. He wants to explore a world without quite committing to it or suffering the consequences of his exploration. Through his flight into the ether of ideas, he avoids the immediacy of both his emotions and his senses, or what von Franz refers to as the feminine principle. Fascinated by the irrational, he is simultaneously scornful, taking a superior attitude toward it. He replaces direct expression with artificial and forced formulations. Von Franz describes Apuleius' flowery and ironic style as the result of a split personality, noting that when someone is split, they are often cut off from the deeper emotions that demand simplicity of expression.

In classical Jungian thought, a man or woman who is identified with the intellect, or the thinking function, is alienated from his or her feeling depths. In the tail of the *Golden Ass*, the fierce antagonism between the dark feminine and the masculine intellect reaches its apogee within the first 'inserted' story within the novel, a tail told by travelers who Lucius comes upon on his journey to his mother's homeland. In this story within a story, the great Socrates, founder of Western philosophy and epitome of the inquiring intellect, a man renowned for his emotional detachment and the wisdom that is believed to come from such a detachment, suffers a gruesome fate. Set upon by robbers while traveling on the countryside, Socrates was later briefly sold into slavery and then released. He found shelter in the home of an old, drunken, sex-crazed witch named Meroe, whose name meant wine, and later became her servant. Von Franz comments that this is typical of the great goddess figures of antiquity when they appear in their negative aspect. Such goddesses often castrate their lovers or turn them into animals. In this tale Socrates suffers a similar fate, for Meroe and her sister Panthia plunge a knife into his throat and heart, then stuff his throat with a sponge and stop his bleeding with a magic spell, leaving him moribund for days before his eventual death. His friend Aristomenes, who is with him, suffers a less dire fate: The two women merely urinate in his face and leave him at the scene of the crime, presumably to be accused of having committed it.

Von Franz (1970 [1992]) interprets the story as a symbolic expression of Lucius' own psychological state and sees it as an expression of the sort of fate that can come across a man like Lucius, or any and "every man who represses his emotions and with them his anima, his feminine element" (p. 27). It is the metaphoric fate of men who worship intellect at the expense of feeling that they suffer such a demise.

The fantasy life of the *puer* type is exceedingly rich, but as one might imagine, its richness seems inversely proportioned to its connection to the real world. He or she is inwardly great and outwardly impoverished, overgrown with fantasies of life not lived, like the asteroid B-612 of Saint-Exupery's little prince that is overrun by baobabs. They have taken root within him and he is entangled within their branches, "caught up in the realm of the archetypal representation" (Von Franz, 1970 [2000], p. 145), and he consequently underestimates real-life experiences. In lieu of this, he:

> Walks about in a cloud of fantasies, fantasies which in themselves are interesting and full of rich possibilities, full of unlived life. You feel that such a person has a tremendous wealth and capacity but there is no possibility of finding a means of realization, and then the tree—the inner wealth—becomes negative, and in the end kills the personality. This is why the tree is frequently linked up with the negative mother symbol, for the mother complex has that danger.
>
> *(Von Franz, 1970 [2000], p. 60)*

Or, as Donald Kalsched (1996) has described the schizoid dissociative defense, "archetypal fantasy takes over and replaces imaginal engagement with the outer world" (p. 38), and a rich inner fantasy life develops. Worse yet, the eternal youth confuses one world with another and, again like Saint-Exupery's little prince, confuses the drawing of sheep with real sheep.

The potential value of puer's flight into the abstract realm of fantasy and idea depends largely on his ability to return. Like many mythic themes and characters, in Jungian thought, 'flight' has both a positive and negative value and is understood to have both adaptive and maladaptive qualities. Whether the former or the latter prevails depends largely upon whether the puer figure is able to land adeptly or if, like Icarus, he plummets to earthly disaster. The flight into fantasy or intellect, if later grounded in action, will have served its purpose. His journey into the abstract realm of ideas can be little more than a cowardly escape from the sordid realm of the earthly mother with all of the troubling feelings she evokes, or it can be a successful attempt to establish a more mature relationship with them. In an ideal outcome, the youth manages a return to a world in which he acts, rather than merely imagining action, and decides, rather than remaining stuck in the eddies of indecision. In a less ideal outcome, the escape remains permanent, offering at best the illusion of healing integration yet "the whole integration takes place up in the sky and not on the earth, not in reality" (Von Franz, 1970 [2000], p. 47). Or, to borrow a metaphor from children's fiction, too often he fails to "enclose fantasy narratives in realistic frames" (Gilead, 1991, p. 280).

Von Franz (1970 [1992]) uses an apt analogy for the eternal youth's lack of presence in the here and now: Those individuals possessed by the archetype "walk about in a transparent plastic sack and only look out of it. There is no immediate friction with reality, no real touch with life" (p. 39). Intellectualism and aestheticism are two forms this transparent sack can take. Both forms provide the eternal youth a way to think himself out of immediacy, to postpone any action in the here and now, any confrontation with the material world. In the case of Lucius, the protagonist of *The Golden Ass*, one calamity after another befalls him, yet he remains strangely distant and emotionally unresponsive. Through a metaphor evocative of a similar image used by Guntrip (1992), that of "a plateglass wall between the patient and the world" (p. 63), Von Franz (1970 [2000]) writes:

> If you are in a glass house, you can see and be aware of everything that goes on outside, but you are cut off from the smells, the temperature, the wind and so on. All such perceptions are excluded, and therefore the feeling relationship to the outer world or to the inner world.
>
> *(p. 212)*

Cut off, his perceptions excluded, and lacking a felt relationship to a lived world—what Husserl would have called the *Lebenswelt*—that is evermore beyond his grasp, he opts for "pseudo-philosophy and pseudo-intellectualism" (Von Franz, 1970 [2000], p. 171). What makes his philosophizing 'pseudo' is not his lack of intelligence but the fact that it is inspired less by a love of wisdom than a love of abstraction, sophistry, and aesthetics.

Wisdom always has some element of the empirical and pragmatic, which is precisely what his intellectualism lacks. Wisdom is also attuned to feeling, but because he suffers from a "destroyed feeling function" (Von Franz, 1970 [1992], p. 50), his feelings are kept at a distance by way of intellectual irony. Writing on another puer figure, the protagonist of Bruno Goetz's *A Kingdom Without Space*, Von Franz (1970 [2000]) tells us that "having escaped into complete intellectualism, he has not suffered in life. He has not lived a normal, human life, so that unlived life catches up with him" (p. 231). Such is "the typical trick of the intellectual, onto whom all the unlived life and all the betrayed feeling-relationships fasten" (Von Franz, 1970 [2000], p. 232).

It is not difficult to see Derrida's critique of Husserl's notion of *lived experience* as another iteration of the eternal youth's glass house. Metaphorically, the eternal youth puts life in quotes as well, so that it is safely confined within punctuation, prophylactically textualized. In doing so, he inevitably conflates life with its representation and subsumes the former under the latter. Deconstruction construes a gaping maw into which the *Lebenswelt* disappears, a chasm that consumes experience and renders life unlived (i.e., absent any pre-reflective and purely perceptual element). It is a variant of puer's provisional life as eternally provisional interpretation. This is because they are rooted in a common mythos.

Likewise, the eddies of indecision within which the eternal youth endlessly spirals share a filial relation with a term of art befitting this attitude. The term is yet another instance of Derrida transmuting a mythic motif into a philosophic framework. The motif is perhaps most clearly epitomized in the Greek and Roman traditions through the figure of Ocnus, who appears in *The Golden Ass* in the tale of Amor and Psyche. Psyche, traveling through Hades, comes across the old man Ocnus, whose name means hesitation. He tirelessly, ceaselessly winds and unwinds a black and white chord. He "occupies himself incessantly with an endless chain of opposites in the unconscious and with the spinning of a yarn from the opposites, so that he never comes to any deed or any breakthrough" (Von Franz, 1970 [1992], p. 128). Ocnus, like a person compelled to weigh every pro and con of a given situation, can never tally all the pros and cons because there are always more yet to come, and he can therefore never decide and never act. Derrida's transmutation of this mythic figure takes the form of the term *undecidability*, which refers to the particular ordeal of being faced with an impossible decision.

The term will be only briefly described here as it relates to von Franz's portrayal of the eternal youth. It first appeared in Derrida's textual theory and was later redeployed in his political and legal philosophy. It is not unusual for Derrida to resurrect certain terms to grant them new life in different contexts than that of the originally intended. In its first appearance, the term—as with others within the deconstructive lexicon like *ghost*, *pharmakon*, *hymen*, etc.—alluded to something that cannot conform to either side of a binary opposition, words that seem to disrupt an either/or logic. Is a ghost present or absent? It is difficult to decide. Drawing attention to such undecidability formed part of his overarching attempt to trouble dualisms, to make it difficult to decide between the black yarn and the white yarn of Ocnus.

Sensitive to the criticism that deconstruction offered little to political, legal, and ethical thought, Derrida returned to the theme of the undecidable in an attempt to offer a more politicized version of deconstruction (Bates, 2005). He needed to demonstrate that it was applicable to real-life concerns and was more than a novel, perhaps even frivolous and potentially destructive means of approaching texts. It was not merely "a quasi-nihilistic abdication before the ethico-politico-juridical question of justice" (Bates, 2005, p. 19). His redeployment represented a move toward what has come to be known as *applied* postmodernism. As David Bates (2005) writes in *Crisis Between the Wars: Derrida and the Origins of Undecidability*, "Derrida's political turn was no doubt motivated by the escalating attacks on deconstruction by those who saw its emphasis on indeterminacy, instability, and polysemy as a threat to moral and political commitment" (p. 2). It appeared to such attackers that it lacked any foundational principles and was, as such, amoral and apolitical. The attacks upon deconstruction in this regard parallel von Franz's description of a personality type that eschews commitment and action, preferring to replace it with speculation. Apparently, the critics of deconstruction noted something similar. Had Von Franz (1970 [2000]) written on Derrida, perhaps she would have said, as she did of the puer aeternus, that for deconstruction ideas are "executed only in reflection and on a philosophical level" (p. 46). They are not applied. Derrida sought to demonstrate otherwise.

In response to his detractors, he entered the political and legal fray more overtly, claiming that, despite appearances, genuine political action must, in fact, be preceded by deconstruction if it were to happen at all. And the undecidable, despite appearances, was "not merely the oscillation between two significations or two contradictory and very determinate rules" (Derrida, 1992, p. 24) not a mere vacillation between a black and a white chord, so to speak. It was also an obligation to decide in the face of this oscillation.

Each case brought before a court of law begins with the initiative to read, to interpret, and to calculate. Making any decision or rendering any verdict requires that a person must first experience doubt and a momentary suspension of judgment. Any case brought to a court must be, furthermore, by definition, unique and singular. It does not conform perfectly to established codes. Yet, despite the "heterogenous and unique singularity" (Derrida, 1992, p. 24) of a given legal case, a decision must involve subjecting this singularity to the universal dictates of laws and rules. Such is the obligation of any legal ruling, which subjects the distinctive and idiosyncratic, the particular and individual to the order of the invariant, homogeneous, standardized, and uniform. Yet one *must* decide. One must cut deliberations short despite such oscillations and thereby subject a unique singularity to a generalized order.

Undecidability, furthermore, is an ordeal, a necessary one that forms part of deconstruction's questioning and meta-questioning that, in fact, must be applied to legal and political texts to reveal the mystical foundations of their authority: To reveal that laws are not laws because they are just, but simply because they are laws. There is a moment, we are told, in which a decision seems to be impossible. Yet, taking account of rules and law, one is obligated, compelled by duty, to give oneself up to the impossible decision. As Derrida (1992) says, "a decision that did not go through the ordeal of the undecidable would not be a free decision, it would only be the programmable application or unfolding of a calculable process" (p. 24). Any decision worthy of the name must be preceded by the experience of indecision.

As he pointed out, this deconstructive meta-questioning was, in effect, what was already happening: Recent developments in critical legal studies were themselves an inevitable response to deconstructive readings coupled with a desire,

> not to remain enclosed in purely speculative, theoretical, academic discourses but rather . . . to aspire to something more consequential, to change things and to intervene in an efficient and responsible, though always, of course, very mediated way, not only in the profession but in what one calls the *cité*, the *polis* and more generally the world.
>
> *(Derrida, 1992, pp. 8–9)*

So, deconstruction precedes intervention in the world but does not preclude it. One does not need to remain forever undecided, there in the antechamber of theory and discourse. After a time, one can enter a more consequential realm.

In this movement from discourse to world involving a redeployment of the term undecidability, Derrida (1992) explains that "there is never a moment that we can say in the present that a decision is just" (p. 23). The phrasing may sound familiar by now. 'There is never a moment' is the sentence stem of many a Derridean affirmation. It is the meta-argument underlying all successive arguments. And it is a tell, a hint that we are in the presence of an archetype's gravitational pull. As the reader might suspect by now, the impossibility of just decisions functions by virtue of the same logic as the impossibility of presence: The logic of never, the logic of the infinite with its absence of limits. According to the dictates of its rationale, justice never arrives and never can. *How can it?* Von Franz might ask, given that the eternal youth's intellectualism permits pondering without limits and even considers it to be an end in and of itself. Such is the psychology of the not yet. It does not *want* to reach the moment when reflection wanes and the decisive moment arrives.

There are other parallels here that deserve comment as regards the limitless logic of never: (1) In establishing that the undecidable precedes decision—in the same way that différance precedes presence—Derrida is once again, though now in a legal context, arguing precedence. (2) Once again, what is more determinative, more constitutional, what in effect is more foundational, by virtue of coming first, is a word that works by way of negation: The *dif* of différance and the *de* of deconstruction are akin to the *un* of undecidable. All these prefixes denote lack, opposition, or negation. (3) In the same way that presence is itself undermined by a fundamental otherness, subverted by an alien element, as we saw in Derrida's critique of Husserl, decisions regarding justice are undermined by the specter of injustice. Justice is always yet to come. Just as the trace serves to hollow the present, the undecidable vacates "from the inside every assurance of presence, and thus every criteriology that would assure us of the justice of the decision" (Derrida, 1992, pp. 24–25). (4) Derrida (1992) claims that deconstruction is from the outset engaged in the "infinite demand of justice" (p. 19), and by way of the appeal to the infinite, once again, he (1992) invokes the logic of never, just as when he speaks of the desire for justice as a "responsibility without limits" (p. 19), telling his reader that deconstruction always "strives to denounce not only theoretical limits but also concrete injustices" (p. 20). (5) The infinite demand is made infinite by appeal to the *not yet* or the *yet to come* which, paradoxically, always already has been: "Justice remains, is yet, to come *à venir*, it has an, it is *à -venir*, the very dimension of events irreducibly to come. It will always have it, this *à -venir*, and always has" (Derrida, 1992, p. 27). (6) Immediacy is rendered problematic, especially as it relates to the infinite: "Just decision is always required *immediately*, 'right away.' [Yet] it cannot furnish itself with infinite information and the unlimited knowledge of conditions, rules or hypothetical imperatives that could justify it" (Derrida, 1992, p. 26). Just as the finite present cannot serve as an origin of sense, it cannot serve as an origin of just decisions.

A charitable interpretation of such parallels might claim that they are the result of an admirable consistency or a much-vaunted philosophical rigor. But an interpretation more adept at perceiving mythic motifs clothed in philosophic frameworks sees the imperative of the archetype, echoes of which resound in the phrases *never a moment* and *every criteriology*. They echo as well in Derrida's (1992) belief that the ordeal of the undecidable, once past, "if that is possible" (p. 24) in no way guarantees that justice has been done. On the contrary, it is always yet to come and always already never was. There is no moment, as far as one can tell, during which a decision could be called presently and fully just, and the absence of full justice, like the absence of full presence, undermines fully its possibility.

There are no just decisions in the here and now, yet one must decide. As a consequence, it would seem, even after the fact, once a decision is made, "the undecidable remains caught, lodged, at least as a ghost—but an essential ghost—in every decision, in every event of decision" (Derrida, 1992, p. 24). Its phantasmal presence, like the ghost of Hamlet's father, returns anew to undermine certitude. In fact, it never really leaves. It can never be banished, just as Ocnus can never quite decide, even after he has. Even when the eternal youth decides finally to enter time and space, a consequential realm beyond the sphere of his abstractions and theories, he does so in the name of an indecision that haunts him. This basic temporal inequity that relinquishes justice to the land of never yet grants undecidability a persistent presence, albeit a ghostly one, is simply evidence of an impossible want, a double bind that demands decision yet precludes justice.

## References

Alderman, B. (2016). *Symptom, symbol, and the other of language: A Jungian interpretation of the linguistic turn*. Routledge.

Bates, D. (2005). Crisis between the wars: Derrida and the origins of undecidability. *Representations*, *90*(1), 1–27. https://doi.org/10.1525/rep.2005.90.1.1

Bennington, G. (2010). *Not half no end: Militantly melancholic essays in memory of Jacques Derrida*. Edinburgh University Press.

Derrida, J. (1967 [1978]). *Writing and difference* (A. Bass, Trans.). University of Chicago Press.
Derrida, J. (1973). *Speech and phenomena, and other essays on Husserl's theory of signs.* Northwestern University Press.
Derrida, J. (1976). *Of grammatology* (G. C. Spivak, Trans.). Johns Hopkins University Press. (Original work published 1967)
Derrida, J. (1981 [1982]). *Positions* (A. Bass, Trans.). University of Chicago Press.
Derrida, J. (1982 [1986]). *Margins of philosophy* (A. Bass, Trans.). University of Chicago Press.
Derrida, J. (1992). Force of law: The "mystical foundation of authority". In D. Cornell, M. Rosenfeld, & D. G. Carlson (Eds.), *Deconstruction and the possibility of justice* (pp. 3–67). Routledge.
Dickens, C. (1853 [2003]). *Bleak house*. Penguin Books.
Dillon, M. C. (2003). The Madonna imago: A new interpretation of its pathology. In J. Phillips & J. Morley (Eds.), *Imagination and its pathologies* (pp. 133–146). MIT Press.
Dougherty, C. (2006). *Prometheus*. Routledge.
Gilead, S. (1991). Magic abjured: Closure in children's fantasy fiction. *PMLA, 106*(2), 277–293. https://doi.org/10.2307/462663
Guntrip, H. (1992). *Schizoid phenomena, object relations and the self.* Karnac Books.
Jung, C. G. (1933). *Modern man in search of a soul.* Harcourt.
Jung, C. G. (1953). Two essays on analytical psychology. In *The collected works of C. G. Jung* (Vol. 7, R. F. C. Hull, Trans.). Princeton University Press.
Jung, C. G. (1959). Aion: Researches into the phenomenology of the self. In *The collected works of C. G. Jung* (Vol. 9.2, R. F. C. Hull, Trans.). Princeton University Press.
Jung, C. G. (1964). Civilization in transition. In *The collected works of C. G. Jung* (Vol. 10, R. F. C. Hull, Trans.). Princeton University Press.
Jung, C. G. (1969). The archetypes and the collective unconscious. In *The collected works of C. G. Jung* (Vol. 9.1, R. F. C. Hull, Trans.). Princeton University Press.
Jung, C. G. (1970). Mysterium coniunctionis: An inquiry into the separation and synthesis of psychic opposites in alchemy. In *The collected works of C. G. Jung* (Vol. 14, 2nd ed., R. F. C. Hull, Trans.). Princeton University Press.
Jung, C. G. (1973). Psychology and religion, west and east. In *The collected works of C. G. Jung* (Vol. 11, R. F. C. Hull, Trans.). Princeton University Press.
Jung, C. G. (1977). The Tavistock lectures, lecture III. In *The collected works of C. G. Jung: The symbolic life: Miscellaneous writings* (Vol. 18, R. F. C. Hull, Trans.). Princeton University Press.
Jung, C. G. (1981). The development of personality. In *The collected works of C. G. Jung* (Vol. 17, R. F. C. Hull, Trans.). Princeton University Press.
Jung, C. G. (1983). *The essential Jung* (A. Storr, Ed., R. F. C. Hull, Trans.). Princeton University Press.
Jung, C. G. (2011). *Memories, dreams, reflections*. Vintage.
Jung, C. G., & De Laszlo, V. S. (1991). *Psyche and symbol: A selection from the writings of C. G. Jung* (R. F. C. Hull, Trans.). Princeton University Press.
Kalsched, D. (1996). *The inner world of trauma: Archetypal defenses of the personal spirit.* Routledge.
Kalsched, D. (2013). *Trauma and the soul: A psycho-spiritual approach to human development and its interruption*. Routledge.
Marlan, S. (2005). *The black sun: The alchemy and art of darkness*. Texas A & M University Press.

Marlan, S. (2020). *C. G. Jung and the alchemical imagination: Passages into the mysteries of Psyche and soul*. Routledge.
Marlan, S. (2022). *Jung's alchemical philosophy: Psyche and the mercurial play of image and idea*. Routledge.
Perera, S. B. (1981). *Descent to the Goddess: A way of initiation for women*. Inner City Books.
Von Franz, M. L. (1970 [1992]). *The golden ass of Apuleius: The liberation of the feminine in man*. Shambhala Publications.
Von Franz, M. L. (1970 [2000]). *The problem of the puer aeternus* (3rd ed.). Inner City Books.
Von Franz, M. L. (1980). *Projection and re-collection in Jungian psychology: Reflections of the soul*. Open Court Publishing.
Whitmarsh, T. (2011). *Narrative and identity in the ancient Greek novel: Returning romance*. Cambridge University Press.
Wood, D. (2001). *The deconstruction of time*. Northwestern University Press.

# 4

# THE ETERNAL NOW AND THE PLEASURES OF DISPLACEMENT

## I

According to deconstruction, it is by way of *repetition* that the trace constitutes presence. Although every now moment is finite and fleeting, the fact that we can recall or anticipate other moments of its kind suggests that it is repeatable. Repetition is what makes *the form that persists* persist. The hollowed now endures because it can be repeated. This logic is certainly open to question, but for the moment what concerns us is that by way of invoking the infinite, Derrida also invokes the eternal. The hollowed now is also an eternal now. The present, as mere form devoid of perceptual content, in its infinite repeatability, persists infinitely, that is to say, eternally.

In Chapter 4 of *Peter and Wendy* (Barrie, 1911) entitled "The Flight," Wendy and her brothers, John and Michael, glide over unending seas toward the isle of Neverland, following Peter's imprecise instructions: "Second to the right, and straight on till morning" (p. 43). But which morning, and to the right of what? The giddiness of flight had lured them into winging their way endlessly around church spires and other tall objects for the sheer pleasure of doing so. What extasy! After all, a short time before they had been astonished to merely levitate and make furtive attempts at circling their London flat before finally gliding out the window. But how short a time? It was hard to tell. Was it their second sea and their third night of flight? It was difficult to be sure. Who could know? All the seas looked the same and the delight of flight was intoxicating as they learned ever more acrobatics, mastering every aeronautic skill except, curiously, that of knowing how to stop, which Peter had never taught them. It was also difficult to know whether one was hungry or sleepy, or just pretending to be one or the other. Chasing birds to snatch food from their beaks for nourishment again and again was exhausting

DOI: 10.4324/b23321-5

and exhilarating, satiating yet famishing. All days seemed the same, blurred by the pleasure of repetition. Peter would appear and disappear, being so much faster and adept in the air, deftly swerving in and out of clouds, even conversing with stars he could fly so high.

Yet upon his returns, Wendy noticed something peculiar. Often, he would not even remember them, or just barely: She would see the scantest glimmer of recognition in his eyes as he was about to pass them and then go on. Once, in fact, she even had to tell him her name. Upon hearing it, Peter whispered, "always if you see me forgetting you, just keep on saying 'I'm Wendy,' and then I'll remember" (Barrie, 1911, p. 46). Peter could not simply trust the evidence of his senses to remind him of who Wendy was. He needed her to repeat her name.

Maria Tatar (2011), editor of the centennial edition of *Peter Pan*, addresses the idea of an eternal present, describing it as a form of eternal amnesia, and in doing so, touches upon numerous themes relevant for the present discussion of deconstruction as a variant of the Neverland tale:

> That Peter has no memory and lives in an eternal present has been seen as the curse of living in Neverland. But because Neverland makes you forget everything, it also opens up worlds of possibilities and allows you to try out everything. In this sense, it begins to resemble Wonderland, for everything is new and arouses curiosity for the elated pilgrims wandering through it. Peter lives each moment to the fullest, reveling in the opportunities it offers and disregarding what was past and what the future holds. His identity remains unstable, for he can freely reinvent himself at any moment, even to the extent of turning into his own adversary.
>
> *(p. 56)*

The hollowed now is easily forgotten. Peter's eternal present is subject to an equally eternal forgetting. This is the curse of living in Neverland, yet it is also its blessing. With forgetting comes the possibility of re-invention, and who has never wanted to re-invent themselves? When presence is an empty form lacking any continuity with past and future other than the most tenuous, what is there to remember? The logic of Neverland amounts to a remembrance of form coupled with an amnesia of content: The abstract present is retained and repeated but it is not the actual presence of anything in particular. Such a hollowed form is plastic, easily shaped and reshaped.

Yet, because the present is merely a form that persists through continuous changes of matter, things do not matter in quite the same way. Thus, in the words of Sarah Gilead (1991), in her seminal essay *Magic Abjured*, "Peter, forgetting the past, is entrapped in an eternal present without emotional or cognitive meaning" (p. 287). Caught in such a present, one that requires its own erasure, its own consignment to oblivion, how could identities not be unstable? How could they not require the repetition of names to provide some sense of continuity, some sense of an enduring identity? And how could Peter's nemesis Captain Hook have any color eyes other than the indelible blue of forget-me-nots?

We have already visited this theme of the repetition of names and the conferral of identity, albeit in another context and clothed in another vocabulary. It bears a resemblance to an issue raised earlier regarding linguistic transcendentalism as described by M. C. Dillon. The logic of the trace in his reading makes it difficult to understand how anything might be identified without the mediation of a signifier: If such a mediation is required, then it would seem that I could not see a cat as a cat or as black if not for the a priori operation of the signifiers 'cat' and 'black' (Dillon, 1998). Similarly, I could not recognize a person without the use of his or her name or, in lieu of a name, some other set of signifiers like 'unnamed person.' This contrasts starkly with what an empiricist might argue: that the abiding nature of an object is what allows us to continue to identify it through time, through successive moments, days, or years.

For Peter, such object constancy or enduring identity requires naming. It does not operate as Husserl, the self-proclaimed empiricist, would have it: by way of perception without the need for intellectual synthesis and the mediation of language. The present moment, a full, synthetic unity of past, present, and future, provides sufficient ground for identification. In contrast, Derrida, by way of the trace, conceives the present as a minimally repeatable form, emptied of perceptual content. Signifiers appear to be a prerequisite for the identification of perceptual themes, which in and of themselves can have no abiding presence. For Peter, the present moment is equally hollowed. The sensate perception of Wendy and her brothers is not sufficient to identify them. He needs names for perceptions to have meaning. He cannot trust the mere evidence of his senses. Wendy can appear to Peter only on the condition of her name. In the land of make-believe, it is words and their repetition that make us believe, an idea that, in a slightly different form, appears in Judith Butler's understanding of gender performativity which will be addressed in a subsequent chapter.

Despite being the curse of Neverland, there is an undeniable appeal to its forgetting, for the world of unstable identities—unstable perhaps because they are not grounded in perception but rather repetition and the movement of traces—is also one of endless possibilities. Neverland offers "ecstasies innumerable" (Barrie, 1911, p. 172), and how could it not? A realm that, by its very definition, disrupts sequence—because it is beyond time—is therefore also beyond *con*-sequence: Although pirates chase lost boys as Indians chase pirates as beasts chase Indians, there is no capture or mortal confrontation, only an endless round of capture deferred and chase forever renewed. Yet the chase and its renewal consist of a relatively meager set of adventures involving a rather limited cast of characters, given the limitless resources that might be inferred by innumerable ecstasies and infinite time. This is because Neverland is a land of eternal return (Tatar, 2011), which, at least in Nietzsche's formulation—from which Derrida drew inspiration—is infinite time coupled with a finite number of possible events. Or, better yet, one might call it a realm of *eternal repetition* that is necessarily inscribed *ad infinitum* into presence itself (Derrida, 1973). But is such an inscription inherent within presence itself or, rather, only a particular kind of presence, an entirely eternal one, abstracted into sheer form without content, and dissociated from both past and future?

The land of forgetting, a land without consequence, is an island in Barrie's tale and, like Pinocchio's Pleasure Island, it is one of innumerable ecstasies. Therein lies its endless charm. It is a utopia—a place that is not a place. Neverland is Nowhereland. How could it be otherwise? Deferral, when infinite, amounts to never. Distance, when infinite, amounts to nowhere. This is what accounts for its innumerable ecstasies, for *ecstasy* is from the Latin *extasis* and the Greek *ekstasis*—from *ek* 'out' and *histanai* 'to place.' Etymologically, ecstasy alludes to a fundamental displacement and the pleasures associated with it. These pleasures are perhaps most clearly epitomized by Peter's response to Captain Hook's query as to who or what he is; Peter responds "I'm youth. I'm joy" (Barrie, 1911, p. 159). We might add to his response that he is not merely the joy of youth, but the joy of youth in perpetuity. Like Tristan, he "wants eternity, for he wants to escape suffering, and suffering is linked to time and space, which modify, distinguish, and separate—'but all joy wants eternity, wants deep, wants deep eternity'" (De Rougemont, 1963, p. 152). Peter is who he is not merely because he is a child, and a joyful one—Wendy and her brothers are joyful children as well. Peter is who he is because he will be a child forever, and since Neverland is also Nowhereland, he will be nowhere forever. His is the delight of living in a realm unhindered by the empirical and pragmatic concerns that come with time and space, one in which the mundane matters of living and the usual laws of causality do not apply. In Neverland "the 'real' laws of existence and of any interest at all in use-value or profit" (Tatar, 2011, p. xli) are suspended.

The Neverland of différance is no less utopic. It is not only timeless and placeless. It also offers the promise of endless pleasure, though not the innumerable ecstasies of pirates chasing lost boys as Indians chase pirates as beasts chase Indians without capture or confrontation. No. Although this Neverland offers the promise of a form of play no less infinite, with ecstasies no less innumerable. It is the limitless *free play* of signification, and just like Peter's ecstasies, it involves the pleasure of displacement. Derrida (1967 [1978]) exuberantly describes this play as "the affirmation of a world of signs without fault, without truth, and without origin" (p. 292). The logic of spatial and temporal displacement brought about by différance results in the absence of a fixed point—a point of both presence and origin, balance and orientation—and this absence makes possible such an infinitely *free play*. Words and our interpretations of words are now open to endless possibilities and texts can mean things that no one would have imagined previously. Because signs that might have alluded to such a point are no longer understood as surrogates substituting for some preexisting thing or meaning, they are no longer restrained by these roles (Derrida, 2007). The absence of a point of presence, and the decentering of terms that once served as the linguistic proxies of this point, renders the realm of interpretation boundless: "The absence of the transcendental signified extends the domain and the interplay of signification *ad infinitum*" (Derrida, 1967 [1978], p. 280).

Play, in this description, is something like the *joie de vivre* of those who understand even life itself as, first and foremost, a text, and embrace life's textuality with a resounding Nietzschean affirmation, and it is the Nietzschean critique of metaphysics, being, and truth that Derrida cites as a prior instance, albeit a less radical one, of what he intends with his conception of free play. Following in the footsteps of the Dionysian inspiration that sought a "de-centred subjectivity, liberated from all constraints of cognition and purposive activity, all imperatives of utility and morality" (Habermas, 1987, p. 94), Derrida's play shares a similar impulse of liberation from such imperatives. It allows him to write in jest, as it were, for "Derrida's own Nietzschean theory of language as 'play' warns us not to take him literally, especially when his statements seem to refer to concrete historical situations such as the present" (p. 137) as his colleague and confidant Paul de Man tells us (1971 [2013]).

This form of play is, in a sense, a response to loss, or at the very least should be understood within this context. On Derrida's account, the hollowed now—demoted from an origin of meaning and sense to a merely formal placeholder emptied of content—marks the place of an irreparable loss. Yet it does not result in a hell of meaninglessness or a disconcerting deprivation of reassuring foundational truths, a nihilistic wasteland, or the sad, guilty nostalgia of Rousseau. On the contrary, it represents an invaluable opportunity for new meaning and sense made possible by the disenfranchisement of the constraints of verisimilitude. It grants a newfound interpretive freedom. When the only legitimate hermeneutics is intra-linguistic, that is to say, one that interprets interpretations and not things (Kearney, 1986), the limitations of 'things in themselves' no longer apply. When the constraints of perception and its primacy are no longer in place, one is at liberty to construe texts in ways heretofore unimagined, although Derrida was quick to note, such a liberty does not imply that one might construe texts in any which way; some interpretations are simply *mis*interpretations (Derrida, 1988).

To speak of free play in terms of both loss and opportunity is, put differently, an acknowledgment that such play is not merely the result of the deconstruction of presence; it is also a means of furthering this deconstruction because "freeplay is the disruption of presence" (Derrida, 1967 [1978], p. 292). It arises from the absence of the transcendental signified and perpetuates "the destruction of onto-theology" (Derrida, 1976, p. 50) and its metaphysics. It is as if, faced with this irreparable loss and the pleasure associated with it, another pleasure was found, or founded, in its stead. The deferred pleasure of presence, one that never was and never could have been, is replaced by another pleasure, one that is infinite and unbounded: the pleasure of free play.

The previous reference to Dionysus is instructive because it helps remind us of the archetype being enacted, that of the eternal youth. Derridean play, insofar as it is the vertiginous pleasure of leaving the weighty matters of truth, utility, and morality behind, belongs to the thematic of flight, which is also that of transcendence, so common in puer myths: Hermes and Cupid are winged; the sun-bound, chariot-riding Phaeton flies, as does the wax-winged Icarus. The more contemporary stories of Mary Poppins and Willie Wonka feature flying as well, a means of escaping life's gravity in both literal and metaphorical senses. And of course, Peter Pan, in the forever-fun land of ecstasies innumerable knows well the euphoric delights of gliding through the air unhindered, as does his spritely winged companion Tinkerbell, whose self-effacing footfalls leave only evanescent traces.

Yet Icarus and Phaeton suffer fatal falls, having failed to heed any constraints on their newfound freedom. Both "experience exhilaration. Icarus flies too high, and Phaethon flies too fast and both too high and too low" (Adams, 2013, p. 125), although they had been warned by their more experienced fathers, Daedalus and Phoebus, respectively, to pursue more moderate courses. Tatar (2011) tells us that "in children's literature, characters are frequently airborne, and flight comes to represent liberation from adult authority and the possibility of adventure" (p. 47, f. n. 25). The history of myth and children's literature would seem to suggest that the distinction between flight that is fatal and flight that is merely fun resides in the relative liberation from this authority: when too great, as in the case of Icarus and Phaeton, disaster ensues. There is a difference between the freedom of flight and the absolute freedom of absolute flight, a difference between freeing oneself momentarily from mundane, earthly limitations and believing that said limitations no longer apply whatsoever. One allows for landing. The other elicits a calamitous crash. Innocence is malignant if it is not open to transformation through experience, and the fact that neither Icarus nor Phaeton heed the voices of experience, those of their fathers, suggests the malign, tragic nature of their innocence. It is an absolute innocence.

One can say of Derrida what commentators have said of Peter Pan: "although he fancies himself free and powerful, his freedom and power remain isolating illusions" (Yeoman, 1998 [1999], p. 141). They are illusions made possible by an absolute innocence common to other flying youth. Because deconstruction interrupts and disables sequence, it risks being without consequence or understanding that actions have consequences. A freedom that is granted by way of a disruption of sequence, a disturbance of chronology, an avoidance and disavowal of the god Chronos, as we will see in the chapters to follow, is also a freedom granted by remaining deaf to the voice of experience.

Then again, it is easy to make a bit too much, or too little, of the connotations of frivolity and jest, spontaneity and creativity that deconstruction's *free play* elicits, easy to suggest that it might be a form of flight ignorant of all limitation, all empirical and pragmatic concerns, although Derrida certainly gives one reason to suspect this, as do many of his interpreters. The term evokes a sense of amusement and diversion in linguistic invention, a luxuriance in semiotic improvisation, a reveling in innovative phonetic amalgamations, puns, and double entendres, all of which Derrida is a consummate master. Yet *free play*, more fundamentally, alludes to a sense of 'wiggle room,' 'give,' or 'loosening' that provides the opportunity for a movement beyond—beyond logocentrism, beyond metaphysics, and beyond humanism as well: In slackening the knot that once tightly bound signifier and signified and loosening the tie that binds terms to their field of reference, Derrida sees an opportunity to move beyond the sort of humanistic thought that, regretfully in his view, still dreams of a reassuring foundation, origin, or center. In this regard, play is a determination to find in the non-center something other than the *loss* of a center (Derrida, 1967 [1978]).

In the Afterword to *Limited Inc.*, Derrida (1988) addresses his critics regarding this tendency to emphasize the connotations of frivolity and jest, as well as the absoluteness of *free play*. With apparent vexation, he assures the reader that he never proposed "a kind of 'all or nothing' choice between pure realization of self-presence and complete freeplay or undecidability" (p. 115), adding that "there is no completeness where freeplay is concerned" (p. 115). Yet this is hard to square with his claim, to give but one example, in *Freud and the Scene of Writing* that "there is no purity of the living present" (Derrida, 1967 [1978], p. 212), just as it is hard to square with the entire line of argument in *Speech and Phenomena* (Derrida, 1973) regarding "the theme or import of 'pure presentation,' pure and primordial perception, full and simple presence" (p. 45n). It is not difficult to locate numerous instances of argumentation that pivot upon the purity of presence and appear to offer the choices that Derrida claims he does not offer.

He goes on to further explain that many of the lexical associations of the French *jeu*, which his translators have rendered as *play*, have been lost, and after delineating these lost associations, explains that the effect of both play and undecidability "is precisely to render all totalization, fulfillment, plenitude impossible" (Derrida, 1988, p. 116). Yet perhaps therein lies the rub, the point of friction between Derrida and his critics: To render *all* totalization impossible is itself a species of totalization or, at the very least, a form of thought that produces its own conundrums. Perhaps Derrida's rendering is another instance of shadow boxing, an instance of criticizing in one's intellectual adversary the very sin that oneself is guilty of. If we take Derrida at his word, we are left with a claim that interpretation is infinitely free, but not totally so, which itself raises questions. Perhaps such questions are the inevitable consequence of trading in such notions as purity, totalization, and the infinite.

Further addressing misunderstandings regarding a form of play that he himself described as "the affirmation of a world of signs without fault, without truth, and without origin" (Derrida, 1967 [1978], p. 292), in *Positions*, Derrida (1981 [1982]) confirms that, prior descriptions of play notwithstanding, "we must have [il faut] truth," but continues by way of qualification that "we must recognize in truth 'the normal prototype of the fetish.' How can we do without it?" (p. 105), he asks. The truth, he reassures us, exists, albeit in some vestigial or phantasmal form that is far from being that of an ultimate arbiter of sense. Rather, it is something akin to a vice or addiction. One might swear it off only to shamefully indulge it yet again, possessed by its magical potency—unless, perhaps, one discerns the symbolism in the talisman: Fetishes, when more thoroughly understood, often loose something of their compulsive, possessive power.

Is truth really the normal prototype of the fetish? Like so many other terms that Derrida disavows, discredits, and deconstructs, he cannot do without it. It must return, as they do, at least in parenthetic form. Or it must return in the manner of an oxymoron like the *non-origin that is originary*. The equivocal status of terms like *truth*, *primordiality*, and *presence* are akin to Roland Barthes (1975) description of a striptease in *The Pleasure of the Text*: "the staging of an appearance as disappearance" (p. 10), or perhaps just the opposite: the staging of a disappearance as an appearance. Substituting the vestigial, phantasmal form of truth for truth as an arbiter of sense is a way of enacting such a tease. It is also prototypical of fetishes, which, as Freud understood, are a way of sustaining incompatible assertions simultaneously without acknowledging their incompatibility. If Derrida affirms a truthless world and yet also affirms a world in which we must have truth, the incompatible affirmations require the truth's fetishization. Such a logic suggests that the fetish is Derrida's prototype of truth and not the other way around.

Play works by the same dispersive, dissociative logic as différance, which for Derrida involves a process of *dis*semination (Kearney, 1986; Derrida, 2021), a dispersal of signs that also suggests a dispersal of seed or semen. Signs disseminate rather than inseminate, spill themselves rather than impregnate. Such is the case when the truth has been reduced to fetish. Metaphorically, différance as desire is the glass pane of a peep show or the condom that sheaths a penis and prevents direct touch. It serves a prophylactic function: Infinite deferral prevents insemination. It is sexual play without consequence. The fetishized truth, as with many fetishes, becomes the object of an autoerotic fantasy. How could it not? When words play upon words within an *intra*-linguistic realm foreclosed to any contact with a world beyond themselves, when play refers to the ecstasy of displacement, one made possible by the absence of a longed-for presence, what should one call it? When play involves the infinite arrangement and re-arrangement of representations that are nothing more than stand-ins for absent presences, simulacra substituting for what has been lost or never attained, *auto-erotic* is an apt descriptor. More colloquially and crassly, though perhaps no less accurately, one might refer to deconstruction's free play simply as a form of intellectual masturbation. It may allow for a faux consummation, but the beloved with whom to consummate is not really there.

How could it be otherwise, if différance is a form of pothos? How can one satisfy the dueling imperatives of such an impossible love, one that must move toward its object and must, simultaneously, remain distant from it? Answer: by way of the "immanent fantasy of the lover rather than the transcendent reality of the beloved" (Dillon, 2001, p. 17), by way of the immanent play of signs rather than a relation to the transcendental signified, the play of words rather than their relation to things themselves. If truth has no transcendent element and yet cannot be relinquished, then it must be purely immanent; it must exist solely within the cryptic enclosure of signs, in fully 'fetishized' form. Yet for any erotic fantasy to arouse desire it requires a certain suspension of disbelief. Just as the image of a lover must be taken to actually *be* the lover it purports to represent, Derrida's phantasmal truth must be taken to actually be what it appears to be, something with a transcendent dimension, something with a reality beyond the phantasmal play of words. The erotic fantasy of deconstruction requires a suspension of disbelief as regards the existence of truth.

Rollo May (1994), in *Courage to Create*, reminds his reader that the original Greek and Hebrew words that meant 'to know' also meant 'to have sexual relations,' and suggests that the etymologies of the words demonstrate that knowledge itself, that truth itself is a dynamic encounter between subject and object, self and other, in which there is often no clear delineation between the two. There is a profound association, an analogy to be drawn between carnal knowledge, that is to say, sexual intercourse and knowledge *per se*. But the auto-erotic logic of deconstruction appears to run contrary to such an understanding. Its understanding of truth as fetish and its seemingly Manichean splitting of language from its ostensible referents suggest that truth can never be carnal, can never be of the *flesh* in quite this sense. The disunion of self and other is too great. Words do not couple, do not copulate with the world, so to speak. They only play with themselves.

In Chapter 3 of Milan Kundera's satiric novel *Life Is Elsewhere* (1976 [1986]), entitled "The Poet Is Born," the reader learns that for the youthful, death-obsessed hero Jaromil, poetry offers a way to soar above his experience. In the following chapter, "The Poet Masturbates," the reader learns of yet another way that Jaromil enacts a similar flight through a certain secret pleasure. These two themes—poetry and masturbation—form the backdrop upon which the theme of the pleasures of displacement is illuminated. Kundera's protagonist lives in two realms, one above and one below. In the latter, he is a mere schoolboy living a monotonous life, no more than a child who must have lunch with his mother and grandmother. Awkward in appearance, timid, red-cheeked with shame, and at times even cowardly, he has few friends, no girlfriend, and feels mortified at the thought of his virginity. But in the other realm, distinctly above this lowly and mundane monotony, he would imagine himself to be one of the *elect*, different, and exceptionally so. There in the world of verse, but also in the world of erotic fantasy, he was able to create a life of artistic and sexual adventure. He could make love to those very women to whom, in the bleak reality of his day-to-day, he would not even dare to speak.[1]

Kundera's description of the way in which poetry in particular is able to serve as a world onto its own will perhaps sound familiar to the reader of the present work, for it involves a question of disrupted reference. He tells us that poetry turns words that would otherwise be fleeting into objects that have an existence above and beyond their ordinary usage. They become aesthetic objects independent of the life events that may have inspired them. Ordinary words merely serve to communicate, "they are subordinate to objects; they are only their signs" but, more importantly, "by means of the poem, words [for Jaromil] had been transmuted into objects themselves and were no longer subordinate to anything" (Kundera, 1976 [1986], p. 59). This fundamental insubordination is no different than the essential pattern described thus far: Deconstruction places words, once subordinate to a world and answerable to it, into a superordinate and privileged position, granting them priority. The world that Jaromil creates through verse, like Derridean free play, ruptures the constraints that verisimilitude might offer. Fittingly, given the cluster of themes that tend to coalesce around eternal youth figures, the young poet had an obsession with certain verbs denoting movement, but especially the verbs 'float' and 'fly,' as well as nouns like 'wings.' In his poems, wings pulsed and beat and even emotions as leaden as sorrow took a 'winged course.'

The independence of the poem allowed Jaromil to enter a hidden world separate from the one inhabited by adults, a second existence of his own creation and bound only by the rules of his imagination. The absence of adults, and particularly parents, is important in this regard. Kundera (1976 [1986]) tells us this is a question of origins, for "the absence of parents is the first precondition of freedom" and "he is free who is unaware of his origin" (p. 121). Such is the spirit and logic of youth in Kundera's reading, and, unsurprisingly, freedom, play, flight, death, mother, and the issue of a *not yet* are all themes equally and intrinsically bound to it.

The latter of these themes, the *not yet*, for Jaromil manifests as an obsession with the future, in particular a revolutionary one that "merged with an equally vague idea of the bohemian freedom of poets" (Kundera, 1976 [1986], p. 100). It was not only a future filled with personal literary glory and erotic prowess but also a Marxian freedom in which the world had moved from a realm of economic necessity to a realm of liberty. In Jaromil's mind, "the liberation of the human imagination entailed the same leap into the realm of freedom as the liberation from economic thralldom" (Kundera, 1976 [1986], p. 116). This is, as Kundera points out throughout the novel, not an unusual association of ideas: Many poets throughout the ages have been political revolutionaries, and in the twentieth century they often carried the banner of a new socialist or Marxist utopia. An unfettered imagination, like the one brought about by the surrealist discovery of automatic writing with its liberation from the confines of grammar and reason, has often segued seamlessly with ideas of political revolution. Both freedom from material needs and freedom of the imagination unchained from economic bondage filled Jaromil's imagination, just as it has filled the imagination of many others.

For him, as with other targets of Kundera's lampoon, the revolutionary future must be totally new, or it will be no future at all. Any revolution must be absolute. The future must be pure, leaving no bourgeois value overturned. The young, Kundera notes, are often emissaries of the absolute and therefore the future they wish to create must be *absolutely* new, having no historic precedence. Everything is all or nothing, life or death, and the political slogans and lines of verse that Jaromil composed were often slogans that rejected millennia of history. He was horrified by the idea that "there was no real difference between yesterday and today, and that the new world was really an illusion" (Kundera, 1976 [1986], p. 234). For him, the coming revolution had to transcend the past with all of its bourgeois conventions, morality, and values.

Yet his fantasy life is also tinged with thoughts of death, a death that paradoxically the young poet can somehow live by evoking it in his mind's eye. Curiously, such a lived death he associates with the eternal embrace of a beloved woman. Such a death in life, Kundera (1976 [1986]) tells his reader, bears "a remarkable resemblance to that period when there is no need to enter the world because one is a world unto oneself, under the sweet arch of mother's belly" (p. 105). Such imagery is found throughout the novel. To live within the imagination is also to live within the mother, under her skirt, within her grasp, or head in her bosom, metaphorically if not literally suckling upon her nipple. Yet to live in the imagination is also a means of trying to escape mother. It is like the schizoid withdrawal from the external 'real' world—where she is—in flight to the inner mental world: *into oneself and out of the body*, to use Laing's phrase.

The life that Jaromil longs for is a life of action, yet this is also what he fears: to act. For Kundera (1976 [1986]), this is the basic situation of immaturity and one way of dealing with this situation is that of the poet who, "banished from the safe enclosure of childhood longs to go out into the world, but because he is afraid of it he constructs an artificial, substitute world of verse" (p. 219). The words evoke von Franz' description of an individual who fails to adapt to reality by making it into merely an idea or something to be lived in fantasy. Jaromil even constructs a substitute identity, an alter ego named Xavier, who he often imagines himself to be while inhabiting the realm 'above' that of his daily experience. It perhaps should be noted here that the original title for Kundera's novel was actually *The Age of Inexperience* and was only changed at the urging of his publishers. Experience is, by definition, what youth lacks.

## II

The realm of play, flight, and ecstasies innumerable in Barrie's tale is, fittingly, an island: a location temporally and spatially distant from the everyday world where every day is marked upon a calendar. Mythic and mystic realms, from Oz to Wonderland to Narnia to Hogwarts, although not literally islands, are certainly metaphorically so. Enchanted towers, as in the tale of Eros and Psyche, or magic gardens, as in the books of Genesis and Ezekiel serve similar functions: They separate a mundane time-bound reality from an enchanted, apparently timeless one. These Neverlands promise immortality, as did Calypso to Odysseus, and are often out at sea and frequently uncharted. They are frequently 'unplottable,' magically hidden from plain sight, conveniently excluded from all maps so as to protect certain secrets and the location of schools of magic.

In a similar vein, such is the case with the land of the transcendental signified, for it is certainly no less distant, and no less of an island, and its precise location is a matter of dispute. Recall Caputo's description of the differential play of signs and the admonition that what you will "never find in the dictionary is a word that detaches itself from these internal relationships and sends you sailing right out of the dictionary into a mythical, mystical thing in itself 'outside' of language, wistfully called the 'transcendental signified'" (Derrida & Caputo, 1997, p. 100). Such a form of sailing, impossible as it may be, would lead one to an isle so transcendent as to be described as mythical, in the sense of being illusory or nonexistent. Yet one might rightly ask, which is the mythical realm—the one outside of dictionaries or the one within? Which is more real, the world of things or of words? Just where is Neverland?

To ask such questions is not merely to quibble over an isolated metaphor. Such questions not only touch upon difficulties regarding what Derrida means by free play but also get at the nub of an issue that has divided scholars, roughly, into two opposing camps, the first of which (Dillon, 1995; Fisher, 2002; Habermas, 1987; Scholes, 1991) sees Derrida as radically textualist in a way that forecloses contact with the 'other' of language. Such critics tend to discern implications of nihilism and abject relativism in such a foreclosure and in the sort of free play that would affirm "a world of signs without fault, without truth, and without origin" (Derrida, 1967 [1978], p. 292). They cite instances in which he appears to bolster their argument through his disavowals of such descriptions of play, as well as his defenses against charges of relativism.

The scholarly camp that opposes this radically textualist, self-enclosed portrait sees his approach not as a *foreclosure* but as an *openness* toward the other of language. If there is a single phrase that might act like a shibboleth to distinguish between these two tribes, it is undoubtedly *il n'y a pas de hors-texte*. One tribe has taken it to mean that 'there is nothing outside the text,' while the other tribe prefers the reading 'there is no outside-text.' The former appeared in the first English translation of *Of Grammatology*. The latter appeared in a corrected edition decades later. The former suggests an enclosure within language, whereas the latter does not. Derrida addresses the first of these two tribes with open disdain in Richard Kearney's *Dialogues with Contemporary Continental Thinkers*:

> It is totally false to suggest that deconstruction is a suspension of reference. Deconstruction is always deeply concerned with the 'other' of language. I never cease to be surprised by critics who see my work as a declaration that there is nothing beyond language, that we are imprisoned in language; it is, in fact saying the exact opposite. The critique of logocentrism is above all the search for the 'other' and the 'other of language'. Every week I receive critical commentaries and studies on deconstruction which operate on the assumption that what they call 'post-structuralism' amounts to saying that there is nothing beyond language, that we are submerged in words—and other stupidities of that sort.
>
> *(Kearney & Ricœur, 1989, p. 123)*

It is totally false, he tells us, that deconstruction suspends reference to 'the other of language.' It is totally true, others tell us, that it does: the entire conception of différance, upon which deconstruction is inspired, is a deferral, a postponement, a suspension. The whole point is that the other of language, "the thing itself, if there is anything at all to it, slips away" (Derrida & Caputo, 1997, p. 31). What are we to make of this impasse?

The emphatic tone of annoyance, Derrida's ceaseless surprise, and the sheer volume of critics who so grossly misconstrue deconstruction for no apparent reason give one pause. Perhaps they are all tells, clues that suggest the presence of an archetype with all of its autonomy, obsessive and possessive power, and affective charge (Jung, 1983). Similarly, the words *always* and *never* suggest a reductive one-sidedness, just as the phrases *totally false* and *the exact opposite* suggest the archetype's polarizing effect. It is when one is most annoyed or in the grips of any strong emotion that the archetype's power is most keenly felt, and one conceives the world in radically dichotomous and mutually exclusive terms. Conversely, one might wonder whether the penchant for radical dichotomies and mutual exclusivity are not both reactions to such inexplicably stupid misunderstandings but, rather, their causes.

There is an inevitable price to be paid for the profligate trading in such absolutes as moments that *never* were and *never* have been; principles that account for the genesis of *all* oppositional concepts; totalizing affirmations that *everything* begins by representation; their no less totalizing negations regarding the nonexistence of perception; and the rendering of *all* totalizations as impossible. It is difficult to see how Derrida's openness to the other of language, to a world that transcends representation, can allow for this 'other' to be determinative. *The perceived world seems to have no say*. Or perhaps it does, but being so remote as to require a search, we cannot hear its distant call.

The difficulty in discerning whether deconstruction represents the height of linguistic idealism utterly foreclosed to, and in denial of, any sort of extratextual reality, any world 'outside the text,' or, on the contrary, represents an uncompromising openness to the extratextual is itself instructive. Perhaps it is simply a false dilemma that offers a false choice, much as does the choice between describing Neverland as nothing but a hell or nothing but a heaven, only a dystopia or only a utopia. Connoisseurs of fairy tales, or those familiar with the bipolar valence of the archetype, know better than to linger too long on such questions, the answer to which frequently is 'both/and' or 'it depends.'

Innocence can grow malignant when deprived of experience for too long. The ecstasies of free play and a joyous world without fault or truth can surreptitiously turn to ennui. Then, utopic longings become dystopic actualities. Such is the principle of compensation that Jung referred to as enantiodromia. The sun reaches its apex and at that very moment, at its greatest height and intensity, it begins its decline toward its eventual eclipse behind the horizon. Things become their opposites. Dreams of absolute freedom become themselves prisons because, "in accordance with the principle of compensation which runs through the whole of nature, every psychic development, whether individual or collective, possesses an optimum which, when exceeded, produces an enantiodromia, that is, turns into its opposite" (Jung, 1989, p. 168). Such inversions almost always occur "when an extreme, one-sided tendency dominates conscious life; in time an equally powerful counterposition is built up, which first inhibits the conscious performance and subsequently breaks through the conscious control" (Jung, 1971, p. 426). What appears to be an absolute foreclosure then appears as an equally absolute opening and often the selfsame intellect that proposes one absolute is oblivious to having proposed its contrary. Such is the psychological law of enantiodromia.

The issue of enclosure that sparks debates as regards deconstruction is not as foreign to Peter's version of Neverland as one might imagine. Neverlands, whether created by the fabulists of children's literature or the savants of philosophical inquiry, inevitably inspire questions of enclosure that are also implicitly ontological: The longer Wendy and her brothers sojourn in Neverland the more they doubt the reality of anything beyond the isle. Increasingly, their life in London with mother and father takes on the semblance of a dream, and their eternally recurrent adventures with Peter take on the semblance of the real. Such Neverlands also inevitably inspire questions regarding time and what might be thought to exist inside of it and outside of it: One can pass what feels like eons in one realm only to find that little or no time has passed in the other, which makes one wonder if time is real at all, or if it is what one thought it was. This question will be addressed further on in a different form in the coming chapter on Derrida's critique of Aristotle regarding the question of whether time exists inside or outside of Being.

Such questions of enclosure are typical of stories that "enclose fantasy narratives in realistic frames" (Gilead, 1991, p. 280); there are moments of inevitable confusion regarding what is *enclosed* and what is *enclosing*, what is inside and what is outside, which is also a doubt as to which world is fantasy and which is real. Is Neverland real and London a mere dream? Or is it the other way around? This equivocation between reality and fantasy exists whether the story is *Peter Pan, The Wizard of Oz*, *Harry Potter*, *Alice in Wonderland*, or *The Never Ending Story*. In a speech delivered to the Royal Literary Fund, Peter Pan's creator, J. M. Barrie (1938), invoked this issue of enclosure as he wondered aloud "whether we are really here or whether this is only a chapter in a book; and if it is a chapter in a book I wonder which of us all is writing it" (p. 13).

Interpreters ask similar questions of enclosure regarding deconstruction: Are we within the text or outside of it? And what does it mean to be 'here'? Each, in their own way, responds to such queries, and in so doing, places himself or herself on one side or another of an enclosing frame: Either we are within the chapter of a book, so to speak, ensconced within a radical textualism or, conversely, we are more fully opened to a world that transcends the text by virtue of the realization of just how utterly transcendent that world is.

Sarah Gilead (1991), in her aforementioned essay *Magic Abjured: Closure in Children's Fantasy Fiction*, describes the device of enclosing fantasy narratives within realistic frames, a device common to children's fantasy fiction, as follows:

> Such a device recurs in many classic works of children's fantasy fiction: the adventurers return home, the dreamer awakens, or the magical beings depart.

> Often the ending completes a frame around the fantasy, reestablishing the fictional reality of the opening. Despite its commonness, indeed its seeming naturalness, the pattern is surprisingly varied in dramatic mode and in meaning. So familiar is the return-to-reality closing, embedded as it is in literary tradition and convention, that the reader's interpretive query is disarmed by the satisfaction of formal expectations.
>
> *(p. 277)*

Reader's of *Peter Pan*, *The Wizard of Oz*, *Harry Potter*, *Alice in Wonderland*, or *The Never Ending Story* know that Wendy, Dorothy, Harry, Alice, and Bastian return home eventually. They return to a world that feels familiar and real to us, although it may not be quite our own: Home may be the rural Kansas of the dust bowl era or London's Kensington Gardens of a century gone by, but these worlds appear to operate by the same laws of cause and effect familiar to us all. The violations of the laws of Newtonian physics, most notably often as regards flight, are no longer possible. The fantastic is enclosed at both beginning and end by the mundane, which acts like two bookends constraining volumes of implausibility.

Such a constraint, such a framing has become an almost hackneyed convention, one that reassures the reader and often serves to neutralize further inquiry, although, as Gilead elucidates throughout the essay, further inspection makes it clear that not all returns are created equal. The protagonists do not merely arrive at the selfsame status quo that they left behind before the adventure. This is because they have changed, albeit each in their own way. Although they return to the familiar, nothing will ever be quite the same again.

Heroines and heroes, as well as the authors who create them, offer a variety of understandings of their return to consensus reality. For some, the return solidifies an understanding of their journey as a salutary sojourn that equips the protagonist with a more fully formed social personality, one that has had the opportunity to experience and tame extremes of anxiety, anger, resentment, and other difficult emotions. Both fantasy and a return from it have clearly formed integral parts of a coming-of-age story. For others, upon return, there is a rejection of the fantasy world and only a partial or equivocal realization of greater insight or psychological development. For still others, there is neither a beneficent socialization nor a rejection of the fantasy world but rather a recognition of its seductive and dangerous force. Each heroine or hero evinces a different degree of 'magic abjured,' that is to say, each reveals a different measure of renunciation, acceptance, and valuation of the fantastic realm from which they have returned. In each case the return is a *bildung*, an education of sorts, although the valorization and understanding of fantasy differs greatly.

Peter Pan is therefore a *bildungsroman*—a coming-of-age story of moral and spiritual education. But this is only so for Wendy and perhaps her brothers but it is not so for Peter. He remains in the stasis of Neverland whereas Wendy does not. She visits there and returns. More importantly perhaps, she *remembers* her adventures. She has internalized Neverland, taking it with her rather than being swallowed up by it. Hers is a hero's adventure following in its basic outline the monomyth discerned by Joseph Campbell (1967): A hero ventures forth from a prosaic world into a region of supernatural wonder where fabulous forces are met and victories won. Then the hero or heroine *comes back* from the mysterious adventure with the power to bestow boons upon others. These boons, in Wendy's case, take the form of stories that she can share with her daughter Jane and a knowledge of things that most adults tend to forget. Yet for her there is also a tragic sense of the dangerous, seductive nature of fantasy (Gilead, 1991). Nevertheless, Wendy individuates whereas Peter does not. Wendy returns and remembers whereas Peter stays and forgets.

It is telling that Peter repeatedly pleads with Wendy to share stories like the ones her mother would tell her in the nursery. He has none of his own to share because he cannot discern past from present from future. For him, there is only one moment, if there is any moment at all, and consequently his ability to discern the basic narrative structure of exposition, rising action, climax, falling action, and denouement is hindered, although he remains hungry for it. His sense of sequence, of the linearity implied by a beginning, middle, and end is absent or disrupted. Peter, unsurprisingly, does not and cannot evolve. For him, there is no bildung, no education or coming of age, no individuation.

How are we to categorize deconstruction in terms of this schema of fantasies enclosed in realistic frames? If the frame is completed, if there is a return to the real, then what is Derrida's measure of renunciation, acceptance, and valuation of the fantastic realm visited? This is a difficult question, if we are to take seriously the two sides of a debate as regards the issue of deconstruction as absolute enclosure within language or as an equally absolute openness to its other. Derrida assures us that deconstruction is not a suspension of reference, which suggests that words *do* in fact reach the 'presences' they purport to represent. Reference, from the Latin *referre* means quite literally 'to carry back.' The very idea of reference implies a return. Yet the logic of différance says that no such return is possible. After all, différance names not only a detour whose aim is to return to presence but also the impossibility of such a return (Derrida, 1982 [1986]). The idea of representation as a return to presentation (an original phenomenon or perception) is what deconstruction argues against: There is no origin to return to. Yet the 're' of representation conveys the sense of *back to the original* or *to return once more*. Deconstruction denies the possibility of Husserl's phenomenological reduction, which is also a return, in this case a return to something *pre-existing* the philosophical distinctions, assumptions, and presuppositions that deconstruction attempts to dismantle. All of this raises the question of *reversibility*, or a return through an enclosing frame, a theme that will be addressed further on in relation to Merleau-Ponty's later work.

Let me try to draw these parallels more clearly, yet with a degree of poetic license: Derrida begins his project by way of incantation. Once upon a time, in a timeless, placeless place there was a magic word of sorts. The word alludes to, or even *is*, something that "*is not*, does not exist" (Derrida, 1973, p. 134). This word that *is not* is also not a concept. Yet it seems to produce certain effects and it even explains why words never quite mean what they seem to mean. By way of this incantation, we are transported—displaced, in our understanding at least, to a realm where perception is not real—or not in the way we thought it was. There, we see through a prism that inverts our most basic sense of temporal unfolding, making the prior be former, and the precedent be subsequent. We come to understand that nothing is really self-evident or ever has been, and that words do not work the way we thought they did. They do not direct us to things or meanings beyond the words themselves. Any *thing in itself* 'outside' of language is but myth and mysticism. Nor do origins exist, not as we thought they did. Also, moments are strung together with the thinnest of traces that are erased before they are even formed. In this realm, empirically demonstrable truths do not apply. Nor do the laws of geometry have their origins in lived experience. Words like *hot* and *cold*, *light* and *dark*, *up* and *down* do not originate in any experience or perception either, rather they are the result of this strange word that is not a word.

Through such an incantation, Derrida passes through a magic portal. But does he return? To me, it seems that he does not, or that the return is somehow botched. He's a bit like Peter Pan knocking at the window of Wendy's nursery, yet he can't get back in, try as he might. On the one hand, in later works, we hear that deconstruction does not preclude reference (a return) and that play is not as free as it had seemed. The flight of interpretation must be grounded, as it were. This suggests a return of sorts as well as a landing. On the other hand, we also hear that truth is like a fetish. The 'other of language' is acknowledged, but it remains some distant place that must be searched for, and the apparent antipathy toward empiricism seems unabated. Does he enclose the fantasy narrative of deconstruction in a realistic frame, or does he enclose realistic frames in the fantasy of deconstruction?

In lieu of deciding between these two readings and in the interest of transferring them from the realm of thought to the realm of psyche, it is perhaps better to simply note that the issue of the enclosing frame and the corresponding ontological questions it inspires form part of the basic thematic of all Neverland stories, whether they are children's tales or the machinations of silver-haired savants. The enclosing frame is an aspect of the archetypal pattern of Neverland, as is the polarizing response that the frame evokes.

The confusion regarding what is enclosed and what is enclosing, what is real and what is dream—whether it belongs to Wendy and her brothers or the critics and advocates of deconstruction—is the same confusion. This is because mythic motifs are, at heart, philosophic motifs, and vice versa: Stories that enclose fantasy narratives in realistic frames are, though dressed in dissimilar guises, also questions of fundamental ontology. They are issues that have transfixed both philosophers and children alike for millennia and continue to do so today. The themes of children's literature are also those of adult speculation regarding ultimate reality because they share the same archetypal provenance. They are grounded in the same human psyche.

Such questions of enclosure, whether those of fantasy narratives in realistic frames, or those of a more philosophical discourse, inevitably summon a magic portal, a place, there on the cusp of reason, or perhaps just beyond its limits: Down the rabbit hole and through the looking glass Alice must travel. The Pevensie children—Peter, Susan, Edmund, and Lucy—step through the wardrobe to reach the chronicled Narnia. Harry and other students of the magical arts meet at King's Cross Station, Platform 9¾ to board the Hogwarts Express. Wendy and her brothers fly to Neverland through a London windowpane. Yet the magic portal is also the frame that encloses the fantasy world within the real. It is both an enclosure and an opening. Such is the paradoxical nature of magic portals, and to say that they are more enclosures than openings is perhaps an error that humans inevitably commit when faced with magic and paradox. Questions unavoidably arise: How can a portal, so diminutive as a wardrobe, open to chronicles as vast as Narnia? How can a windowpane frame a Neverland? How can the prison house of language be the exact opposite?

The relationship between the *enclosed* and the *enclosing*, dream and reality—whether within the realm of children's fiction or within the realm of philosophic reflection—operates according to a similar dynamic: As Neverland grows ever more real, London is but a vaguely recollected dream; as Dorothy approaches Oz, Kansas recedes ever further upon the yellow brick horizon. The risk of traveling to Neverland or Narnia, Wonderland or Oz, is that one might never come back. The risk of the baobabs of asteroid B-612 growing ever larger is that they threaten to engulf the little prince's petite planet entirely. The trees of his inner wealth, as von Franz reminds us, have become negative. His rich fantasy life has impoverished the soil of the real from which it attains its nourishment. Puer risks being left with no ground at all, no material from which his life of fantasy and intellection might grow and flourish.

In a similar fashion, a play without truth or origin risks being left with no ground at all, no matter of which to speak, no substance from which to draw sustenance. A similar relationship exists as regards the schizoid's withdrawal and compromise, which requires that he always be halfway in and halfway out of relationships with others, always hesitating at the threshold of the magic portal and perhaps confused as to whether he is making use of it as an entrance or an exit. His careful psychic economy requires a delicate balance between internal and external worlds, lest he lose all identity or suffer from an unbearable isolation. Laing (1960 [2010]) writes:

> The self, as long as it is 'uncommitted to the objective element', is free to dream and imagine anything. Without reference to the objective element it can be all things to itself—it has unconditioned freedom, power, creativity. But its freedom and its omnipotence are exercised in a vacuum and its creativity is only the capacity to produce phantoms. The inner honesty, freedom, omnipotence, and

> creativity, which the 'inner' self cherishes as its ideals, are cancelled, therefore, by a coexisting tortured sense of self-duplicity, of the lack of any real freedom, of utter impotence and sterility.
>
> *(p. 210)*

Uncommitted to an objective element, freed of reference to things in themselves, Derrida's play exhibits a similar freedom, one unconditioned by the constraints that perception, phenomena, and primordiality might offer. It is infinite interpretive liberty, with no fixed point of origin or orientation. It promises the pleasure of displacement. Yet both pleasure and freedom come at the expense of relevance and the real. As Gilead (1991) notes, sometimes what is "murdered for the sake of freedom appears to be the reality principle itself, which cannot be eliminated permanently" (p. 279).

The flight of semiotic play, if the play is infinite, risks being utterly inconsequential because it is without con*sequence*. That is to say, it is without sequence. It has no sense of time. Play risks triviality when it happens within the absolute vacuum of Neverland. A play that interprets interpretations and not things results in impotence or irrelevance. The play that disrupts presence is a play that is purely frivolous and phantasmal, one that cannot matter because it has lost touch with matter.

If the aforementioned literary motifs are philosophic motifs in another guise, if fantasy narratives in realistic frames are also the questions of fundamental ontology, though merely dressed in different attire, then to what might such magic portals and stories of flight correspond? Does Derrida (1982 [1986]) have the key to such portals? Is this all related in some way to what he calls "the small key that both opens and closes the history of metaphysics" (p. 156), which we will address in the chapter to follow? The ontological questions of the enclosing frame, in more philosophical terms, are undoubtedly related to such perennial themes as time and eternity, immanence and transcendence, inside and outside. It is, after all, the meaning of the *transcendental* signified that is at issue. Just how transcendent is it? And what does this transcendence entail? How are we to understand the undeniable immanence of the term *différance* itself? It is, after all, a word on a page like any other, one that alludes to something outside the web of words.

## Note

1 Similar themes are found in *Step Brothers*, the 2008 (McKay et al., 2008) cinematic and comic masterpiece about two immature, middle-aged men living at home with their parents. During a conversation in a treehouse, Dale (played by John C. Reilly), in response to Brennan (played by Will Ferrell), who expresses admiration for his stepbrother's collection of pornographic magazines from the 1970s, '80s, and '90s replies: 'Yea. It's like masturbating in a time machine!' In the scene we see several themes typical of eternal youth types: elevation above the earth, auto-eroticism, and the desire to exist outside of time.

## References


Adams, M. V. (2013). *For love of the imagination: Interdisciplinary applications of Jungian psychoanalysis*. Routledge.

Barrie, J. M. (1911). *Peter and Wendy*. Charles Scribner's Sons.

Barrie, J. M. (1938). *McConnachie and J. M. B.: Speeches*. Peter Davies.

Barthes, R. (1975). *The pleasure of the text* (R. Miller, Trans.). Hill and Wang.

Campbell, J. (1967). *The hero with a thousand faces*. Meridian Books.

de Man, P. (1971 [2013]). *Blindness and insight: Essays in the rhetoric of contemporary criticism*. Routledge.

De Rougemont, D. (1963). *Love declared: Essays on the myths of love*. Pantheon Books.

Derrida, J. (1967 [1978]). *Writing and difference* (A. Bass, Trans.). University of Chicago Press.

Derrida, J. (1973). *Speech and phenomena, and other essays on Husserl's theory of signs*. Northwestern University Press.

Derrida, J. (1976). *Of grammatology* (G. C. Spivak, Trans.). Johns Hopkins University Press. (Original work published 1967)

Derrida, J. (1981 [1982]). *Positions* (A. Bass, Trans.). University of Chicago Press.

Derrida, J. (1982 [1986]). *Margins of philosophy* (A. Bass, Trans.). University of Chicago Press.

Derrida, J. (1988). *Limited Inc* (A. Bass & S. Weber, Trans.). Northwestern University Press.

Derrida, J. (2007). Structure, sign, and play in the discourse of the human sciences. In R. Macksey & E. Donato (Eds.), *The structuralist controversy: The languages of criticism and the sciences of man* (pp. 247–265). Johns Hopkins University Press.

Derrida, J. (2021). *Dissemination*. University of Chicago Press.

Derrida, J., & Caputo, J. D. (1997). *Deconstruction in a nutshell: A conversation with Jacques Derrida*. Fordham University Press.

Dillon, M. C. (1995). *Semiological reductionism: A critique of the deconstructionist movement in postmodern thought*. State University of New York Press.

Dillon, M. C. (1998). Beyond semiological reductionism. In A. Tymieniecka (Ed.), *The reincarnating mind, or the ontopoietic outburst in creative virtualities*. Analecta Husserliana (The year book of phenomenological research) (Vol. 53, pp. 75–88). Springer.

Dillon, M. C. (2001). *Beyond romance*. State University of New York Press.

Fisher, A. (2002). *Radical ecopsychology: Psychology in the service of life*. University of New York Press.

Gilead, S. (1991). Magic abjured: Closure in children's fantasy fiction. *PMLA*, *106*(2), 277–293. https://doi.org/10.2307/462663

Habermas, J. (1987). *The philosophical discourse of modernity: Twelve lectures*. MIT Press.

Jung, C. G. (1971). Psychological types. In *The collected works of C. G. Jung* (Vol. 6, R. F. C. Hull, Trans.). Princeton University Press.

Jung, C. G. (1983). *The essential Jung* (A. Storr, Ed., R. F. C. Hull, Trans.). Princeton University Press.

Jung, C. G. (1989). Aspects of the masculine. In *The collected works of C. G. Jung* (Vol. 4, R. F. C. Hull, Trans.). Princeton University Press.

Kearney, R. (1986). *Modern movements in European philosophy*. Manchester University Press.

Kearney, R., & Ricœur, P. (1989). *Dialogues with contemporary continental thinkers: The phenomenological heritage: Paul Ricoeur, Emmanuel Levinas, Herbert Marcuse, Stanislas Breton, Jacques Derrida*. Manchester University Press.

Kundera, M. (1976 [1986]). *Life is elsewhere* (P. Kussi, Trans.). Faber & Faber.
Laing, R. D. (1960 [2010]). *The divided self: An existential study in sanity and madness*. Penguin Books.
May, R. (1994). *The courage to create*. W.W. Norton & Company.
McKay, A., Miller, J., Apatow, J., & Ferrell, W. (2008). *Step brothers*. United States; Sony Pictures Entertainment.
Scholes, R. (1991). *Protocols of reading*. Yale University Press.
Tatar, M. (2011). *The annotated Peter Pan*. W.W. Norton & Company.
Yeoman, A. (1998 [1999]). *Now or Neverland: Peter Pan and the myth of eternal youth: A psychological perspective on a cultural icon*. Inner City Books.

# 5

# ARISTOTLE'S IMPOSSIBLE POSSIBILITY

## I

Time is an impossible possibility for Derrida (1982 [1986]), at least as it has been conceived in the Western philosophic tradition. Husserl's understanding of time—founded on the impossible possibility of temporal continuity and temporal atomism, a permeable present that was, nevertheless, impermeable—is, for him, merely another instance of a recurrent flaw. Derrida has given many names to that flaw, all of which, inevitably, imply the apparently impossible coincidence of multiple nows, moments within moments, instances within instances, and blinks of an eye within blinks of an eye. This is the impossible coincidence of a continuous present that must also be, in some sense, discontinuous.

In his essay "*Ousia and Gramme:* Note on a Note from *Being and Time*," in which he offers a deconstructive reading of Aristotle's *Physics IV*, the terms used to describe the impossible coincidence have changed, but the reading that they undergird has not. What he finds wanting in Aristotle is what he finds wanting in Husserl. The latter's blind spot is a variation of the former's. In one, he discerns the unresolved tension between a description of temporal continuity and a vocabulary of temporal atomism. In the other, he focuses upon a similar tension, "that time is continuous according to the now and divided according to the now" (Derrida, 1982 [1986], p. 54). For Aristotle, "time is divisible into parts" (Derrida, 1982 [1986], p. 40), yet he also maintains the inverse hypothesis, that time is not divisible into parts, or 'now moments' (*nun*). Both in Aristotle and in Husserl (as well as Hegel), the now is conceived of as a point, a punctum, a stigmē, and this conception contradicts others that are less pointed or more diffuse. Within Husserl's thought, Derrida identifies an

DOI: 10.4324/b23321-6

ostensibly unspoiled present that is, nevertheless, always already contaminated by moments other than itself; the identity of the present as present is subverted by an alien element. In a similar vein, he points to the fact that "Aristotle affirms that the now, in a certain sense, is the same, and in another sense, is the nonsame" (Derrida, 1982 [1986], p. 54).

Despite the differing conceptions of time and presence in Husserl and Aristotle, for Derrida, it would seem, they are oh-so-similar. Yet these similarities are to be found throughout the historical record, from one iconic thinker to the next. Relentlessly finding identities within differences, he reads the history of Western philosophy as a series of chapters regarding presence and its metaphysics. For him, "there is no alternative concept of time to the metaphysical one. To think outside metaphysics, or to try to, the concept of time must be abandoned" (Wood, 2001, p. 270), and no one as yet, with the possible exception of Derrida himself, has been able to do this, not even Heidegger or Nietzsche, from whom he draws inspiration. Time, presence, and metaphysics all form parts of a story to which Derrida attempts to bring closure. Therein lies the enormity of his project and pretension.

Inspired by a footnote in *Being and Time* in which Heidegger (1927 [1967]) assigns a specifically Aristotelian provenance to the vulgar conception of time (which Hegel later repeats and reconfigures through his dialectical logic), Derrida teases apart the contradictory implications of such a conception that the West has inherited. On his account, the nascent seedlings of not only Husserl's phenomenology but phenomenology as a whole are planted in the Greek soil that Aristotle so assiduously tended. The transcendental subjectivity of which Husserl wrote so extensively—a consciousness sufficiently self-aware (i.e., present to itself) as to be able to investigate its own experience—is already apparent, albeit in nascent form, in Aristotelian metaphysics and epistemology, specifically as regards the question of time. In Husserl this is unambiguous: there is no consciousness without temporal synthesis. Yet, it would appear that his understanding of a protentional, retentional structure of consciousness replicates an Aristotelian understanding, or misunderstanding, of time. But the same can be claimed for the entirety of phenomenology. For Derrida, the idea of consciousness itself is a modification of presence as originally misconstrued in Greek thought and "phenomenology's principle of principles, the principle of presence and of presence in self-presence" (Derrida, 1982 [1986], p. 125) is deeply implicated in a problem elucidated, though not sufficiently resolved, by Aristotle.

The sequelae of this problem ripple throughout history. Thus, Hegel's metaphysics of subjectivity and his "transformation of parousia [i.e. presence] into *self*-presence, and the transformation of the supreme being into a subject thinking itself, and assembling itself near itself in knowledge, does not interrupt the fundamental tradition of Aristotelianism" (Derrida, 1982 [1986], p. 53). Nor does Kant's apperception or Descartes' *cogito*, for that matter. Ultimately, both propose a form of self-awareness grounded in Aristotle's conception of time and presence. In the words of M. C. Dillon (1995):

> As Derrida interprets the tradition, transcendental subjectivity *is* temporality. Husserl identifies consciousness with temporal synthesis in an explicit way. The correlation of consciousness and time under the heading of transcendental synthesis can also be seen as a core thesis in Hegel and Kant. Derrida makes a plausible case that this thesis is incipient, covertly operative, in Aristotle's metaphysics and epistemology: That it is an unthought thought (a fundamental presupposition never explicitly identified as such) which drives Aristotle's thinking.
>
> *(pp. 17–18)*

Aristotle, Kant, Hegel, and Husserl fail to answer the question of time adequately, but the same can even be said of Nietzsche and Heidegger, and their equivocal answers always falter, to a greater or lesser degree, upon conceptions of presence. This is the through line, or the Ariadne's thread, that traverses the labyrinthine history of the West's errant metaphysics according to the Derridean metanarrative.

Even Heidegger's project of *Destruktion*, to which Derrida's deconstruction is so greatly indebted, falters on this issue of presence by way of its notions of authenticity and fallenness which, from Derrida's point of view, still echo the fundamental contradictions at the center of the West's understanding of presence and time (Dillon, 1995): Although Heidegger attempted to jettison the metaphysical baggage bestowed on us by the ancient Greeks, his notion of authenticity was underwritten by a sense of presence as eternal, whereas fallenness was given warrant by presence as temporal. This is, once more, the issue upon which his mentor Husserl and everyone else have stumbled: the divisibility and continuity of presence.

Yet Heidegger correctly diagnosed that "traditional ontology . . . can be destroyed only by repeating and interrogating its relation to the problem of time" (Derrida, 1982 [1986], p. 31), and rightly, it would seem, located the persistent flaw in the tradition as "the impact of Aristotelian ontology and logic" (Derrida, citing Heidegger, 1982 [1986], p. 37), both of which unduly privileged presence:

> Has not the entire history of philosophy been authorized by the "extraordinary right" of the present? Have not meaning, reason, and "good" sense been produced within this right? And also that which joins ordinary discourse to speculative discourse, Hegel's in particular? How could one think Being and time *otherwise* than on the basis of the present, in the form of the present to wit and certain *now in general* from which no *experience*, by definition, can ever depart? The experience of thought and the thought of experience have never dealt with anything but presence.
>
> *(p. 38)*

But what exactly is this persistent flaw? What was Aristotle's logic that unduly granted such an extraordinary right?

The issue of time's continuity and divisibility, which runs through an entire lineage of philosophers from Aristotle to Husserl and beyond, represents only one side of a problem as regards the extraordinary rights of the present. In the case of Husserl, Derrida exploits this tension to undermine concepts like perception and phenomena, as well as the transcendental subject to which these concepts are inextricably bound. In the case of Aristotle, Derrida exploits this tension to undermine the concept of Being. For Husserl, there is no transcendental subject, no perception, and no phenomena without the temporal synthesis that Derrida attempts to deconstruct. For Aristotle, there is no Being without a similar failed attempt at synthesis.

The crux of the issue in Aristotle is "the beingness or nonbeingness of time" (Derrida, 1982 [1986], p. 40). He asks, "[W]hether it is among things that are or things that are not" (Aristotle, 1983, p. 51). According to Derrida (1982 [1986]) Aristotle (and later Hegel), by way of a "fundamentally Greek gesture" (p. 45), understands beingness as eternal presence. To *be* is to be eternally present, yet, clearly, at least some portions of time *are* not: The future is yet to come and the past is no longer. There are elements of time that are not in the here and now. Thus, the idea that time

> either is not at all or [only] scarcely and dimly is, might be suspected. . . . Some of it has been and is not, some of it is to be and is not yet. From these both infinite time and any arbitrary time are composed. But it would seem to be impossible that what is composed of things that are not should participate in being.
>
> *(Aristotle, 1983, p. 41)*

For time to truly be in any sense other than scarcely and dimly—a mere flicker of a barely perceptible flame—every moment, past, present, and future would have to *be* simultaneously. If what is is always present, what do we make of the *has been* and the *not yet*, without which time is inconceivable?

An eternal present implies a sense of time that is "not divisible into parts, or 'now moments' (*nun*)" (Derrida, 1982 [1986], p. 40). An eternal present, because eternal, has no definitive beginning or end. The specter of such a present immediately raises, yet again, the issue of divisibility. The present, understood as eternal, "is not a part, for a part measures [the whole], and the whole must be composed of the parts" (Aristotle, 1983, p. 41). The eternal present cannot be a *point* in time or a segment of it. It cannot be a temporal present, it would seem, one moment in a series of other moments. But time is clearly "resoluble into parts, some [parts] have been, some are to be" (Aristotle, 1983, p. 41). Is the present, is the now a single continuity or multiple units divided from one another? Aristotle expresses doubt: "It is not easy to see whether the now, which appears to be the boundary between past and future, remains always one and the same or is different from time to time" (Aristotle, 1983, p. 41).

Yet the eternal present raises another issue because it defines being: If to *be* is to be eternally present (an idea that, on Derrida's account, is essential to Greek thought) then it would seem that time itself, understood as a succession of individual now moments (*nun* in Greek), would exist *outside* of being. From there arises the quandary as to the beingness or non-beingness of time. The question, most simply put, amounts to something like this: How can the present be fleeting yet eternal, and if being is that which is eternal, how can time's fleetingness *be* at all? It would seem that moments (plural), which are capable of enumeration or measurement (i.e., divisible) *are* not. Yet Aristotle equivocates on this issue: "*On the one hand*, time, as the number of movement, is on the side of non-Being. . . . But, *on the other hand*, time is not non-Being, and non-Beings are not in time" (Derrida, 1982 [1986], p. 62). The upshot of Aristotle's equivocation is similar to that of Husserl's: On Derrida's account, the issue of divisibility versus continuity undermines the latter's claim that something is perceived. The same issue in Aristotle undermines whether time *is*—whether it can be said to be or reside in Being. Derrida (1982 [1986]) states the two horns of the dilemma as follows:

> This first phase of the *aporia* involves thinking time in its divisibility. Time is divisible into parts, and yet none of its parts, no now, is *in the present*. Let us pause here before considering the other phase of the *aporia* on the beingness or nonbeingness of time. There Aristotle will maintain the inverse hypothesis: the now is not a part, time is not composed of *nun*.
>
> *(p. 40)*

Because such contradictions remain unresolved, the extraordinary right of the present—eternal yet temporal, continuous yet divisible—is not warranted and what it attempts to underwrite—whether Being or transcendental subjectivity—cannot claim it as a grounding principle. Yet, inevitably, this is what happens and always has. There is a fundamental contradiction at the very heart of the Western philosophic tradition, and it runs throughout every conceivable iteration of it, and some form of it manifests in every usage of the verb *to be*. The magnitude and importance of this contradiction cannot be underestimated. If Derrida's critique of a metaphysics of presence is correct, then an entire system of thought that has buttressed an entire civilization for millennia is systemically and irremediably flawed.

On his reading, the duplicitous thinking of this metaphysics is at work whenever anything like sense, essence, meaning, or archē is invoked because they are all terms that seek their ground in presence:

> The meaning of time is thought on the basis of the present as nontime. And this could not be otherwise; sense (in whatever sense it is understood: as essence, as

the meaning of discourse, as the orientation of the movement between archē and telos has never been conceivable, within the history of metaphysics, otherwise than on the basis of presence and as presence. The concept of sense, of meaning, is governed by the entire system of determinations that we are pointing out here, and every time that a question of meaning is posed, it must be posed within the closure of metaphysics.

*(Derrida, 1982 [1986], p. 51)*

On Derrida's account, thinking time on the basis of presence as non-time, in other words, thinking temporal presence as eternal presence, has governed an entire system of sense and meaning, an enclosure known as metaphysics.

This is an apt image, that of an enclosure, given that Aristotle's attempt to reconcile temporal and eternal presence—as well as the question of time's being or non-being—conveys this sense of enclosure. It is by way of a circular line (the *grammē* of the essay's title) that Aristotle attempts to overcome the logical deadlocks arising from his speculations, which he himself has acknowledged. Time, he suggests, is analogous to a circle. By way of the circle, the passing moment—a moment with a beginning and an end—and the eternal now—with neither beginning nor end—are combined (see Figure 5.1):

**FIGURE 5.1** A simple circle used by Aristotle as a heuristic device

The analogy is elegant in its simplicity and serves as a heuristic device for resolving multiple aporias and reconciling apparent contradictions. It also offers Aristotle a way of elucidating relations between such binaries of time and space, potentiality and actuality, origin and telos, as well as others.

The Greeks understood circles to be symbolic of the infinite. Aristotle uses the idea of a circular line—which can be understood as a series of points—to reconcile the dueling conceptions of presence as finite, measurable, and temporal yet also infinite, indivisible, and eternal. It is by way of what Derrida (1982 [1986]) calls a "dialectical manipulation of the concept of *gramme*" (p. 54) that Aristotle attempts to make sense of his own contradictory affirmations regarding presence and time.

The spatial depiction of a line allows for multiple 'now moments' (*nun*) to be thought in simultaneity. Each point along the circle is like a moment in time, a temporal now, yet each point exists simultaneously with others and this simultaneity is analogous to eternity. Although we may be at a particular point in the circle, just as the hand of a clock might point at a particular number on its face, this point forms part of the circle's simultaneity—there are other numerical points on the clock face that exist, though they are not being indicated by the hand. Through the circle, the real, eternal now, and the irreal, temporal now, the being and non-being of time dovetail and harmonize. Or so is the intent.

> Since the now is an end and a beginning of time, but not of the same time, being the end of past time and the beginning of future time, time will be like the circle—the convex and the concave are in what is in a sense the same—so too time is always at a beginning and at an end. And for this reason it is thought always different, for the now is not the beginning and the end of the same thing; otherwise opposites would hold simultaneously and in respect of the same thing. And so time will not give out, for it is always at a beginning.
>
> *(Aristotle, 1983, p. 50)*

The metaphysical tradition that Derrida seeks to undermine has defined the temporal and the eternal in mutually exclusive terms, and the circular line, the *gramme* is an attempt to explain their paradoxical relations. Through this analogy, time's essential divisibility and indivisibility are represented, allowing the unreal, ephemeral now to reside permanently within the eternal now (Dillon, 1995). The now, a moment that is the fundamental constituent of time, is a finite moment, with beginning and end, yet because it is never the same beginning and end, it is always beginning and always ending. It is, in a sense, both open and closed, infinite and finite, temporal and eternal, much in the same way as a circular line is both convex and concave.

But the circular line is not merely a temporal metaphor, it is also a spatial one, in the most literal sense. Lines occupy space, and because of this, they raise questions and potentially provide answers as to the relations of time to space: The spatialization of time by way of the analogy of the line allows for thinking of temporal and eternal presence together, but it also necessitates thinking of time and space in a similar fashion. It manages the spatialization of time that cannot be consistently thought within Aristotle's ontology. The line, by 'spatializing' presence, reminds us that presence is not merely a now but also a here. Something that is present is here. Each point on a line is a moment, but also a place, and just as we can be at a particular point in space while other points do not cease to exist, so too might this be the case with points in time, speculates Aristotle, although this raises its own contradictions. If such were the case, "then events of a thousand years ago will be simultaneous with those of today and none will be either previous or subsequent to any other" (Aristotle, 1983, p. 42).

Thinking about time through the spatial metaphor of a circular line allows for a certain simultaneity or co-presence. Different points in space can exist at the same time. Time, it would seem, does not allow for this. It is defined by succession. But because the circle allows for thinking simultaneity and succession together, it also allows for thinking of time and space together. The circular line allows for the coincidence of succession proper to time and the simultaneity proper to space. Yet it also serves to unite both of these binaries with one another: It simultaneously shows the succession proper to time (the temporal present) and the simultaneity (the eternal present) proper to space.

But the image of the circle, it would seem, does not ultimately satisfy Aristotle, for whom such a spatial representation of time is inadequate: The relationship between points on such a circular line cannot be the same as that of points in time. Points on such a circular line do not destroy one another, while points in time appear to do so: The future is a constant erasure of the present as the present is an erasure of the past. If this were not the case, then all moments would coexist simultaneously, which Aristotle believes to be impossible. For Derrida, Aristotle's own rejection of the conciliatory circle is yet more evidence of the irresolvable contradictions that riddle philosophy's understanding of presence, and through it, the temporality of being.

The spatialization of time by way of the analogy of the circle merely makes all the more evident the impossible coincidence of the succession proper to time and the simultaneity proper to space. Derrida contends that the metaphysical tradition, of which Aristotle is the quintessential exemplar, defines succession and simultaneity as mutually exclusive, yet must think of them together to sustain the extraordinary right of the present. Thus, Derrida (1982 [1986]) concludes that "time is a name for this impossible possibility" (p. 55). Similarly, this same tradition defines time and space as mutually exclusive, yet must think of them together to sustain this right. For something to *be*, it must be present in time and space simultaneously, yet the circle that attempts to reconcile the two, thinking them together, clearly fails. And such circular reasoning, on Derrida's (1976) account, replicates itself throughout history, even in the circularity of Heideggerian hermeneutics.

Aristotle attempts another reconciliation, less graphical than lexical, not a circular line but a word, an attempt that Derrida, not surprisingly, casts doubt upon. He (1982 [1986]) claims that

> The entire weight of Aristotle's text comes down upon a word so small as to be hardly visible, and hardly visible because it appears self-evident, as discreet as that which goes without saying, a word that is self-effacing, operating all the more effectively in that it evades thematic attention. That which goes without saying, making discourse play itself out in its articulation, that which henceforth will constitute the pivot [*cheville*] (*clavis*) of metaphysics, the small key that both opens and closes the history of metaphysics in terms of what it puts at stake, the clavicle on which the conceptual decision of Aristotle bears down and is articulated, is the small word *hama*. . . . In Greek *hama* means "together," "all at once," both together, "*at the same time*."
>
> *(p. 56)*

By now, it should come as no surprise that what Derrida takes aim at in his critique of Aristotle is a word that denotes togetherness and simultaneity. Such is the divisive logic of *différance*, which seeks to cleave and split everything that might be conceived of as 'together.' Its operative logic is that there is no 'at the same time' or 'at the same place.'

So much depends on this sense of togetherness and simultaneity introduced by Aristotle through such a small, self-effacing word. That little word *hama*, although it has hardly been noticed by others, is of such epochal importance. Like the pea beneath a hundred mattresses that disturbs the sleep of any true princess, on Derrida's account, hama disturbs the philosophic slumber of an entire tradition: Aristotle, throughout *Physics IV*, explores the multiple dilemmas in thinking of time (chronos), and the relation of time and space, but in the end, he resolves none of them, and subsequent generations have passed down this genetic defect. Despite sustained reflection,

> the unity and identity of the now are problematical. 'If in fact the now is always other, and if none of the parts in time which are other are simultaneous (*hama*). . . and if the 'now' which is not, but formerly was, must have ceased to be or been destroyed at a certain moment, the 'nows' too cannot be simultaneous (*hama*) with one another, but the preceding now must always have been destroyed.'
>
> *(Derrida, 1982 [1986], pp. 53–54)*

This little word embodies the fundamental contradiction of the West's thinking on time: the coexistence of moments that must be possible, yet is not. *Hama* is an insistence that, despite this impossibility, it *is* possible. In the insistence on a simultaneity that it cannot conceptually justify, Derrida discerns merely attempts at what the symbolic, analogic representation by way of the circle both attempts and fails to do.

Yet an astute observer might note that this failure of simultaneity bears a striking resemblance to another simultaneity, one that has already been addressed and is equally, perhaps even more self-effacing. In fact, "erasure belongs to its structure" (Derrida, 1982 [1986], p. 24). It is the simultaneity of the trace, which must "disappear in its appearance" (Derrida, 1982 [1986], p. 24); that is to say, both disappearance and appearance must both occur *all at once*, or *at the same time*. This would seem to present a contradiction no more and no less resolvable than those that Derrida so lucidly discerns in others. Is the trace not itself a possibility no less impossible than Aristotelian time? Is the pivot of metaphysics not also the pivot of his anti-metaphysics?

## II

A mythic figure has been looming in these pages, without quite being named as often as warranted. The figure is senex: He is the personification of Aristotle's impossible possibility, this is the sequence that deconstruction disrupts, and it is also the metaphysical heritage that it attempts to dismantle. Although this strategic disruption of sequence or temporal unfolding is a way of putting the primordial mother in quotes, in mythic terms, it is also a conflict with father time. Time is the eternal youth's antithesis, his shadow adversary with whom he duels, the Captain Hook with whom Peter Pan crosses swords. The specter of immanent death that time elicits is the natural antagonist of Peter's dream of immortality.

The two interpretations of the eternal youth's fundamental antagonism—one with the primordial mother, the other with the temporal father—do not conflict as much as it might appear. They are merely two aspects of a psychological complex that is, by definition, complex. These two mythic figures with which the eternal youth is most often associated represent two poles within Jungian and post-Jungian thought regarding the puer aeternus. They also represent the pre- and post-Oedipal dimensions of this complex. The former—the pairing of the eternal youth with the primordial mother—I have already addressed, whereas the latter—the conflict with father time—has been waiting, fittingly, in the shadows. Now is his moment to emerge from the penumbra.

Derrida (1982 [1986]) tells us in *Margins of Philosophy* that "there is no chance that within the thematic of metaphysics anything might have budged, as concerns the concept of time, from Aristotle to Hegel" (p. 39), and there is no reason, that I know of, to doubt him. In fact, part of the impetus for this book is that I do not. The thematic has not budged and the conceptual problems of conceiving presence that Derrida, Heidegger, Aristotle, and others have elucidated are real. Much time has passed, yet time is still the issue, and its conception is still a problem. Perhaps this is because the thematic of metaphysics is also the thematic of a human psyche that changes less with time than we might imagine, a psyche that wrestles with the same conundrums through multiple eons, untying Gordian knots only slowly if at all, one that tirelessly traverses Aristotle's circular logic, producing only minor variations upon this basic form. The thematic of metaphysics, and particularly as it relates to the question of time, is also a psychological thematic, and an archetypal one, as its unbudging character suggests.

In his seminal book *Senex and Puer*, Hillman (2005) construes the problem of the puer aeternus personality as one of an archetypal split, a conflict between two mythic figures that are, at root, one. The two figures are personified concepts of temporal, divisible presence, on the one hand, and eternal, continuous presence, on the other. Yet they are so much more than this because the archaic idiom of the imagination does not articulate itself merely in allegory, and therefore such figures are not just stand-ins substituting for philosophic abstractions. On the contrary, they represent the styles of consciousness and psychological patterns that give rise to these abstractions. Human beings see through the eye of time and see through the eye of the eternal, yet when the two eyes do not move in unison, our binocular vision is lost, and with it, any sense of depth. Our world is flattened, and we see double.

In Hillman's reading, youth and senescence, eternity and temporality are to be found in the everlasting agon between political calls to freedom and revolt, on the one hand, and the insistence on law and order, on the other. They can be found as well in the desire to break with tradition or to abide by it, as well as preferences for capriciousness or consistency; chaos or order; improvisation or structure; beginnings or endings, blossomings or harvests; the nascent or the aged, egalitarianism or hierarchy.

Saturn and Mercury are two astrological incarnations of these innately human attitudes, and when we are in a mercurial mindset, for us "nothing is given and everything can be transformed; all limits may be overcome and conditions may be altered through re-learning" (Hillman & Slater, 2005, p. 42). This is contrary to our "saturnine attitude of fateful limits set by character traits where psychic disposition is congenital" (Hillman & Slater, 2005, p. 43). We are within a senex mindset when we prefer the old and the tested over the new and the novel. The optimism of naivete versus the pessimism of experience; the loosening of impulse versus the hardening of habit; intemperance versus temperance; speed versus slowness; heterodoxy versus orthodoxy—all such oppositions can easily fall under the rubrics of puer or senex attitudes, which can "manifest in physical, social, linguistic, aesthetic and spiritual modes" (Hillman, 2021, p. 11). Puer and senex are categories of the imagination, each with their own ethos and mystique.

We are always shaded by both of their hues to one degree or another, yet at times we might appear monochromatic. We suffer from the simplicity of our psychic palette—our unidimensional and selective vision that perceives by way of a highly limited spectrum. Then, it is difficult to make sense of anything at all. Our perception of depth is lost. Bereft of balance as our values become skewed and off kilter, we tilt to one side or the other, unaware that each side of the archetypal dyad serves to counterbalance the other. Each informs and complements its seeming opposite:

> Without the enthusiasm and eros of the son, authority loses its idealism. It aspires to nothing but its own perpetuation, leading but to tyranny and cynicism; *for meaning cannot be sustained by structure and order alone*. Such spirit is one-sided, and one-sidedness is crippling. Being is static, a pleroma that cannot become. Time—called euphemistically 'experience' but more often just the crusted accretions of profane history—becomes a moral virtue.
>
> *(Hillman & Slater, 2005, p. 47)*

The temporally minded require the perspective that the infinite and eternal provide. Eternal expectation needs time-bound consequence to inform it. Puer brings new life to a dying order (Yeoman, 1998 [1999]). Senex brings order to new life. The two archetypal figures are symbiotic.

On Hillman's reading, the negativity of the negative puer—his maladaptive or pathological guise—resides precisely in his being split off and dissociated from, even antagonistic to, his seeming opposite, the senex or old man. His imaginative flights of fancy, his perpetual pondering in lieu of action, his indecision and failure to make anything at all come to full fruition, his lack of any pragmatic understanding of the world or an empirical approach to it, and other traits typical of this figure are the products of a divorce from his senex self. Likewise, the negativity of the negative senex lies in his alienation from his own eternal youthfulness: If he does not drink from the fountain of youth, senex becomes parched, a desiccated and tyrannical ogre, a rigid and brittle patriarch, a reactionary rear guard, demon king, or Captain Hook. Such a senex figure lives in a world that is oppressively governed by a reality principle that allows for no play, no wiggle room, no exuberant freedom. Yet the two figures, in fact, form a single, albeit "two-headed archetype, or a Janus-Gestalt" (Hillman & Slater, 2005, p. 39), and the negativity of each resides in their mutual estrangement from one another. Father time and eternal youth are shadow versions of one another and, for this reason, are paired as antagonists in innumerable tales, including Peter Pan (Tatar, 2011).

Hillman, quite likely, would have acknowledged Aristotle's failure, his inability to give a reasonable account of the conundrums of time's divisibility and continuity, its relation to Being, etc. He would have acknowledged the failure of Aristotle's logos—his words and logic—but perhaps he would have been a bit more sympathetic to the philosopher's attempt to reconcile the contradictions of this logos by way of a circle, which is to say, by way of symbol and analogy, given that, like Husserl (Kearney, 1986) he believed the truth of the real is most fully attained through the symbolic. This is, on his account, precisely why we need symbols—to make sense when mere logic cannot, to bridge the gaps that mere reason cannot fill: "Paradox and symbol express the co-existence of polarity, the fundamental two-headed duality that is both logically absurd and symbolically true" (Hillman &

Slater, 2005, p. 41). This is a resonant phrase and one that warrants further comment: *logically absurd and symbolically true*. It is Hillman's own pivot of metaphysics, to use Derrida's phrase, or perhaps it is better described as a pivot of metaphor, an acknowledgment of the paucity of rational explanations, as well as an attempt to shore them up by way of analogy. Symbols throw or cast disparate elements together, and in this respect, they are like *hama*, which brings together, all at once, all at the same time. In this respect, they are also impossible possibilities.

For Hillman, the curative salve that might heal the *puer-et-senex* split lies in the recognition that the two poles of the archetype were originally united in a single whole, and even, in a sense, still are. Behind and beneath their shared antipathy, eternal youth and father time are secretly allied. There is a fundamental identity at the heart of their difference, and even the simple recognition of their split condition is an act of healing. In lieu of the disjunctive rationalism of the ego, which only serves to deepen the split, intensifying the suffering and illness of an archetypal rupture, Hillman offers an approach grounded in the imaginative capacity of the soul and the healing power of the mythic imagination, one that embraces the paradoxes of mythic images with their capacity to express the logically absurd yet symbolically true. Such an approach is necessary because "the binary oppositions, the polar coordinates, cannot be healed through an effort of mind and will, since the willful mind is the splitting instrument" (Hillman & Slater, 2005, p. 65).

Divided from his other half, the puer aeternus is "that structure of consciousness and pattern of behavior that . . . refuses and struggles with the senex—time, work, order, limits, learning, history, continuity, survival and endurance" (Hillman & Slater, 2005, p. 187). The embodiment of the aforementioned themes of limitation, law, and logic is the god that the eternal youth dismisses at his own peril. He is Saturn, Zeus, Daedelus, Yawheh, and Jehovah, to name but a few of his incarnations. His temporal dimension is perhaps most clearly epitomized in Chronos, father of Zeus and cruel cannibal of his own progeny. He is the personification of the relentless progression of moments that consumes us all eventually, from whom we derive the words chronological, chronic, and chronology. This is the archetypal image of puer's problem with time and his belief that authority is built upon mystical (i.e., illusory) foundations. Or, perhaps more precisely, it is one manifestation of it, one exemplar of a more general senex consciousness that "is particularly temporal, structuring its vision in terms of the chronic" (Hillman & Slater, 2005, p. 281). Consequently, puer's displacement in time—his eternal *not yet*, nostalgic longing for what was, and difficulty with simple presence in the here and now—all correspond, mythically speaking, to a conflict with senex. Because of this conflict, the now moment is not possible, or must be staved off, postponed indefinitely.

This figure, the proverbial, white-bearded father time, scythe in hand, embodying the tireless march of the sequential and its demarcation into discrete units of definitive endings and beginnings, is who puer sets himself against—by precluding endings, completion, and fulfillment through his eternal *not yet*, or undermining beginnings and births by way of his reductive *always already*. Yet the very logic of a split archetype, and of an identity at the heart of difference, would suggest that senex is not only who puer sets himself against, it is also who puer, in some sense, already is. Indeed, it would be hard to argue that deconstruction is anything other than an approach that is 'particularly temporal, structuring its vision in terms of the chronic,' that is to say, in terms of a senex consciousness of temporal unfolding, even if (or perhaps because) it seeks to undermine this unfolding; Derrida's entire critique rests upon an analysis of time and an exceedingly acute awareness of it, and his idea of repetition suggests the sort of temporal divisibility or atomism that is a senex quality. Yet senex is also a figure of continuity, which we have thus far associated with a continuous, unending, eternal present. The deep antipathy and complicity within the split archetype are both there in plain view: Deconstruction undermines temporality by way of temporal notions. Its relation to the metaphysical tradition that it seeks to undermine is one of hostile dependency. Delay and deferral, as well as the movement of the trace, imply temporality in the very act of attempting to undermine it. They are said to precede it (i.e., be more primordial) yet are temporal themselves. The deconstructive argument lives on borrowed time; it appeals to the very sense of temporal unfolding that it attempts to discredit. It borrows the sense of unfolding bequeathed by the very tradition that it critiques in order to make its critique. It is always indebted to the present moment, which it sees as specious. Such is the logic of the split archetype, and in many ways the logic of myth and symbol:

> myth is the language of ambivalence; nothing is only this or that; the Gods and dancers will not stand still. They allow no sharp pictures of themselves, only visions. Besides, as Kluckhohn has paraphrased Lévi Strauss: ". . . mythical thought always works from awareness of binary oppositions toward their progressive mediation. That is, the contribution of mythology is that of providing a logical model capable of over-coming contradictions."
>
> *(Hillman & Slater, 2005, p. 65)*

On this account, the unbudging quality that Derrida rightly identifies as regards time and presence is overcome only by way of mythical thought. Our only hope is the imagination.

When ideas are returned to their psychic, archetypal ground, when the willful, splitting mind allows itself a return to imaginative depths, the symptomatic and symbolic dimensions of our abstractions can be engaged because their more fully human provenance has been acknowledged. Then, we can see *différance* as an ancient form of longing known as pothos. It is a disposition of the soul that codifies in the sphere of ideas a particular state of mind enthralled by the *not yet* and mesmerized by the beyond. Writing on the puer aeternus, Hillman notes that the beyond is

> the flag under which he sails, whether *horizontally* beyond . . . . or temporally beyond which lies in the future and demands ever-increasing acceleration, or

> psychologically beyond, that drive to deliteralize, deconstruct and see through every limiting denotation, every reductive explanation, every barrier of law, logic and religion
>
> *(Hillman & Slater, 2005, p. 174)*

On his reading, the yen for the beyond forms part of the very same archetypal impulse as the impulse to deconstruct, the drive to discredit intended meaning, and the will to overcome all obstructions of law and logic. If he is correct in this and, furthermore, the parallel drawn in the present text between puerile desire and semiotic deferral is valid, then we would expect to find the eternal youth's antipathy toward limitation, law, and logic at work within deconstruction; what both the eternal youth and deconstruction set themselves against—the nemeses and specters that they struggle to overcome and defeat—should be akin.

They should be akin and indeed they are: Senex is the principle of order, structure, and abstraction, limits, authority, and borders. He is heavy, leaden, dry, and hierarchical. Not only does this figure represent what is old, but also what is changeless. When he is in harmony with his own puerile self, his ever-creative youthfulness, he appears in the more benevolent, though always ambiguous guise of a wise old man. When he is not, he is the hardening of consciousness, the calcification of habit, the stiffening of the body into the inevitable immobility of the tomb and the eventual stasis of stone. So close to the grave, he is grave in mood and the laws that he confers, etched on stone tablets as well, are equally static. In this hardened form, his morality is a code often void of spirit or love, a law without mercy, inflexible in principles too firm and entrenched, too unalterable and immutable. This hardness can also be ithyphallic, represented as an erect penis. When divorced from his youthful self, he is tradition without its needed renewal. His knowledge is void of wisdom, inflexible in its certainty, yet brittle and in constant need of defense. As the image of patriarchal authority grown authoritarian, if utterly divorced from his youthful half, he represents oppressive laws built on spurious foundations and ossified tradition with scant relevance to the present. As the image of the past divorced from the present, he is the mythic embodiment of a metaphysical heritage that is little more than an antiquated set of prejudices arbitrarily and unjustly imposed.

A reading of deconstruction that envisions a story of mythic dimension and import conceives the seeming irreconcilability of time with eternity and the 'problem' of presence not merely as a philosophical conundrum: It is not something that needs to be resolved solely with an effort of the intellect, argued for or against, and accepted or rejected only by virtue of the plausibility of an argument—such an approach would only serve to further entrench the sterile conflict that is in need of resolution. Rather, it seeks to recognize that this irreconcilability is between two archetypal sensibilities that share a common root. From this perspective, the philosophical conundrum is but one aspect of a psychological conflict, as is the apparent irreconcilability of the finite with the infinite and the immanent with the transcendent. It stems from a fissure at the level of experience, an alienation of archetypal dispositions intrinsic to the human condition. Placing the conflict within the realm of psyche is an acknowledgment that "metaphysical ideas are hardly independent of their complex roots; so ideas can be foci of sickness, part of an archetypal syndrome" (Hillman & Slater, 2005, p. 120).

Under the influence of this particular syndrome, both sides of the puer-et-senex dyad are prone to their own forms of tyranny. The eternal youth, who may be a prince, struggles to overcome the old and often corrupt King. But the King's tyranny can just as equally be mirrored by that of the prince's. When the puer-et-senex dyad is split, they both represent tyrannies of absolutes: absolute freedom or absolute constraint, absolute play or absolute responsibility, absolute becoming or absolute being. When the dyad is split, the eternal youth can be nothing more than "eternal Becoming never realized in Being, possibility and promise only" (Hillman & Slater, 2005, p. 55).

Such is the case when a person is possessed by a mythical deity. By its very nature, the one-sidedness of archetypal possession knows no limitation. When we are within its grasp, the archetype "becomes charged with a force that acts as an irresistible *vis a tergo* to whatever view or idea or tendency our intellect may choose to dangle enticingly before our desiring eyes (Jung, 1969, p. 94). The intellect privileges certain principles, aspects, or characteristics to the point of excluding all that might countervail them. In the case of deconstruction, we might name them as indeterminacy, instability, absence, polysemy, deferral, etc. Through these principles, they threaten an established moral, political, and cultural order, the conceptual edifice of an entire civilization on Derrida's account. Such is, and perhaps will always be, the eternal youth's role: To undermine the foundational principles of preceding generations and Hillman's reading would suggest that this is both necessary and potentially catastrophic.

Because of the tyranny of absolutes that archetypes often impose, the eternal youth without the counterbalancing principle of father time results in a no more desirable state than that of a deeply entrenched orthodoxy, the order of the corrupt king. This youth, but one side of a Janus-faced duality, when estranged from his senex self, knows no truth because truth is the daughter of time—*Veritas filia temporis* (Hillman & Slater, 2005). Truth is what is gained from experience, but experience is a mere abstraction to those who have little of it, or who retain only traces of what they do possess. But is such a disposition sustainable? Can one live without a sense of truth, without a sense of origin or end, without any belief in constants or abiding principles? Is such an attitude practical, viable, or is it, like the attitude of Icarus, doomed to fail because it refuses to recognize the laws of physics, because it insists on flight as absolute flight and play as absolute play?

Deconstruction takes aim at the corrupt King by claiming that all of the names related to fundamentals, to central guiding principles, are mere *nomina*, mere names. They cannot convey any truth other than that of the aberrant metaphysics of past generations. In this sense, its archetypal attitude toward history is skeptical and incredulous: History has been mistaken, not just in some peripheral, insubstantial way, but fundamentally, constitutionally so. History, from this perspective, is seen as a history of oppression, something to be overcome, but only after having put it on trial and found it guilty. It has been deeply, systemically flawed in its thinking, and it is the same pervasive flaw over and again, the same aporia. But there is the possibility of escape, there is a strategy: différance. With this word (that is not a word) an entire ontology, one that has defined our historical epoch, and the entire edifice of Western metaphysics, is made to tremble (Derrida, 1973, 1982 [1986]). Ironically, this attempt to transcend history, to break free of the illusory presences and all that might be said to be archetypal is itself a type and an archaic one, that of the eternal youth:

> Our polarities—senex and puer—provide the archetype for the psychological foundation of the problem of history. First, in the conventional sense, puer and senex are history as sequence and transition, as a process through time from beginning to end. And second, history as a problem in which I am caught, for which I suffer and from which I long to be redeemed, is given by the same pair as Father Time and Eternal Youth, temporality and eternity, and the puzzling paradoxes of their connection. To be identified with either is to be dominated by an archetypal attitude towards history: the puer who transcends history and leaps out of time, and is as such a-historical, or anti-historical in protest and revolt; or the senex who is an image of history itself and of the permanent truth revealed through history.
>
> *(Hillman & Slater, 2005, p. 35)*

Seen in light of this description, deconstruction expresses a longing for redemption from the travails of history, and its protest and revolt is a perennial one. Puer, in his transcendence of time, is the archetype of the unconditioned and uncaused and, as such, represents *creatio ex nihilo* (Hillman, 1997), which is, in effect, what Derrida is striving for, a form of thought unconditioned by a history that precedes it (Wood, 2001).

But the dominion of senex consciousness is not merely that of time and history. It is also the realm of the opposites: In his incarnation as Kronos, senex is the god of the opposites and in no other mythic figure is duality so fundamental (Hillman & Slater, 2005). The senex tendency to conceive in terms of polarities, dualisms, oppositions, and dichotomies—the black and the white—belongs to a general thematic of discrimination and discernment, judgment and judiciousness that strives to cleave right from wrong, virtue from vice, and truth from error. Even his virility is cleaved in two, oscillating between extremes. He is represented by images of the ithyphallic—the erect male member—on the one hand, and images of castration, sometimes of his own male children, sometimes of himself through the symbolic castration of an impotence that comes with age.

Deconstruction is perhaps, above all else, a deconstruction of just such senex binaries. By way of its obsessive focus upon the differential and deferential play of signs, it undermines any sense in which said binaries may be primary phenomena, rooted in sense impressions (Habermas, 1987) or in a layer of prelinguistic meaning that language merely expresses but does not create (Richardson & St. Pierre, 2005). From the mythic perspective that deconstruction inhabits, these binaries are particularly nefarious and must be overcome. This is, in fact, an ethical imperative, a necessity, and "to do justice to this necessity is to recognize that in a classical philosophical opposition we are not dealing with the peaceful coexistence of a vis-à-vis, but rather a violent hierarchy" (Derrida, 1981 [1982], p. 41). This hierarchy, with its presumed violence, unduly privileges one term over another by way of an illusory belief in the self-presentation of meaning (Johnson, 1981). But are the privileges truly unwarranted or is this belief itself merely the expression of an age-old motif, the youthful belief in the absolute and arbitrary injustice of prior generations? Is this belief the true fount of James Hillis Miller's (1987) claim that a millennium of peace and justice for all humankind might be ushered in by the act of deconstructive reading?

If each archetypal figure has its ethic, then the ethic of puer sets itself against this polarizing senex tendency, which is understood to be brutal in its rigidity, restrictive in its formality, and oppressive in its hierarchy. After all, for the eternal youth, "two is the beginning of the end" (Barrie, 1911, p. 1) and the end is what must be avoided. Then again, when the puer-et-senex archetype is split, such a polarizing tendency *does* become just that: A calcified tradition, an unyielding and merciless law, a despotic sovereign that admits no contradiction, a fundamentalist truth that will tolerate no counterargument. For good reason, puer's ethic is to overturn hierarchy and undermine entrenched order. His moral code is that codes are not moral. The act of codification, the establishment of taboos, and the formalization of law and edict all represent little more than structural inhibitions to be overcome, given that structure itself has a negative value: It hinders, imprisons, suppresses, represses, and confines. Even the most seemingly fundamental of oppositions—light and dark, central and peripheral, masculine and feminine, up and down—that some might see as fundamental to the human psyche (Jung, 1953) or fundamental to our existence as embodied beings (Lakoff & Johnson, 1999) are understood to be illusory (Johnson, 1981), mere machinations of a corrupt, senescent orthodoxy.

Each archetypal figure also has a mystique that shrouds its ethic, a numinous aura that surrounds its precepts. Derrida (1992), consciously or otherwise, knew this well. In his description of the *undecidable*, he contrasts the mystical foundation of authority, the one that supports the laws and axioms, principles and practices of legal systems, with "another sort of mystique" (p. 25), to which deconstruction is allied, a form of "justice, which isn't law, [that] is the very movement of deconstruction at work in law and the history of law" (p. 25). Such is puer's mystique, which defines itself in opposition to law insofar as this is an embodiment of senex authority. Derrida (1992) was correct when he claimed that "it was normal, foreseeable, desirable that studies of deconstructive style should culminate in the problematic of law" (p. 7). This is a natural culmination. It is foreseeable because it has been seen before, time and again. The archetypal disposition that values indeterminacy and instability, that drives to deliteralize and see through every limiting denotation and reductive explanation, inevitably finds something problematic in entrenched orthodoxy and authority, whatever the established moral, political, or cultural order may be. It is not surprising that deconstruction places its dissociative logic right in the crevice between law and justice rather than, as one might expect and would be more intellectually consistent, the one between justice and injustice. Nor is it surprising that in cleaving law from justice, deconstruction identifies itself with the latter rather than the former.

The undecidable is more than the ordeal of indecision as was described in pages prior, more than an obligatory antechamber through which one must pass before a final decision is made. The essay in which the term is given a new political and legal potency is entitled *Force of Law: The "Mystical Foundation of Authority"* (Derrida, 1992) and the title speaks clearly to the mythic antagonism that I am defining here. The entire essay pivots upon the distinction between these two mystiques, as if there were an absolute difference between justice and law, as if a Venn diagram portraying the two in no way overlapped. Such is the case when the archetype is split.

For Derrida (1992), "since the origin of authority, the foundation or ground, the position of the law can't by definition rest on anything but themselves, they are themselves a violence without ground" (p. 14). The groundless violence of the law, on his account, exists *by definition*. But whose definition is this? Let us remind ourselves. For deconstruction, nothing is quite self-evident because evidence is always already rendered non-evidential. Derrida's critique of phenomenology begins by undermining the very sense of *seeing* that, for Husserl, is the ultimate legitimizing source of all rational assertions. The word *evidence*, from the Latin *ex* plus *videntem*, in its most primary sense means *that which is seen*. Derrida defines the law as groundless violence only after having established the inadmissibility of any and all evidence. In a court without evidence, admittedly, the position of the law, *whatever that may be*, must be arbitrary. Having already preemptively denied the grounds for *any* ruling, no ruling can possibly be just.

The force that opposes this groundless authority of law is a justice that precedes it and exceeds it. The name of this force, unsurprisingly, is deconstruction: "Deconstruction *is* justice" (Derrida, 1992, p. 15) because it is an always unsatisfied appeal to more justice, one beyond its current manifestation and codification in law. Law is always an *imposition* of a universal upon the particular. Before the law, the singularity of a case must be subjected to the "generality of a rule, a norm or a universal imperative" (Derrida, 1992, p. 17), and deconstruction, which always works to suspend the validity of axiomatic truths, undermines this imposition. Legal decisions are always in opposition to the logic of différance which requires remaining forever open to possibilities rather than taking a definitive stance. Drawing attention to undecidability, the ordeal of having to decide upon one or another legal interpretation, is itself an act of justice. Deconstruction is like an appellate court that must rule that no verdict is beyond a reasonable doubt because reason itself is always doubtful.

The logic by which deconstruction determines the groundless violence of law and the inadmissibility of evidence is the same logic that claims that philosophical binaries are not given but derivative. They are not nature, but second nature. Thus, Derrida's critique, as Barbara Johnson writes in her introduction to Derrida's *Dissemination*:

> reads backwards from what seems natural, obvious, self-evident, or universal, in order to show that these things have their history, their reasons for being the way they are, their effects on what follows from them, and that the starting point is not a (natural) given but a (cultural) construct, usually blind to itself.
>
> *(Derrida, 2021, p. xv)*

Accordingly, the task of undoing such binaries, demonstrating that they are the mere machinations of a metaphysics of presence or logocentrism, is a genealogical one. Deconstruction operates by discerning the descent of a seemingly self-evident binary shedding light upon its lineage within a historical record. This, it would seem, is sufficient to undermine any sense of it being given, universal, or natural. Pointing to the existence of a construct within historical time, and within culture, vitiates the sense in which it may also allude to something given, as it were, by the nature of things. By this method, the factual is made artefactual, rendered a relic. What is given, rather, is given by authorities that "have not dropped from the sky; they are contingent formations, constituted products" (Caputo, 1987, p. 145). Deconstruction "dogmatically stops before any inherited determination of justice" (Derrida, 1992, p. 20) in order to interrogate it, precisely on the grounds that it has been inherited. It stops to interrogate a heritage, and this is its dogma. It is the quality of being historical, temporal, placed within a chronology, the quality of being senescent and artifactual that undermines what previously appeared to be self-evident, universal, or timeless. It is by reference to such senex qualities that deconstruction proceeds to dismantle the validity and truth of any authority expressed in oppositional terms. But the critique is as deficient as it is implacable.

Yet the passage cited earlier is noteworthy not merely because it speaks to the *how* of the eternal youth's deconstruction of limiting law and logic. It is noteworthy because it epitomizes not only the opposition between puer and senex, but their secret collusion as well. It illustrates both the split in the archetype, and its underlying unity: Ironically, critiques of binary thinking, by virtue of their critical stance, must themselves always rest upon a binary, a *not this but that*, or, in this case, the idea of "not a natural (given) but a (cultural) construct" (Johnson, 1981, p. xv). Following Hillman's thinking, it would seem that the split within the archetype requires that cultural construction and natural givenness be opposites that absolutely and utterly preclude one another.

Yet because of the complicit unity of the archetype, as puer's opposition to senex binaries grows stronger, so does his own set of binaries. What he places in the foreground, so as to fix it plainly within the sights of his analytic quiver, becomes the background, or the milieu, within which he operates. The more he attempts to deconstruct polarities, the more he polarizes. Such are the puzzling paradoxes of the relation between these mythic figures. In a state of *chronic deferral*, he is simultaneously most puer and most senex. This same complicity and collusion, as they manifest within deconstruction, are also evidenced by the fact that, as critics and supporters (Garver, 1977; Johnson, 1981; Sweetman, 1997), as well as Derrida (1967 [1978]) himself have noted, his critique relies upon the language, the rhetorical gambits, the phraseology, and the metaphors of the very metaphysics that it so relentlessly attempts to undermine. It relies upon the very terms, like presence and absence, that it will later deconstruct. Pointing this out is not merely a way to highlight a philosophic inconsistency, one that perhaps all of us are guilty to some degree. At a deeper level, it is to point out the puzzling paradox of the puer-et-senex connection, the mind-bending inevitability that each side of the archetypal dyad will always implicate itself in the other, that time and eternity, seeming opposites, imply one another.

The secret collusion between the two halves of the archetype is also made manifestly apparent in multiple performative contradictions. Such contradictions arise when the propositional content of a claim contradicts the presuppositions of its assertion. The content of the claim as regards the transcendence of the signified would seem to make any meaningful reference to it impossible, as well as render its signification insignificant: If I refer to a transcendental signified, I appear to perform the very act of reference that the signified's utter transcendence must preclude. I make reference to something in the act of stating the impossibility of doing so. In a similar vein, the statement that dífférance is not a word contains the word 'dífférance' itself. One can argue that this is not what is meant: There is a word 'dífférance' that alludes to something else that is not a word but rather something like a dynamic or quality. *That* is what is meant. But it is this form of allusion that is disallowed by the argument: Words can only lead us to yet more words. Such contradictions are not incidental but systemic, in the sense of being foundational. They are endemic and cannot be glossed over.

The aforementioned genealogical approach lays bare an *aporia*, an ostensible logical impasse, that deconstruction is inexorably drawn to, one that, in fact, it must be drawn to by virtue of the unhealed split of the archetype. For Derrida, the question of truth is never dissociable from the question of time (Currie, 2013), or more specifically, two seemingly dissimilar aspects of time. From a deconstructive standpoint, any truth that is more than a mere pragmatic fiction "requires the coincidence of finite consciousness (or finite temporal synthesis) with absolute consciousness (time itself or eternity)" (Dillon, 1995, p. 18). The consciousness of an individual, historically contingent human being, located in time and space, must concur with something truly incomparable—the eternal or, to paraphrase Caputo's figurative language, that which has dropped from the sky. Yet this concurrence is thought to be impossible. It is forever and always already deferred; finite, sequential time with its serial progression of moments is incommensurate with the absolute time of eternity. And because this is the case, so the argument goes, the movement between archē and telos, potentiality and actuality, is equally impossible, as is an entire system of sense and meaning (Derrida, 1982 [1986]).

Finite representation cannot correspond to a reality that transcends it. What undergirds Derrida's critique and any claim to truth made under its auspices, is a cleavage between the temporal and the eternal, the finite and the infinite, the immanent and the transcendent. Time is irreconcilable with eternity. Senex is split from puer aeternus, and the split makes truth impossible, at least the form of truth proffered by a certain metaphysical heritage.

## References

Aristotle. (1983). *Aristotle's physics, books III and IV* (E. Hussey, Trans.). Clarendon Press.

Barrie, J. M. (1911). *Peter and Wendy*. Charles Scribner's Sons.

Caputo, J. D. (1987). *Radical hermeneutics: Repetition, deconstruction, and the hermeneutic project*. Indiana University Press.

Currie, M. (2013). *The invention of deconstruction*. Palgrave Macmillan.

Derrida, J. (1967 [1978]). *Writing and difference* (A. Bass, Trans.). University of Chicago Press.

Derrida, J. (1973). *Speech and phenomena, and other essays on Husserl's theory of signs*. Northwestern University Press.

Derrida, J. (1976). *Of grammatology* (G. C. Spivak, Trans.). Johns Hopkins University Press. (Original work published 1967)

Derrida, J. (1981 [1982]). *Positions* (A. Bass, Trans.). University of Chicago Press.

Derrida, J. (1982 [1986]). *Margins of philosophy* (A. Bass, Trans.). University of Chicago Press.

Derrida, J. (1992). Force of law: The "mystical foundation of authority". In D. Cornell, M. Rosenfeld, & D. G. Carlson (Eds.), *Deconstruction and the possibility of justice* (pp. 3–67). Routledge.

Derrida, J. (2021). *Dissemination*. University of Chicago Press.

Dillon, M. C. (1995). *Semiological reductionism: A critique of the deconstructionist movement in postmodern thought*. State University of New York Press.

Garver, N. (1977). Derrida on Rousseau on writing. *The Journal of Philosophy*, *74*(11), 663–673. https://doi.org/10.2307/2025768

Habermas, J. (1987). *The philosophical discourse of modernity: Twelve lectures*. MIT Press.

Heidegger, M. (1927 [1967]). *Being and time*. Blackwell Publishing.

Hillman, J. (1997). *The myth of analysis: Three essays in archetypal psychology*. Northwestern University Press.

Hillman, J. (2021). *Archetypal psychology*. Spring Publications.

Hillman, J., & Slater, G. (2005). *Senex & puer*. Spring Publications.

Johnson, B. (1981). Introduction. In J. Derrida (Ed.), *Dissemination* (pp. vii–xxxiii). University of Chicago Press.

Jung, C. G. (1953). Two essays on analytical psychology. In *The collected works of C. G. Jung* (Vol. 7, R. F. C. Hull, Trans.). Princeton University Press.
Jung, C. G. (1969). The archetypes and the collective unconscious. In *The collected works of C. G. Jung* (Vol. 9.1, R. F. C. Hull, Trans.). Princeton University Press.
Kearney, R. (1986). *Modern movements in European philosophy*. Manchester University Press.
Lakoff, G., & Johnson, M. (1999). *Philosophy in the flesh: The embodied mind and its challenge to Western thought*. Basic Books.
Miller, J. H. (1987). *The ethics of reading: Kant, de Man, Eliot, Trollope, James, and Benjamin*. Columbia University Press.
Richardson, L., & St. Pierre, E. A. (2005). Writing: A method of inquiry. In N. K. Denzin & V. S. Lincoln (Eds.), *The Sage handbook of qualitative research* (3rd ed., pp. 959–978). Sage.
Sweetman, B. (1997). The deconstruction of Western metaphysics: Derrida and Maritain on identity. In R. T. Ciapalo (Ed.), *Postmodernism and Christian philosophy* (pp. 230–247). Catholic University Press.
Tatar, M. (2011). *The annotated Peter Pan*. W.W. Norton & Company.
Wood, D. (2001). *The deconstruction of time*. Northwestern University Press.
Yeoman, A. (1998 [1999]). *Now or Neverland: Peter Pan and the myth of eternal youth: A psychological perspective on a cultural icon*. Inner City Books.

# 6

# GENDER PERFORMATIVITY IN THE LAND OF MAKE-BELIEVE

## I

The word *gender* comes from the Proto-Indo-European root *gene*, which means to birth or beget. Consequently, it forms part of an associative and etymologic cluster of ideas inseparable from motherhood, with all of the correlate notions thus far delineated, not the least of which is that of an origin. To have a gender is to have an origin, to have a mother. To claim that gender has no original, in this regard, is like claiming that a non-origin is originary: a prima facie contradiction. To be gendered is to be born or begotten, to be engendered, defined by an originary moment. To be born is a beginning and as such it is inextricably related to primordiality, with all of its adjacent connotations. This associative, etymologic cluster furthermore comprises the idea of *nature,* derived from *natus*, also indicative of birth, from which we derive words like *natal*, *nascent*, and *native*, all words that can be traced back to the root *gene*, as can the word *genitals*. Such semantic associations all gathered around *mother* are subsequently linked to the idea of matter, as previously outlined, a linking that, explicated earlier, is not limited to the West.

Of course, if, in fact, différance is a non-origin that is originary, as deconstruction would have it, then by a similar reasoning, gender might be an imitation for which there is no original (Butler, 1996 [2011]). If "the present in general is not primal but, rather reconstituted" (Derrida, 1967 [1978], p. 212), then certainly gender likewise can be reconstituted without recourse to originals. If gender is not as primordial as the aforementioned etymologic associations suggest, then perhaps it is derived from the sort of surrogate 'primordiality' that one puts in quotes. Perhaps, like Derrida's trace, its seeming primordiality is based on repetition. This is how the trace constitutes presence, so why can't repetition constitute gender in a similar vein? This appears to be the logic behind Judith Butler's (1996 [2011])

DOI: 10.4324/b23321-7

understanding of gender as performance, which is, above all else, a matter of repetition, a "reiterative and citational practice by which discourse produces the effects that it names" (p. xii). Such reiteration even produces 'sex' and 'materiality.' As noted earlier, *eternal repetition* is also the logic of Neverland. In that realm, although pirates chase lost boys as Indians chase pirates as beasts chase Indians, there is no capture or mortal confrontation—that would bring an end to the fun. Nor is there a starting point for these recurrent conflicts. There is only an endless round of capture deferred and chase forever renewed. It is repetition without origin or end.

Another Neverland, or perhaps it is the same, the one that is constituted by différance, creates itself through a disruption of sequence, a cheating of time as conventionally understood, and a similar disruption of sequence is to be found in the works of Judith Butler, although her own disruption attempts to avoid a clear affirmation of the priority of any language or protolanguage. Nevertheless, hers is also a dis-temporal logic in which the before comes after and presence is made absent. Or perhaps we should say that at times it does. In many ways Butler's reasoning appears to be yet another variation of Derrida's account of a moment demoted from an origin of meaning and sense to a merely formal placeholder emptied of content. Although perhaps it is more accurate to say that both thinkers are repeating variations of a pattern that belongs more to the human condition than to any particular thinker.

Gender as performance is gender deconstructed. It relies on the same disruption of sequence. To deconstruct the gender binary is to deconstruct one of the most foundational and one of the most archetypal binaries in human thought. Because he considered it so foundational, in Jung's psychology, this binary has a name of its own: *syzygy*, which Jung (1959) uses to refer to the masculine and feminine principles that are bound together in the human psyche. Because it is so foundational, the issue of gender also attracts the ire of those antagonistic to foundations and binaries. Because it is so self-evident, the gender binary of male and female is anathema to those who question the very concept of the self-evident. It is perhaps in the arena of gender that the eternal youth's qualms with both the primordial mother and the temporal father are most apparent because the gender binary epitomizes the origin that the youth would rather escape from or deny, as well as the ineradicable dualism that he or she so fiercely opposes.

It should come as no surprise, then, that eternal youths are often androgynous, insofar as androgyny is a form of disrupting this foundational binary. It is to be expected that in Peter Pan, "gender confusion manifests itself in covert ways throughout the text," as Maria Tatar (2011) points out (p. 177, f. n. 3). Androgyny forms part of the general theme of eschewing definition and the finitude of form that characterizes the eternal youth. It is an aspect of the desire to be potentially anything rather than actually something. This penchant for confusion and aversion for definition is shared with queer theory, a foundational text of which is certainly Judith Butler's *Gender Trouble* (Lawford-Smith, 2022; Stock, 2021) a claim made by the author herself in her 1999 preface to the book (Butler, 1990 [2007]). To 'queer' language is to do just that: break down accepted definitions and confuse meanings. Such queering owes much to deconstruction, which has been a prominent influence on queer theorists generally (Joyce, 2021; Sullivan, 2003) and Butler specifically (Brunskell-Evans, 2020).

But the androgyny of the eternal youth is of a particular type, one more intent on rejecting the binary than embracing its paradox, or perhaps simply one that has yet to recognize the inevitability of the binary. Pre-pubescent, it is still virginal, less a synthesis than an undifferentiation, not the actualization of a paradoxical relationship of defined oppositions, a boon of psychological maturity as androgyny often is, but the amorphous indistinction of potential yet to manifest. Wendy describes this androgyny well when she speaks of fairies as those "little sillies who are not sure what they are" (Barrie, 1911, p. 176). This androgyny is prior to the separation and later synthesis of psychic opposites. As pre-pubescent, it is that which exists before the moment of ripening and fertility. In its pathological guise, it is a resistance to this ripening, a fierce insistence on remaining undefined and beyond categorization.

Butler, a philosopher by training, has had an enormous influence on third-wave feminism and gender theory. In the introduction to the present volume, following Michele Lamont (1987), I made an observation about Derrida that also applies to Butler: Her cultural impact, perhaps far more than the innumerable citations of her writings, may have less to do with the intrinsic value of her work and more to do with an appeal to a preexisting desire or imperative. She gives voice to something that was already there, something that sought expression and found its proxy. In this regard, it is less relevant the extent to which Butler draws from Derrida, although this is perhaps the case to a degree often overlooked—she is more often associated with Michele Foucault. What is more relevant is that she is influenced by the same archetypal readiness "to produce over and over again the same or similar mythical ideas" (Jung, 1953, p. 69).

As to similarities, whereas Derrida inverts the relationship between signs and perception, granting primacy to the former, Butler *appears* to invert the relationship between signs and the body, also granting primacy to the former, although the primacy is attenuated by caveats, provisos, and equivocations that would seem to make for a duplicitous argument. At times, she appears to argue that representation must precede presentation, though she adds a twist or two, or perhaps even three. Whereas Derrida posits a protowriting without a present origin, without an *archē*, Butler posits a discourse without an *originally* sexed body. The strategy of making the secondary into something primary, and the derivative into something constitutive, plays itself out in Butler's writing in multiple ways, although the arena has changed and the strategy is directed at another opponent: The generalized system of schemata to be dismantled no longer goes by the name of a *metaphysics of presence*, but rather a *metaphysics of substance*, one that, on her account, is responsible for the production of the category of sexed bodies. One author undermines the notion of an abiding presence, while the other undermines the notion of an abiding substance. Another form of this disruption of sequence is to no longer see gender as a consequence of sex, a behavioral and cultural elaboration of a biological fact. The undermining of the female/male binary takes place by way of what Judith Butler calls a strategic displacement (1990 [2007]). When terms like *woman* and *man* no longer refer to any such abiding substances, then what is left is a repetition of forms—the terms have been hollowed out. Such abiding substances are fictive constructions brought about by repetitive behavior: For Butler, gender is always a *doing*.

Both philosophers, each in their own way, construe seemingly self-evident binaries as non-evidential, understanding them as machinations of a pre-existent, unfounded intellectual order, one whose very existence must be called into question, interrogated, and found deficient. In *Bodies That Matter* (1996 [2011]), published three years after her groundbreaking work *Gender Trouble: Feminism and the Subversion of Identity* (1990 [2007]), Butler (1996 [2011]) writes:

> The body posited as prior to the sign, is always *posited* or *signified* as *prior*. This signification produces as an *effect* of its own procedure the very body that it nevertheless and simultaneously claims to discover as that which *precedes* its own action. If the body signified as prior to signification is an effect of signification, then the mimetic or representational status of language, which claims that signs follow bodies as their necessary mirrors, is not mimetic at all. On the contrary, it is productive, constitutive, one might even argue *performative*, inasmuch as this signifying act delimits and contours the body that it then claims to find prior to any and all signification.
>
> *(p. 6)*

Typically, we understand the body to be something that presents itself to us and is later represented by us. Because humans are bodies that perceive other bodies, we have words to reflect this fact and words to reflect different types of bodies. In this sense, the body exists prior to the sign, prior to the language that represents it. Language has a mimetic, representational relation to the body, or so it would seem. This has been the classical conception. But for Butler, judging solely from the paragraph above, it is the passage from body to sign, the process of signification, that *produces* the body that was thought to exist prior to this passage. What one thought was prior is actually subsequent, an effect, or better yet, an aftereffect. In rendering the secondary into something primary, the derivative has become something constitutive, an origin. The new origin is discourse, signification, language, and signs. It is no longer the material body.

As regards the sex of these bodies, delimited and contoured as they are by this signifying process, Butler (1990 [2007]) claims that sex does "not qualify as a prediscursive anatomical facticity" (p. 11). It is not that we encounter a sexed body, one of a sexually dimorphic species that, by virtue of that fact, must belong to one side or another of a binary, that is to say, must be either female or male. Rather, it is the signifying process, the putting into language that creates "the binary framework for both sex and gender [which] are considered throughout as regulatory fictions that consolidate and naturalize the convergent power regimes of masculine and heterosexist oppression" (Butler, 1990 [2007], p. 46). For Butler, because the scientific language that describes the sex binary arises from within the milieu of culture and language, it is possible that biology itself is constructed. What masquerades as natural fact is, to the contrary, a fiction, born of the same oppressive power regimes that, in her mind, characterize culture. Sex "is not a simple fact or static condition of a body, but a process whereby regulatory norms materialize 'sex' and achieve this materialization through a forcible reiteration of those norms" (Butler, 1996 [2011], p. xii). As addressed in the previous chapter, pointing to the existence of a construct within historical time and within culture appears to invalidate the sense in which it may also allude to something given by the nature of things. By this method, the factual is made to appear merely artefactual.

In its most fundamental aspects, Butler's critique of a metaphysics of substance *is* Derrida's critique of a metaphysics of presence, though dressed in another attire, one better suited for her gender-bending intent and adorned with all of the Foucauldian accessories that one might expect: references to power, bodies, inscriptions, regimes, confinement, discipline, regulatory norms, etc. This fact does not require a direct influence of one author on the other, although such an influence is certainly there. For Butler (1990 [2007]), "sex appears within hegemonic language as a *substance*, as, metaphysically speaking, a self-identical being" (p. 25), and this raises the same issues for her as it does for deconstruction as regards presence and the illusion of a self-identical sign: For deconstruction, no such sign exists. The two elements of the sign, signifier and signified, are non-identical and each iteration of a sign is non-identical to every other. For Butler (1990 [2007]), the illusion of a substantive being is "achieved through a performative twist of language and/or discourse that conceals the fact that 'being' a sex or a gender is fundamentally impossible" (p. 26) by virtue of a similar logic that claims that any presence denoted in language is impossible or vacuous. Language creates the illusion of a 'there' that is *actually* there, or at least one that can be reached. But no such there exists. How could it, when the very concept of 'actuality'—with all of its historic connotations of presence—has already been discredited?

The illusion of a substantive being is a trick of sorts, one that retroactively installs material bodies as the seemingly primary givens that biology appears to dispassionately describe. Butler (1996 [2011]) tells us:

> "Materiality" designates a certain effect of power or, rather, is power in its formative or constituting effects. Insofar as power operates successfully by constituting an object domain, a field of intelligibility, as a taken-for-granted ontology, its material effects are taken as material data or primary givens. These material positivities appear outside discourse and power, as its incontestable referents, its transcendental signifieds. But this appearance is precisely the moment in which

> the power/discourse regime is most fully dissimulated and most insidiously effective. When this material effect is taken as an epistemological point of departure, a sine qua non of some political argumentation, this is a move of empiricist foundationalism that, in accepting this constituted effect as a primary given, successfully buries and masks the genealogy of power relations by which it is constituted.
>
> *(pp. 9–10)*

It would seem from the above passage that Butler's point is as clear as she will ever make it: Materiality, the apparently primary given of an empirical field of study like biology is not what it appears to be because it is actually an insidious *effect of* discourse and power, which would seem to suggest that discourse precedes matter in a similar way that signs precede phenomena for Derrida. But as soon as the reader seems to grasp Butler's argument, in fact even before this happens, as if anticipating objections, she appears to withdraw it by way of proviso. In a footnote to the above citation, she (1996 [2011]) clarifies that "this is not to make 'materiality' into the effect of a 'discourse' which is its cause; rather, it is to displace the causal relation through a reworking of the notion of 'effect'" (p. 192). Having read numerous Butlerian texts, it is difficult for me not to see such a 'reworking' as a prime example of the very sort of insidiously effective dissimulation that she herself derides. This reworking appears to suggest that empirical reality itself is a form of oppression.

Even before this footnote addended to the above passage, in the opening lines of *Bodies That Matter*, Butler (1996 [2011]) has told her reader explicitly that she will *not* be "claiming that discourse causes sexual difference" (p. xi), merely that such differences are indissociable from it. This is the nub of the issue. Nor is it the case that "the body is simply linguistic stuff or, on the other [hand] that it has no bearing on language" (Butler, 1996 [2011], p. 37). She is, in effect, trying to avoid making the sort of argument that might be vulnerable to the same critiques that have been launched at Derrida. It is important, then, for her to argue that it is *not* that language takes precedence, but rather that language is so entwined with matter, so entangled with the matter of the body, that we cannot take the body as simply given in an unproblematic way. Rather, it is as if the two are inextricably *fused*. We cannot extricate ourselves from language (and therefore discourse and power) in order to grasp materiality in and of itself (Butler, 1996 [2011]). The machinations of language, protolanguage, signs, or what have you are not an origin, but neither is matter.

She explains in this same footnote that "power is established in and through its effects, where these effects are the dissimulated workings of power itself" (Butler, 1996 [2011], p. 192). But an astute reader might ask, *who or what is dissimulating here?* Who or what is this agent called 'power'? How can the effects of power also be what establishes it to begin with? And what discourse, or whose, is acquiring such an insidious effect? Is the true concealment that of an empiricist foundationalism—one that surreptitiously creates a chimeric object domain it will later take to be incontestably given and undeniably real? Or is it Butler (1996 [2011]) herself who is, by way of referencing a "dissimulation [that] operates through the constitution and formation of an epistemic field" (p. 192), the person who is, in fact, covertly referencing her own dissimulation, her own formation of a field, one called queer theory? Does the discipline of biology, as an agent of power, with all of the oppressive connotations bestowed upon it, create an object domain of which the sexual binary forms a part, or is Butler establishing her own domain, her own epistemic field, her own branch of studies, with its own cleverly disguised and insidiously effective power/discourse regime? If we allow for this latter prospect, perhaps being a sex or a gender is not an impossibility, as she contends, but rather a matter of self-evidence, a primary given, and it is Butler's own performative twists of language that attempt to conceal the fact. This, to my mind, seems more plausible.

An oft-cited passage from Lewis Carroll's *Through the Looking Glass* (1981), might help shed light on such questions as performative twists of language, agents of power, and discourse regimes:

> 'I don't know what you mean by "glory,"' Alice said.
> Humpty Dumpty smiled contemptuously. 'Of course you don't—till I tell you. I meant "there's a nice knockdown argument for you!"'
> 'But "glory" doesn't mean "a nice knock-down argument,"' Alice objected.
> 'When I use a word,' Humpty Dumpty said in rather a scornful tone, 'it means just what I choose it to mean—neither more nor less.'
> 'The question is, said Alice, 'whether you can make words mean so many different things.'
> 'The question is,' said Humpty Dumpty, which is to be master—that's all.
> (p. 103)

Echoing Humpty-Dumpty in a more contemporary language, we might ask which is to be the agent of power and whose discourse regime is to take precedence, that of biology or that of Butler and similar theorists. The latter, it would seem, as hopefully will be made even clearer further on, would like words to mean many different things that they have not traditionally meant. Their performative twists have implicitly posed Alice's question, and in so doing, revealed its political consequences. Can words like 'man' and 'woman' be used in the way they would like, and who will be the master who makes this decision?

Butler's two block quotations above, which suggest a simple inversion of the body/sign dichotomy, follow an introduction in which she distances herself from the sort of typical linguistic constructivism that they seem to suggest, a linguistic monism that would reduce everything to merely a question of language. She rightly notes that such a constructivism tends to lead toward one or another unsatisfactory presumption: Construction either operates deterministically, granting no place to human agency, or it presupposes a voluntarist subject fully responsible for construction. It requires that we be either puppets or gods. Neither of these are satisfactory. The former, which presumes that discourse constructs the subject, is merely a reversal of the claim that the subject constructs discourse, yet construction, on her account, must mean more than such a simple reversal of terms. Weary of some of the inevitable difficulties implicit in construction, Butler opts for what she calls *materialization*, which rests more upon the idea that although bodies are not the direct effect of discourse, they are certainly indissociable from it. Butler (1996 [2011]) writes:

> What I would propose in place of these conceptions of construction is a return to the notion of matter, not as site or surface, but as a process of materialization that stabilizes over time to produce the effect of boundary, fixity, and surface we call matter. That matter is always materialized has, I think, to be thought in relation to the productive and, indeed, materializing effects of regulatory power in the Foucaultian sense. Thus, the question is no longer, How is gender constituted as and through a certain interpretation of sex? (a question that leaves the "matter" of sex untheorized), but rather, Through what regulatory norms is sex itself materialized? And how is it that treating the materiality of sex as a given presupposes and consolidates the normative conditions of its own emergence?"
>
> *(pp. xviii–xix)*

If, for a moment, we leave aside the circular definition of matter as a process of materialization, it is still a bit perplexing to suggest that replacing the idea of matter as a surface with the idea of some obscure process that makes matter into, yet again, a surface, is somehow clarifying or edifying. Butler seems to be making not merely a distinction without a difference but an indistinct distinction, leading the reader to indifference. One is reminded of Nietzsche's (1978) observation: "They all muddy their waters to make them appear deep" (p. 128). What appears to be important is that matter is not construed *first* as a given. It may come to be given only through some sort of congealing, stabilizing process involving power and discourse.

Caveats, provisos, footnotes, and subterfuge aside, the net effect of her argument remains to render the matter of bodies, especially sexed bodies, as no longer given prior to discourse. Matter *must* be compromised by discourse and not merely reflected by it, in much the same way that différance must not only inhabit presence but actually *constitute* it. In both cases, conclusions are less determined by argument than by a primary imperative that guides the argument. As discussed earlier, such an imperative forces a person to bend logic to fit a conclusion, twist syntax to hide agency, and place the reasoning mind at the service of an unreasoned compulsion. Enthralled by the archetype and following its edict, one finds a way to arrive at the desired belief, often while projecting one's own intellectual foibles onto the object of critique.

In the absence of sexed bodies, or in the presence of bodies that have only been sexed fictitiously by the reconceptualized effects of discourse, Butler radically reconceives the question of gender and its relation to sex. It is through this reconceptualization that Butler intends to cause the 'trouble' and 'subversion' alluded to in the title of her most influential work to date. The trouble is this: If sex is no longer a biological fact independent of construction, then gender is not culturally constructed upon a primary given. Gender is not the culturally determined software and sex is not the biologically determined hardware. This creates a problem for anyone, feminist thinkers first and foremost, who wants to maintain the culture/nature dichotomy as a way to undermine the idea that biology is destiny, the belief that sex dictates certain social meanings for women.

But on Butler's reading, a split in the feminist subject, a split in the very idea of what a woman is, suggests that the cause of being the gender 'woman' is not the biological fact of being female. So, the selfsame framing of the sex/gender relationship in terms of a biology/culture distinction, intended to further women's liberation, unwittingly introduced the possibility that gender is *not* the cultural expression of biological sex at all. In fact, "the construal of 'sex' no longer as a bodily given on which the construct of gender is artificially imposed" (Butler, 1996 [2011], p. xii) changes everything. The understanding that gender was in some form dependent upon sex appears, in this light, equivocal and misguided. Since sex is no longer grounded in matter, understood as an epistemological starting point, gender is no longer grounded in sex. On the contrary, bodies 'assume sex' in agreement with regulatory social norms entrenched by a heterosexual imperative: Threats of punishment for homosexual desire and the pervasiveness of the heterosexual ideal work together to 'sex' bodies. Despite the troubling, Butler (1996 [2011]) reassures her reader that

> the category of women does not become useless through deconstruction, but becomes one whose uses are no longer reified as "referents," and which stand a chance of being opened up, indeed, of coming to signify in ways that none of us can predict in advance.
>
> *(p. 5)*

The term *women*, having been deconstructed, can still have a meaning, but no one can predict what that meaning might become. No one can know what the term will refer to. This is, in a sense, both absurd and prescient, few would have predicted at the time of publication of the words above that the question *What is a woman?* would have come to the forefront of academic and political debate.[1]

Such a decoupling of core understandings is infinitely exploitable. If discourse is so indissociable from bodies as to require a rethinking of what is meant by 'matter,' then bodies cannot matter in the same way as they previously did. If both sex and gender are equally constructed, or perhaps materialized through twists of language, concealing the fact that being a sex or a gender is fundamentally impossible, then is it not possible that sex is actually a subset of, or even caused by gender? If

Butler can meddle with what might be called 'the order of operations' regarding the equation of bodies and signs, bodies and discourse, why not meddle with the order of sex and gender so that the former becomes an effect of the latter? After all, the whole process of materialization, on her account, requires a reworking of the notion of 'effect.' Who is to say that sex is not the cultural expression of gender? Gender, now no longer the effect of sex, can become its cause, thereby establishing its own primacy and privilege:

> If gender consists of the social meanings that sex assumes, then sex does not accrue social meanings as additive properties but, rather, is replaced by the social meanings it takes on; sex is relinquished in the course of that assumption, and gender emerges, not as a term in a continued relationship of opposition to sex, but as the term which absorbs and displaces "sex," the mark of its full substantiation into gender or what, from a materialist point of view, might constitute a full desubstantiation.
>
> *(Butler, 1996 [2011], p. xv)*

On Butler's account, sex is absorbed and displaced by gender and thereby desubstantiated. It is relinquished. To substantiate, from the Latin *substantia*, meaning "being, essence, material," in modern usage refers to the act of giving substance or form, to embody something, but it also denotes the establishment of something by way of proof or evidence. In her attempt, then, to desubstantiate sex, we see a familiar pattern: An attempt to undermine both matter and evidence by way of *dis* (as in displace) and its variant *de*.

The result is somewhat of a muddle, resulting in the assertion that "the distinction between sex and gender turns out to be no distinction at all" (Butler, 1990 [2007], p. 10), no distinction at all, except when such a distinction is needed for sex to be displaced. By way of a rhetorical strategy similar to Derrida's, one that eviscerates primordiality only to later employ it in another guise, Butler deconstructs sex yet still uses the term with all of the denotations and connotations that she has previously deconstructed. Her *de*substantiation might also be construed as a *tran*substantiation. This is a religious term. Those who are struggling to grasp Butler's logic might be reminded of this term from Catholicism. It denotes a process by which, it is believed, the substance, if not the appearance, of the bread and wine of the Eucharist becomes Christ's real presence. But such a transubstantiation in gender theory, one might argue, lacks the benefit of being understood as a symbolic or religious belief. It is one thing to consciously adopt a religion and enact its sacraments. It is quite another thing to adopt one unawares.

## II

What is the reader to make of all this? The deconstruction of both sex and gender sets the stage for gender performativity, a concept that, with varying degrees of misappropriation and misunderstanding, has had a remarkable impact upon our popular conception of what is meant by 'gender.' As J. Hillis Miller notes, Butler's gender performativity is, in fact, a variation of Derrida's theory of performativity. There is a filial line that runs through Butler, who "appropriated Derrida's modification of Austin's speech act theory and married it, under the impetus of feminism and nascent queer theory, to something more or less alien to Derrida's work, namely Foucault's *Discipline and Punish* and his *History of Sexuality*" (Miller, 2007, p. 224). But the filial line appears riddled with genetic anomalies. Descendants bear only scant relation to their forebears, and parentage at times remains in doubt. In other words, despite professed lineage, what is meant by *performativity* differs from one writer to another more than it does not.

One of the grandfathers in this family tree, along with John Searle, is by all accounts the British philosopher J. L. Austin (1975), who, in his book *How to Do Things with Words*, introduced the idea of a *performative utterance*: A speech act that does not merely *describe* something but *does* something. He points out that certain uses of language serve neither to represent nor to structure reality. They bring it into being. The most paradigmatic and oft-cited example of such a performative utterance is marriage vows. When I say 'I do' within the context of a marriage ceremony, I am not merely describing what I am doing, I am actually doing it. Within appropriate circumstances and specified social contexts, what Austin calls *felicity conditions*, simply saying something brings about a situation that had not existed beforehand. In the act of saying 'I do,' I become married. 'I do' is, in this context, a *performative*: An utterance in which to say something is to do something, which Austin contrasts with a *constative*, an utterance that is assertive or descriptive, correctly or incorrectly, of a set of facts. A constative is. A performative does. It brings about what it says. It is an *illocutionary* or intentional act. Making a bet or promise, christening a ship, saying 'I quit,' giving an order or warning, or apologizing, can also function as performatives.

If I say the words 'I promise' while reporting another person's speech, as an actor in a play, while reading a poem, or as the punch line to a joke, then the words may not be performatives at all. Context and intent are crucial. Without them, the 'abracadabra-like' quality of a performative is not in force. From the Aramaic phrase *avra kehdabra*, which means "I will create as I speak," abracadabra is perhaps a good phrase to remember the denotations if not the connotations of what is meant by *performative* in Austin's original sense of the term. A performative utterance creates what it speaks, but only under certain circumstances that Austin exhaustively attempted to describe.

The filial line of the performative then passes through Derrida, who appropriated Austin's notion, altering it fundamentally in the process. The alteration involves a theme familiar to the reader by now, that of iterability or repetition, first introduced in reference to the idea of semiotic spacing: The fact that each time a sign is repeated, although it may appear identical from one instance to another, its meaning cannot be. Iteration is alteration because the repetition of a sign is always dependent upon an interval, a spatial and temporal gap that amounts to a change of context. Furthermore, context is boundless, infinite. Yet iteration and citationality are the necessary conditions for any code: Words must be repeatable, capable of being cited, quoted, referenced, used in identical form in non-identical contexts. These observations apply to performatives as well, notes Derrida (1988). In fact, repetition and citationality are, in some sense, even *more* paradigmatic of performatives:

> Every sign, linguistic or nonlinguistic, spoken or written (in the current sense of this opposition), in a small or large unit, can be *cited*, put between quotation marks; in doing so it can break with every given context, engendering an infinity of new contexts in a manner which is absolutely illimitable. This does not imply that the mark is valid outside of a context, but on the contrary that there are only contexts without any center or absolute anchorage [ancrage]. This citationality, this duplication or duplicity, this iterability of the mark is neither an accident nor an anomaly, it is that (normal/abnormal) without which a mark could not even have a function called "normal." What would a mark be that could not be cited? Or one whose origins would not get lost along the way?
>
> *(Derrida, 1988, p. 12)*

On this line of thought, one consequence of the fact that such repetition, iterability, and citationality imply transformation is that a performative utterance cannot have a unified, identifiable meaning or determinate content. It has no absolute anchored meaning. Performatives are subject to the same issues of displacement as other signifiers and, even when understood in context, suffer from a degree of indeterminacy, given that "context is never absolutely determinable . . . [and] determination can never be entirely certain or saturated" (Derrida, 1988, p. 3).

Yet this is what Austin's notion of a performative requires: determinate context. A series of circumstances or 'felicitous' conditions must be in place: A set of social conventions, a clear understanding of what is at stake, and the roles being played by all people involved. The words 'I do' will marry no one without the clergy or notary public present, or without required witnesses, and the meaning of these words acquires power as well from certain recognizable conventions and accoutrements: walks down an isle, the passing of the bride from father to groom, the various ceremonial duties of groomsmen and maids of honor, the exchanging of rings, the cutting of cake or smashing of glasses, the use of bouquets, dresses, and tuxedos, all of which help to clearly indicate the special meaning and importance of the event. All of this, and more, make up what Austin (1975) calls the *total speech act.*

Yet Derrida's entire approach is to draw attention to the fact that context is always incomplete, always shifting, always yet to be fully defined. There is no totality. All we really have is the repetition of words amid this semiotic shifting, and because this is the case, the specter that such felicitous conditions have not been met haunts every presumed performative. Butler (1997) takes a similar approach when, in the introduction to *Excitable Speech* and in reference to the total speech act that defines performatives, states that "there is, however, no easy way to decide on how best to delimit that totality" (p. 3). On Derrida's account, given that there is then no clear delimiting of context, there is no clearly discernible difference between a performative and a constative utterance, no clear-cut difference between an utterance with an abracadabra-like quality and one that merely attempts to assert or describe. Much like, for Butler, the distinction between sex and gender turns out to be no distinction at all, except when expedient, the distinction between performative and constative, for Derrida, is no distinction at all, except when it needs to be. Like just about every other binary that he encounters within the texts of others, if not his own, the performative/constative binary is one that he seeks to challenge.

We have encountered the idea of an *anchorage*, albeit by another name, in a previous chapter depicting the limitless free play of signification. Free play, the pleasure of displacement brought about by différance, results in the absence of a *fixed point*—a point of both presence and origin, balance and orientation. This absence is what makes such an infinitely free play possible. Because signs that might have alluded to such a point are no longer understood as surrogates substituting for some preexisting thing or meaning, they are no longer restrained by these roles. This absence of a fixed point that makes free play possible is also the absence of anchorage that makes Austin's understanding of a performative, utterly dependent on context, into a boundless performance, one of unconditioned freedom, an idea that Derrida puts forth in his essay *The University Without Condition* (2002).

In attempting to define the determining factors of such a determinate context, six of which Austin finds indispensable although not sufficient, he names *intention* as one of them. For performatives to function, the intention must be clear. If I speak with irony or in jest, for example, this may undermine the performative effect of an utterance. If I am not clear as to the meaning of the words I am speaking, or if I speak them under duress, then this will undermine their performative function. But the idea of intention offers an opening for the deconstructive method. Performative communication requires the communication of an intentional meaning, a wanting to say something, but Derrida's entire approach undermines the possibility that such a wanting can ever be satisfied or that intention can ever be present as conventionally understood. Intention is, after all, just another name related to the fundamentals and principles—much like essence, existence, substance, or subject—that deconstruction calls into question. It is a lynchpin in the metaphysics to be dismantled, one that requires the "conscious presence of the intention of the speaking subject in the totality of his speech act" (Derrida, 1988, p. 14). But such a presence and such a totality are precisely what deconstruction denies.

Having undermined the intention and context necessary for the performative/constative distinction and having thoroughly deconstructed Austin's speech act theory, Derrida nevertheless proceeds to appropriate it, although distorting it in the process. At the heart of this distortion is the contention that performative speech acts are *not* constituted by intention but rather by the structure of language itself, specifically its repeatability. As Butler (1996 [2011]) writes, "Derrida argues that the binding power that Austin attributes to the speaker's intention in such illocutionary acts is more properly attributable to a citational force of the speaking, the iterability that establishes the authority of the speech act" (p. 214).

Austin's *How to Do Things with Words* (1975) becomes, in Butler's hands, a question of how 'doing things' *are* words. The notion of *speech as act* becomes *act as speech* once it has been reconstrued by Derrida and later (mis)appropriated by Butler (1996 [2011]), for whom "every act is itself a recitation" (p. 187). It is a signifier, and like all signifiers, it can be repeated. In fact, it is only through repetition that it can have meaning. Performativity is a repetition of acts, but both acts and repetition must be seen through the prism of the Derridean notion of iterability: The absolute, unequivocal repetition of a sign, or any meaningful utterance (like a recitation) is an impossibility—because the very act of repetition is transformative. Replace the word *sign* with the word *act* in a Derridean text, and you will approximate Butler's notion of the performative. In Butler's (1996 [2011]) words, performativity involves "the citing of a prior chain of acts [signs] which are implied in a present act [sign] and which perpetually drain any "present" act [sign] of its presentness" (p. 187). Such a statement is remarkable as regards both its parallels and its obscurity. As regards the obscurity, one can say of the logic of performativity what Derrida (1973) said of the logic of différance: it is "difficult and uncomfortable" (p. 142).

Perhaps more importantly are the parallels: Butler's 'perpetually drained present' is a variant of Derrida's—and the eternal youth's—hollowed now. Her understanding of gender as an imitation for which there is no original is a version of the origin story that denies origins or displaces them. For Derrida, there is a form called 'the present' that persists through the continuous changes of matter by way of repetition. For Butler, there is a form called 'man' and a form called 'woman,' but they are like traces of repeated behaviors granting the illusion of something more abiding and substantial: Genders present themselves, perform themselves again and again, but what appears and reappears is only that—an apparition, a vacuous form. They are genders hollowed of sexed bodies, like a now hollowed of perception and primordiality.

The "power regimes of masculine and heterosexist oppression" (Butler, 1990 [2007], p. 46) that her writing seeks to undermine plays a similar role as that of the metaphysical heritage and the unjust imposition of law that Derrida relentlessly indicts. They are all, in a sense, the same senex ogre. Her notion of performativity, which is also construed in Lacanian terms while evoking the same specter of absence and the oblivion of forgetting, forms part of the same mythic configuration that the present work attempts to elucidate: The repetition of acts is the repetition of what cannot be remembered or recovered, and as such, it is a variation of the theme of the eternal youth's irreparable loss, the loss of something that was, curiously enough, never possessed or never existed to begin with. For Butler, gender performance allegorizes a loss it cannot grieve. It enacts a melancholia in response to something that was never possessed yet cannot be let go of (Butler, 1996 [2011]).

Yet the loss also provides an opportunity, for free play in one case, for a performance or 'performativity' with parodic, subversive intent in the other. Derrida's limitless *free play* of signification and Peter Pan's ecstasies both involve the pleasure of displacement, and so does Butler's gender play. Derrida (1967 [1978]) exuberantly describes this play as "the affirmation of a world of signs without fault, without truth, and without origin" (p. 292), and for Butler there is a similar affirmation, one involving gender without the truth of sexed bodies. Many of these themes, familiar to the reader by now, find stark relief in *Bodies That Matter*:

> Is there an original authority, a primary source, or is it, rather, in the very practice of citation, potentially infinite in its regression, that the ground of authority is constituted as perpetual deferral? In other words, it is precisely through the infinite deferral of authority to an irrecoverable past that authority itself is constituted. That deferral is the repeated act by which legitimation occurs. The pointing to a ground which is never recovered becomes authority's groundless ground.
>
> *(Butler, 1996 [2011], pp. 70–71)*

Butler's writings are notoriously difficult and murky in their conceptualization. When the theme is performativity, she often seems to be merely speaking an Austinian dialect in a deconstructive accent so as to communicate simple ideas while giving the impression of saying something far more complex. Performativity does, however, occasionally make its appearance upon the stage of her prose without the sophist's regalia that imbues it with an aura of philosophic complexity. In some essays, she expresses herself with a modicum of clarity, as in *Performative Acts and Gender Constitution: An Essay in Phenomenology and Feminist Theory* (Butler, 1990), in which she informs the reader that "the acts by which gender is constituted bear similarities to performative acts within theatrical contexts" (p. 521). Just as actors on a stage think of their bodies as the 'instruments' through which they perform their craft, bodies outside this context are also involved in the crafting of identities, the creation of characters, the fictions we take to be real. Both on and off the stage, we create the illusion of a self through stylized action. We *'do'* the body as much as we *are* the body. For such a style of thought, to 'present' as a gender, to appear as one, is to be one. One might think of this as yet another variation of deconstruction's demotion of presence from an origin of meaning and sense to a merely formal placeholder emptied of content, a mere simulacrum.

From this perspective, gender is a corporeal style, a dramatic act witnessed by an audience. In truth, it is less fact than act, but one that requires constant repetition to procure its reality, one that must be "renewed, revised, and consolidated through time" (Butler, 1990, p. 523). A skeptical reader might ask whether such prolonged repetition, which always presumes an audience as the word 'performance' suggests, is required because what is being repeated is a fantasy. It is a fantasy that can only pretend to be something more than fantasy through being repeatedly witnessed by others, mirrored and therefore validated by others.

Derrida's deconstruction of the context needed for performative speech offers Butler a way to erase the line between stage and audience, but it is hardly needed. One can appreciate without it that such a line is more porous than often acknowledged. Perhaps none of us ever really leaves the theater. We take it with us: We are always making believe and making others believe, and in so doing, we bring fictional characters into being. We 'constitute' them. But what is more questionable and more telling is that for Butler gender is real *only* to the extent that it is performed. Furthermore, it is through this performance that the social fiction of an interior gendered self is produced. Stripped even further of its academic attire and stated with maximum economy so that even Ockham would approve, one could say that for Butler *gender is what you pretend to be and pretending makes things real.* Just as J. M. Barrie (1911) said of Peter Pan that "to him make-believe and true were exactly the same thing" (p. 75), one might say these words of Butler as well.

But as children know, even pretending has certain rules. For Butler, gender performances are governed by punitive and regulatory social conventions. They are ritualized productions, and the ritual is "reiterated under and through constraint, under and through the force of prohibition and taboo, with the threat of ostracism and even death controlling and compelling the shape of the production" (Butler, 1996 [2011], p. 60). For her, it is hardly by chance that the most paradigmatic example of a performative speech act is the heterosexual marriage ceremony. After all, on her account, it is a socially sanctioned and idealized heterosexist imperative that has written the script of gender performance. What has historically governed, consolidated, and naturalized gender has been the power regimes of masculine and heterosexist oppression. Yet understanding that the authority of such a scripted exchange rests solely on its repetitive, ritualized nature offers an opportunity to subvert its dictates, to undermine its presumptive force, to find loopholes in its law.

Butler's thinking as regards sex follows similar lines, and why wouldn't it, given that she has already established that the term *sex* can easily be absorbed and displaced by gender? Both sex and gender equally partake of a phantasmal existence brought about by repetitive incantation. As if casting a spell, she writes:

> Is "assuming" a sex like a speech act? Or is it, or is it like, a citational strategy or resignifying practice?
>
> To the extent that the "I" is secured by its sexed position, this "I" and its "position" can be secured only by being *repeatedly* assumed, whereby "assumption" is not a singular act or event, but, rather, an iterable practice.
>
> *(Butler, 1996 [2011], p. 71)*

It is not enough, apparently, to establish one's sex only once and leave it at that. An insecurity about one's sex must be, again and again, salved by the balm of repeated assumption. If assuming such a position means seeking recourse to a norm, then it is a question of simply repeating the norm, mimicking some preexistent form. If gender is an act rehearsed again and again until it congeals into believability, then why not sex? After all, it is the sedimentation of gender norms over time that "has produced a set of corporeal styles which, in reified form, appear as the natural configuration of bodies into sexes which exist in a binary relation to one another" (Butler, 1990, p. 524). This specifically *binary* relation is the direct result of a heterosexual normative regime that has as its strategic aim the maintaining of both gender and sex within a binary frame and *nothing* about this framing is simply given by the nature of things: "Sex, gender, and heterosexuality are historical products which have become conjoined and reified as natural over time" (Butler, 1990, p. 525).

Echoing Barbara Johnson's description of deconstruction in pages prior, we can say that Butler reads backward from what seems natural, obvious, self-evident, or universal, in order to show that ideas have their history, their reasons for being the way they are and their effects on what follows from them. Their starting point is not a natural given but a cultural construction that is blind to itself. For her, "there is no nature, only the effects of nature: denaturalization or naturalization" (Butler, 1996 [2011], p. x). Just as for Derrida (1967 [1978]) "the present in general is not primal but, rather reconstituted" (p. 212), sex is not primal but reconstituted, and to think otherwise is to remain blind to the culture, history, or language that creates the illusion of something self-evident or natural: "Whether gender or sex is fixed or free is a function of a discourse which, it will be suggested, seeks to set certain limits to analysis or to safeguard certain tenets of humanism as pre-suppositional to any analysis of gender" (Butler, 1990 [2007], p. 12). Like Derridean free play—interpretation without fault, truth, or origin, Butler's (1990 [2007]) performativity of gender is made possible only by the omission of the truth of sex as origin. The fiction that is sex, once "released from its naturalized interiority and surface, can occasion the parodic proliferation and subversive play of gendered meanings" (p. 46).

Thankfully, for her, discourses evolve and regimes can be disrupted. The oppressive binary that had mistakenly been attributed to nature, biology, or the evidence of direct perception can be overcome now that its performative nature has been revealed. Gender identity as a stylized repetition of acts can be disturbed by interfering with the relation between acts, resulting in a "different sort of repeating, in the breaking or subversive repetition of style" (Butler, 1990, p. 520). A person can disrupt the rhythm of expectation, go off script, recite one's lines in an odd tone of voice, interpret the assigned gender role in a way that defies expectation. One can even offer a *parodic* performance, and indeed parody is a central means of causing the gender trouble that Butler promotes. Parody: The imitation of a style for comic effect so as to make something ridiculous or ludicrously inappropriate; the mimicry of an original form for the sake of mockery—it is not difficult to understand why parody might be chosen as a means to erode gender orthodoxy, or that drag might be focused upon, as Butler often does, as a means to elucidate this parody. It is well known that humor has a corrosive effect on authority. No tyrant can stand being laughed at. So, to poke fun, to mockingly reenact, to spoof, lampoon, distort, and exaggerate are the oft-used weapons of those living under a tyranny, real or imagined, and the 'tyranny' of the gender binary is no different.

But 'parodic performativity' does not merely describe the *content* of Butler's strategy of causing trouble; it describes the very form by which this content is put forth. There is something parodic in the very form of her argumentation. One can easily imagine it as a spoof on intellectualism, a distortion and exaggeration of philosophy's pedantic tendencies, a willful invocation of obscurity, a comical mimicry of its conventions, a stylized repetition of what a neophyte considers philosophy to be. It also echoes von Franz' description of the faux intellectualism of the eternal youth. It is difficult to escape the sense that Butler conceives philosophy itself as a purely performative act. Like a student still finding her way through the halls of higher education, her style suggests a sophomoric belief that complexity and obscurity equal a cogent argument firmly grounded, as well as a naive faith that repeating multisyllabic words, or stuffing a bibliography with innumerable and unnecessary references might grant the illusion of truly 'doing philosophy.' Much of her writing appears to be a subversive repetition of the style of philosophic thought, one that exaggerates what students might take to be the discipline's most salient characteristics. In short, her style is a parody of philosophy, a risible caricature of what is meant by the word.

Unsurprisingly, the identity created through repetitive performance is not a stable one. On the contrary, it is tenuous and always in need of renewed rehearsal and ritualized reproduction. Only in this way can "bodily gestures, movements, and enactments of various kinds constitute the illusion of an abiding gendered self" (Butler, 1990, p. 519). Nor is this identity a locus of agency. The repetition that created it "is not [even] performed by a subject; this repetition is what enables a subject and constitutes the temporal condition for the subject" (Butler, 1996 [2011], p. 60). Put simply, the actor is created through acting. Much like Derrida tells us that repetition does not merely *inhabit* the present but *constitutes* it, Butler tells us that the repetition of stylized acts is not merely *an aspect of* an identity, a fundamental characteristic of it, repetition *creates* the identity and even a sense of self-willed subjectivity, which she understands as a retroactive construction, something established *after* or through performance. Acting like a self creates the self retroactively:

> Gender cannot be understood as a role which either expresses or disguises an interior 'self,' whether that 'self' is conceived as sexed or not. As performance which is performative, gender is an 'act,' broadly construed, which constructs the social fiction of its own psychological interiority.
>
> *(Butler, 1990, p. 528)*

The fiction of a certain psychological interiority, the constitution of identity through performance, the instability of the self thereby created, the abiding self as a mere fiction, the 'I' secured only through repetition, the lack of agency and dependence on mimicry—these ideas are presented in the context of philosophical claims, but they are also undeniably psychological portraits.

Previously, I described how deconstruction replaces Husserl's account of perceptual constancy with a constancy attributed to the play of signifiers, the trace, and protowriting. This play allows for a seeming constancy of objects over time, an apparent perceptual and temporal unity without attribution to any actual presence. Butler's understanding of a metaphysics of substance operates by a similar logic, and this has profound implications for how she understands identity. For her, it is not only discourse but also the repetition of behavioral norms, which themselves function like the words of a discourse, that allows for the sense of an abiding identity. In contrast, for Husserl, it is perception that allows us to confer an enduring identity and infer the abiding presence of persons and things, although they appear at different times and places. This includes a person's own self-identity. As Merleau-Ponty (1964) noted, none of this involves an intellectual synthesis requiring mediation by way of language.

But for deconstruction signifiers in one form or another are a prerequisite for the identification of perceptual themes, which, in and of themselves, can have no abiding presence. Empiricism, in contrast, holds that we perceive natural groupings, things that resemble each other in some way, even without names for them. This perceptual affinity inspires a linguistic identification of objects bearing similar properties. Perceptual identification precedes linguistic identification. Butler muddies the issue with her insistence on a process of 'materialization' that does not claim the priority of signifiers. Nevertheless, her argument claims that natural kinds or differences (like sexual dimorphism) are indissociable from them, inseparable from the language used to communicate such differences. They are still required for identification. This, in effect, is what leads to the strange idea that a word like *woman* might signify who knows what and that it need not mean simply an adult human female. The term is no longer grounded, first and foremost, in the evidence that perception provides. The point of this brief digression is simple: Identity grounded in perception as opposed to identity grounded in language and performance renders radically different understandings of self and other.

Peter Pan, as we have already seen, has an affinity with the latter approach. When he fails to perceive just who exactly Wendy is, he whispers to her, "always if you see me forgetting you, just keep on saying 'I'm Wendy,' and then I'll remember" (Barrie, 1911, p. 46). He could not trust the evidence of his senses. To identify Wendy, he needed the repetition of a name. But there are many more such affinities between Butler's Neverland and J. M. Barrie's tale as regards themes like *naming, identities, forgetting, pretending, ecstasy, loss, imagination*, and even *motherhood.*

Barrie's island is a land of identity subversion and instability where not only signifiers must thread together the otherwise disparate moments of disparate selves, performance does as well. Repetitive performance is what makes one believe in the land of make-believe where to pretend is to be. Furthermore, what applies to fictional islands like Neverland applies to Butler's own rhetorical island: "As places cut off from the rest of the world, they all provide a site for reflecting on identity or reinventing the self" (Tatar, 2011, p. 21, f. n. 26). Cut off and unmoored from the demands of biology, Butlerian gender theory offers similar possibilities of reflection and reinvention, yet it never returns to 'the rest of the world,' where sexed bodies are undeniably real regardless of their performances.

Gender as performance or 'performativity' in particular suggests a reading in terms of the eternal youth's penchant for conflating pretend worlds with real ones, whether this manifests as the belief that the drawings of sheep are little different than the animals themselves, as in *The Little Prince*, or as Peter's belief that make-believe and true are exactly the same thing (Barrie, 1911). This penchant for such conflation is precisely what makes Peter different from the other lost boys, who know when they are, or are not, pretending. But make-believe is in fact so real to him that he even grows fat after eating make-believe meals, a possibility that is no less and no more plausible than Butler's ill-defined, quasi-magical 'materialization,' which has an equally perplexing relation to physical bodies. Her fusion of matter with discourse and her displacement of the causal relations between the two through a reworking of the notion of 'effect,' seem to suggest, if not explicitly state, such inexplicable causal relations. The confusion of real and pretend worlds is also why Peter grows enraged when others break out of their make-believe roles. The two worlds must remain one and the same, and to break character is a reminder that they are not. Peter needs to be mirrored in his delusion.

If, for Derrida, to pretend is merely to pretend to pretend, then perhaps a similar conflation is at work. The idea of being immersed in a fiction becomes an intellectually incoherent concept: One is always immersed, or never. Does it even matter? After all, 'always' and 'never' are just another binary to be deconstructed. The line between stage and audience has been erased. Perhaps it is the audience performing for the actors' entertainment. Who knows? When all of the special circumstances and clearly defined social contexts, all of Austin's carefully delineated felicity conditions, have been summarily set aside, the theater collapses. Everything becomes a question of play, performance, and masquerade. We are no longer visitors to Neverland, but its residents. Play, performance, and masquerade are themes that run throughout *The Little Prince* and Kundera's *Life Is Elsewhere* as well. In the latter work, Jaromil creates an imagined world through poetry, where statements are true by virtue of their utterance, but also creates this imagined world through erotic fantasy and masturbation, an act by which he procures the illusion that even virgins like him can have sexual prowess.

Pretending is the acceptance of pretense, and if we accept the pretense of representation that precedes presentation, then we can pretend a world without fault, without truth, and without origin. In effect, we can pretend whatever we wish, because decisive moments in which our pretensions might be put to the test simply never come. They never can.

Derrida's free play, Butler's performativity, and Neverland's make-believe are all made necessary and possible due to a seemingly irreparable loss, a love made hungry, whether it is the loss of a referent, a pre-discursive body, or a mother. Could it be that all of these terms allude to the same or similar loss? Is there not, at the very least, a parallel worth drawing attention to and exploring? In Neverland, Peter Pan makes the rules, and rule number one is that everyone is forbidden to speak of mothers. The deep ambivalence toward mothers is perhaps best evidenced by an episode involving the lost boy named Tootles. Encouraged by Tinkerbell and believing that Wendy was a bird flying overhead, he shot her. Upon realizing that he had shot a girl and not a bird, and a girl who was, or so they thought, coming to take care of them as a mother would, white-faced and distraught, he spoke of a recurring dream: "When ladies used to come to me in dreams, I said, 'Pretty mother, pretty mother.' But when at last she really came, I shot her" (Barrie, 1911, p. 69). This symbolic matricide encapsulates the ambivalence toward mothers, simultaneously desired and refuted, that characterizes Barrie's isle on which 'Mother Wendy,' as she is called, serves as a surrogate mother for not only the other lost boys but also the pirates and redskins as well. It also encapsulates a semantic confusion surrounding the term: No one in Neverland seems to know what the word mother really means. Who or what is a mother? Peter Pan, for whom the word *thimble* means *kiss* and *kiss* means *thimble*, is the most confused of them all.

Wendy's surrogacy is evidence of ambivalence: a need for a mother coupled with a rejection of a mother. A similar ambivalence within deconstruction, as well as Butler's queer theory, is also expressed in both doubling and surrogacy: The primordiality of perception doubled by the primordiality of différance, in the former; the matter of biology doubled by the process of 'materialization' in the latter. From a Jungian perspective, these doublings suggest a troubled relation to the mother archetype. Mother, and therefore matter, is a problem. In a brief passage found in a footnote from *Gender Trouble*, Butler encapsulates the issue in a manner useful for the argument at hand. She (1996 [2011]) writes:

> In Derrida's consideration of the form/matter distinction in *Positions*, he suggests as well that matter must be redoubled, at once as a pole within a binary opposition, and as that which exceeds that binary coupling, as a figure for its nonsystematizability.
>
> Consider Derrida's remark in response to the critic who wants to claim that matter denotes the radical outside to language: "It follows that if, and in the extent to which, matter in this general economy designates, as you said, radical alterity (I will specify: in relation to philosophical oppositions), then what I write can be considered 'materialist.'"[23] For both Derrida and Irigaray, it seems, what is excluded from this binary is also produced by it in the mode of exclusion and has no separable or fully independent existence as an absolute outside.
>
> *(p. 13)*

Matter must be redoubled, we are told. But why? Such production and exclusion of matter, philosophically tenable or not, suggests an ambivalence that merits a psychological reading, one that strengthens the argument I am putting forth here as regards the eternal youth's eternal ambivalence toward mother.

Both the charm and the curse of Neverland are that it forces one to forget everything, almost in the very instance of its occurrence. Its logic, like that of deconstruction, requires erasure, obliteration to achieve oblivion. Its freedom is paid for in memory. It is also paid for in stability and continuity. Without a thread holding past, present, and future together, Peter's "identity remains unstable, for he can freely reinvent himself at any moment, even to the extent of turning into his own adversary (Tatar, 2011, p. 56. f. n. 4). A similar instability requiring endless performance to solidify itself applies to Butler's understanding of identity as well. Iterability and performativity, absent the grounding functions of reference and biology, cannot provide the stability required to live in a world where one is subject to the laws of time and space. Could it be that any understanding of identity that does not first ground itself in something pre-discursive or pre-linguistic is inevitably unstable? Is it perhaps the case that denying continuity, an abiding presence or substance, leads to a dissociated identity? Could dissociative logic lead to dissociated selves and vice versa? Is this logic not the root cause of the belief that psychological interiority is a fiction, that the constitution of identity happens through performance, and that any abiding self is a mere fiction dependent on mimicry?

Jung undoubtedly would have had much to say regarding such questions. Perhaps he would have pointed out that to ground identity in performance is to identify with the persona, the mask that each of us wears, intent on making a desired impression upon others. The persona, on his account, is a "system of relations between the individual consciousness and society, fittingly enough a kind of mask, designed on the one hand to make a definite impression upon others, and, on the other, to conceal the true nature of the individual" (Jung, 1953, p. 192). With admitted hyperbole, he even went so far as to suggest that the persona is exactly what one is *not*, although it may be what oneself and others believe oneself to be. The persona is a bit of a ruse, and if a person identifies too closely with this ruse, it has dire consequences, namely deindividuation, for "the aim of individuation is nothing less than to divest the self of the false wrappings of the persona on the one hand, and of the suggestive power of primordial images on the other" (Jung, 1953, p. 174).

There is a deceptive clarity in the persona's false trappings, and it can act like a barricade against the more shadowy realm of the inner world. After all, the persona is witnessed by others who act like notaries, attesting to the reality of its performance. It is there for all to see. But the barricade cannot last, and reliance on it appears to provoke the suggestive power that Jung alludes to. There is an inverse relationship between identification with the persona and awareness of the psychological powers within. This way of conceiving in terms of inverse relations is typical of Jung's thinking and forms part of his overall theory of the compensatory dynamics forever at play within the psyche. One is always subject to the autonomous forces of the psyche, but their autonomy and potential danger grow to the extent that they are ignored. Independent interior processes grow stronger when disregarded. Small nagging thoughts, brief flutters of emotion, fleeting, and almost imperceptible fantasies gain power when overlooked. As the psychoanalytic adage says, *what you resist persists*. In fact, it *insists* on being recognized. Subliminal initially and reaching consciousness only gradually, although they are capable of simply erupting forth into consciousness, such autonomous forces can often appear as strange, utterly foreign content. Yet the eruption only *seems* precipitous. It may have been slowly gaining strength for years (Jung, 1953). The internal processes may have been simmering long before reaching a sudden boil that manifests by way of symptoms, actions, opinions, affects, fantasies, and dreams that overtake the individual unexpectedly, all of which have symbolic meaning and some of which may have parallels in mythic and religious iconography. Many of these internal processes are also foisted onto the external world by way of projections, which "change the world into the replica of one's own unknown face" (Jung, 1959, p. 9). When one identifies with the mask, the face it covers is nevertheless seen, although not as one's own. It is seen on the faces of the other actors on life's stage.

There is a deep irony in grounding identity in the persona (or performativity) because such an approach only helps a person hide from themselves. It is the antithesis of true self-knowledge.

> The construction of a collectively suitable persona means a formidable concession to the external world, a genuine self-sacrifice which drives the ego straight into identification with the persona, so that people really do exist who believe they are what they pretend to be.
>
> *(Jung, 1953, p. 193)*

Replace the word 'pretend' with 'perform,' and you arrive at a rough approximation of Butler's thesis: To perform is to be. To perform is to bring into being. The subject does not merely act; it is created exclusively through the act. For her, "repetition is not performed by a subject; this repetition is what *enables* [emphasis added] a subject and constitutes the temporal condition for the subject" (Butler, 1996 [2011], p. 60). Repeated performances have an abracadabra-like quality to them. They invoke and conjure as if by incantation. Such is the magical logic of pretending.

From a Jungian perspective, an identity founded on the performative is vulnerable to possession by the contents of the personal and collective unconscious, the suggestive power of primordial images. It invites possession and beckons disaster. As Jung writes,

> *To the degree that the world invites the individual to identify with the mask, he is delivered over to influences from within* [emphasis added]. "High rests on low," says Lao-tzu. An opposite forces its way up from inside; it is exactly as though the unconscious suppressed the ego with the very same power which drew the ego into the persona. *The absence of resistance outwardly against the lure of the persona means a similar weakness inwardly against the influence of the unconscious* [emphasis added].
>
> *(Jung, 1953, p. 194)*

The ego of insufficient strength, an identity unduly fragile, is torn between inner and outer demands, whereas one that is able to mediate the competing demands of inner and outer, of the persona's false wrappings on the one hand, and the suggestive power of images arising from the depths on the other, is able to avoid this fate. Individuation requires one to navigate carefully between Scylla and Charybdis. To do otherwise "means error, aberration, illness" (Jung, 1953, p. 196). It is antithetical to individuation as "the process by which a person becomes a psychological 'in-dividual,' that is, a separate, indivisible unity or 'whole'" (Jung, 1969, p. 275).

Von Franz describes the aforementioned de-individuating tendency specifically as it relates to the eternal youth in terms of unconscious collectivization. The more one believes oneself to be utterly unique, the possessor of an inimitable identity, the more one becomes merely a type, not an individual at all. The person we call a puer aeternus is someone who has succumbed to the suggestive power of the primordial type that goes by this name, he or she is an eternal youth at odds with mother and father in predictable ways.

> Precisely because the puer entertains false pretensions, he becomes collectivized from within, with the result that none of his reactions are really very personal or very special. He becomes a type, the type of the puer aeternus. He becomes an archetype, and if you become that, you are not at all original, not at all yourself and something special, but just an archetype. . . . One can foretell what a puer aeternus will look like and how he will feel. He is merely the archetype of the eternal youth god, and therefore he has all the features of the god: he has a nostalgic longing for death, he thinks of himself as being something special, he is the one sensitive being among all the other tough sheep. He will have a problem with an aggressive, destructive shadow which he will not want to live and generally projects, and so on. There is nothing special whatsoever. The greater the identification with the youthful god, the less individual the person although he himself feels so special.
>
> *(Von Franz, 1970 [2000], p. 121)*

I would add to this description that one can also foretell a good deal of what such a person will think. Intellects, even brilliant ones capable of complex, sophisticated arguments, can be easily co-opted by archetypal imperatives.

In the case of the archetype of the puer aeternus, there is an imperative to discredit prior authority and couch it in the most condemnatory of terms, highlighting its violence and oppression, as well as an imperative to construe that which is given or immutable as not given and changeable. There is an entire mythology at work that, when understood, gives the reader a clue as to how such authors can be read, a means of foretelling what positions they will inevitably take even when no coherent rationale might warrant it. Reading a Butlerian text and looking for the myth within the theory, one can more easily discern the figure of a boogeyman of sorts, a senex monster, seemingly omnipresent, wielding his regulatory fictions and power regimes with an uncanny, almost magical power.

Reading with myth in mind also acts like a pinprick to the inflated rhetoric that can, at times, be intimidating or lead one astray. The hypervigilant reader, intent on tracking Butler's argument, can often be lulled into a hypnotic stupor by the effort of a judicious reading, only to be startled by her abjectly false and risible conclusions, which themselves function as tells or clues that something is at work behind or beneath the argument. Reading through a mythic lens, understanding her as a proxy for a mythic (recurrent, typical) disposition, allows one to acknowledge the literal falsehoods contained within her work while perceiving perennial patterns in veiled forms. The far-fetched conclusions are but instances of an idée fixe, arrived at by way of a pretzel logic: If the desired conclusion is that a binary is fictitious, even one as self-evident as that of female and male, one will create the needed argument. The reasoning mind will simply become the lackey of an unreasoned compulsion. Witnessing this, one is tempted to ask: Just how far will an intellect go, *in extremis*, to avoid acknowledging what is self-evident?

One-sidedness, as we have seen, is symptomatic of the gravitational pull of the archetype. Under its sway, we become unduly reductive, framing our thoughts by way of a *nothing but* attitude. Just as one can see in Derrida's deconstruction this reductive attitude at work, one can witness it in Butler. The former claims that from the moment that there is meaning, there are nothing but signs with "no determined or invariable substratum" (Derrida, 1973, p. 146). The latter claims that gender is mere performance without the substratum of a sexed body, one that might have at least some say in how gender is performed. Or perhaps, in the case of the latter figure, we might say that the substratum of a sexed body is actually the substratum of a body fused with discourse. Either way, the absence of anything truly bedrock that might sustain, but also limit, both play and performance grants the illusion of an infinite freedom, a limitless flight, which also suggests the sort of limitless psychological inflation that, for Jung, left one vulnerable to the suggestive powers of primordial images, or primordial narratives.

## Note

1 Yet the question *What is a woman?* has certainly come to the forefront of both political and academic discussion as I write this. It is the title of an online documentary film directed by Justin Folk (2022) released in 2022 by conservative commentator Matt Walsh. Philosopher Kathleen Stock, whose book *Material Girls* (2021) offers an excellent counterargument to queer theory and gender theory influenced by Butler, resigned from her position as professor of philosophy at the University of Sussex in 2021 under political pressure resulting from her views. That same year, journalist Helen Joyce published her book *Trans: When Ideology Meets Reality*, which was met with significant commercial success. The book addresses this same question and clearly sets out the dramatic cultural and legal implications of the denial of biological sex and its reduction to social construction. The academic Germaine Greer (2015), a major figure in 'second wave' radical feminism, defied a campaign to prevent her from speaking at Cardiff University. She addressed the incident in a 2015 interview with the BBC in which she stated that transgender women (i.e., biological men) are not women, which provoked yet further controversy. Many other instances of the political and academic debate regarding the definition of words like *woman*, including legislative changes regarding the legal definition of terms like *gender*, *gender identity*, and *sex* could be mentioned here, although they are outside the purview of this book.

## References


Austin, J. L. (1975). *How to do things with words*. Oxford University Press.

Barrie, J. M. (1911). *Peter and Wendy*. Charles Scribner's Sons.

BBC. (2015). *Germaine Greer: Transgender women are "not women"—BBC Newsnight* [Video]. YouTube. https://www.youtube.com/watch?v=7B8Q6D4a6TM

Brunskell-Evans, H. (2020). *Transgender body politics*. Spinifex Press.

Butler, J. (1990). Performative acts and gender constitution: An essay in phenomenology and feminist theory. In S. Case (Ed.), *Performing feminisms: Feminist critical theory and theatre*. Johns Hopkins University Press.

Butler, J. (1990 [2007]). *Gender trouble: Feminism and the subversion of identity*. Routledge.

Butler, J. (1996 [2011]). *Bodies that matter: On the discursive limits of sex*. Routledge.

Butler, J. (1997). *Excitable speech: A politics of the performative*. Routledge.

Carroll, L. (1981). *Alice's adventures in wonderland & through the looking-glass*. Bantam Classics.

Derrida, J. (1967 [1978]). *Writing and difference* (A. Bass, Trans.). University of Chicago Press.

Derrida, J. (1973). *Speech and phenomena, and other essays on Husserl's theory of signs*. Northwestern University Press.

Derrida, J. (1988). *Limited Inc* (A. Bass & S. Weber, Trans.). Northwestern University Press.

Derrida, J. (2002). *Without alibi* (P. Kamuf, Trans. & Ed.). Stanford University Press.

Folk, J. (Director). (2022). *What is a woman* [Online Documentary]. The Daily Wire.

Joyce, H. (2021). *Trans: When ideology meets reality*. Oneworld Publications.

Jung, C. G. (1953). Two essays on analytical psychology. In *The collected works of C. G. Jung* (Vol. 7, R. F. C. Hull, Trans.). Princeton University Press.

Jung, C. G. (1959). Aion: Researches into the phenomenology of the self. In *The collected works of C. G. Jung* (Vol. 9.2, R. F. C. Hull, Trans.). Princeton University Press.

Jung, C. G. (1969). The archetypes and the collective unconscious. In *The collected works of C. G. Jung* (Vol. 9.1, R. F. C. Hull, Trans.). Princeton University Press.

Lamont, M. (1987). How to become a dominant French philosopher: The case of Jacques Derrida. *American Journal of Sociology*, *93*(3), 584–622. https://doi.org/10.1086/228790

Lawford-Smith, H. (2022). *Gender-critical feminism*. Oxford University Press.

Merleau-Ponty, M. (1964). *The primacy of perception: And other essays on phenomenological psychology, the philosophy of art, history, and politics* (J. M. Edie, Trans.). Northwestern University Press.

Miller, J. H. (2007). Performativity as performance/performativity as speech act: Derrida's special theory of performativity. *South Atlantic Quarterly*, *106*(2), 219–235. https://doi.org/10.1215/00382876-2006-022

Nietzsche, F. (1978). *Thus spoke Zarathustra: A book for none and all* (W. Kaufmann, Trans.). Penguin Books. (Original work published in four volumes between 1883 and 1885)

Stock, K. (2021). *Material girls: Why reality matters for feminism*. Fleet.

Sullivan, N. (2003). *A critical introduction to queer theory*. NYU Press.

Tatar, M. (2011). *The annotated Peter Pan*. W.W. Norton & Company.

Von Franz, M. L. (1970 [2000]). *The problem of the puer aeternus* (3rd ed.). Inner City Books.

# 7

# KAIROS & EROS

## Time and Desire

### I

Envisioned as myth and returned to their experiential ground, the conceptual underpinnings of deconstruction speak to a fundamental human dilemma—that of entering time and space completely, which is what Peter Pan cannot do. Such an entrance forces us to acknowledge our mortal limits. Because Chronos represents our entry into the temporal aspect of existence, he also represents the humanization that this entry implies. This humanization requires a certain reconciliation to his brutality and a relinquishment of the *not yet* that holds us back from the deeper suffering of human experience. Puer-et-senex dynamics offer much to meditate upon regarding Jung's distinction between neurotic and authentic suffering: When split, these figures speak in mythic terms of the very avoidance of the "suffering necessary to come into being—necessary for innocence to gain experience" (Kalsched, 2013, p. 20). When in the grips of such avoidance, the eternal youth would rather stay in Neverland, which is to say, the flying youth would rather never land. He would rather never allow transcendent potential to become immanent manifestation, never allow it to be sullied by tangible incarnation in the here and now. He is, after all, "the best, the highest, the most precious *in potentia*" (Jung, 1970, p. 166) and landing, becoming earthly, subject to time's passing, which is to say, subject to the authority of Chronos, entails a painful loss of both potential and omnipotence.

It is worth noting here the deeper meaning of the word *human* that has been bequeathed to us by our own linguistic tradition. Etymologically, the word is related to the Latin *humus*, meaning earth or soil. Our species name is rooted in the earth. Furthermore, to land, to come down from the heights of exuberant flight, is often experienced as a *humbling*, and this word too is rooted in that same *humus*. To be humbled is to come back down to earth, yet this is what is most difficult for the

DOI: 10.4324/b23321-8

eternal youth. He suffers the fall of Icarus or Phaeton. Like the winged Tinkerbell or Hermes, he always prefers flight. The former figures fail to acknowledge limitation, flying too high or too low, dismissing the cautionary voices of Daedalus and Phoebus, respectively, and they crash as a consequence. Translated from the idiom of myth to that of philosophy, we might say that they deny a 'determined or invariable substratum,' for this is exactly what the earth is: a substratum, an underlying support. They deny a 'center or absolute anchorage' to use a Derridean phrasing; they deny any ground. Like Butler, they dismiss such warnings as mere 'empiricist foundationalism' never fully understanding the importance of empiricism or foundations.

Ultimately, such a painful loss of potential and childlike omnipotence is also an acknowledgment of mortality. Time, for all of us, runs out. It puts an end to our limitless deferral. Chronos eats his children. Time clips Cupid's wings. None of us *can* be all that we *could* be. This is simply the nature of being. This is a given—the bitter lesson of finitude. Yet the loss of potential and omnipotence and the acknowledgment of mortality is also what is needed to become *actual*—in the dual sense that cognates of this word profess in other languages, the dual sense of being both real and present. But, as Von Franz (1970 [2000]) notes,

> if you give yourself to reality, you will be disillusioned and the end of it will be that you will meet death. If you accept life, you really, in the deepest sense of the word, accept death, and that is what the *puer* does not want.
>
> *(p. 156)*

Gilead (1991) pierces the heart of this dilemma when she tells us that the "true paradox of the 'never' in Neverland is in its double meaning of stark denial—on the one hand, the refusal of the self to conceive of its own end and, on the other, the absolute reality of death" (p. 286). The true paradox of 'never,' as regards deconstruction, is in its own duplicitous denial—on the one hand, the refusal to conceive of words arriving at a transcendental signified and, on the other, the absolute reality that they must do so, lest language, and life, be meaningless.

Somehow, we are again faced with the question of the magic portal, which is also the question of the finite and the infinite, the temporal and the eternal. All children visit the land of never, but only some return. Wendy and her brothers do. Peter does not, nor do Derrida and Butler. The eternal youth, when split from father time, is the one who refuses to cross the threshold back into the fraudulent realm of adults (Yeoman, 1998 [1999]). Or, perhaps, as long as he does not cross this threshold, the realm of adults remains fraudulent. Its authority remains arbitrary, as arbitrary as we are told is the relationship between signifier and signified, or the discipline of biology and the material bodies it names. So, he suspends earthly manifestation, finding countless pretexts and quasi-logical arguments to do so, often of stunning complexity and virtuosity. He never fully enters life but remains locked in a crypt—and is therefore cryptic: One guesses at his intent as one marvels at the shear genius and audacity of his sophistry, itself required by his inability to address life directly. He can only reference it indirectly. It can only be "life" in quotations, a *Lebenswelt* rendered purely textual, or a biology—the logos of life—reduced to the power regimes of masculine and heterosexist oppression. With cunning obliquity, he eschews restriction and limitation. Being bound, being pinned down, circumscribed, and constrained threatens his grandiosity, and through the prism of this threat he perceives the absolute corruption of convention, orthodoxy, authority, and all commonly held assumptions.

The eternal youth, if he remains eternal and does not cross back through the portal, remains within one variation of the schizoid withdrawal, a peculiar compromise at the core of his problematic (Kalsched, 2013). This compromise allows one to never be quite here or quite there, never fully present or fully absent, never entirely alone or entirely with others (Guntrip, 1992). In a similar vein, Derrida can claim that language never quite reaches the transcendental signified, yet it somehow does so, just enough, for him to make the point that it does not. The typological conventions of quotation marks, italics, parenthesis, and the crossing-out of terms are further illustrations of this compromise; the doublespeak of *sous rature* allows him to refer without referring, and mean without meaning, thus fulfilling the dueling imperatives of pothos, the double bind of an impossible desire. Deconstruction attempts to erase the metaphysical, and therefore senescent, connotations of the terms it uses. "Truth" must become "~~truth.~~" Yet its functional denotation must remain. Many terms of art that serve as infrastructure for the deconstructive project—différance, hymen, pharmakon, arche-trace, supplement, etc. are, on Derrida's account, not concepts at all but attempts to undermine the binary logic of the conceptual. Perhaps he is right that they are not concepts. Perhaps they are mere symptoms of the need to be neither here nor there, neither with someone nor without.

Derrida (1973) claimed that "différance is neither a word nor a concept" (p. 130). It cannot be otherwise as long as the archetype is split, as long as one is within the archetypal syndrome that Hillman describes. If one were to acknowledge that différance is, in fact, both a word and a concept, it would enter space and time in a way that would corrupt it; it would be of a particular place and a particular moment. It would not be utterly transcendent—beyond time and space—but in some sense immanent—within time and space. Then it would exist within a historical record. It would be subject to the same sort of genealogical approach that ostensibly strips words of the pretense of being given by the nature of things. It would be merely an earthly manifestation, not dropped from the sky, just a word, coined by a particular thinker at a particular historical moment, in a particular cultural milieu. Then, "the subterranean operation of transcendental *différance*" (Caputo, 1987, p. 145) would be rendered immanent, mundane, and the particular method by which Derrida "interrogates entrenched authority, the established powers that be, that pretend to be, that pretend to be present" (Caputo, 1987, p. 145) would be called into question—as itself an entrenched authority, as an established power pretending to be present. If différance is, in fact, both a word and a concept, then the metaphysics of presence—the senex worldview with all of its traditions, laws, orthodoxy, and authority—would be validated.

If différance were understood as both a word and a concept, then some semblance of identity between signifier and signified, words and their meanings would have to be acknowledged. The coherency of the concept of the *sign*—that most metaphysical of notions (Derrida, 2007)—would have to be conceded. The necessity of Aristotle's *hama* (togetherness and simultaneity), and his circular, uroboric logic would have to be acknowledged. If this were to happen, then the fault attributed to the reigning metaphysics of presence would be revealed as a dubious one, and Derrida's critique would lose its revolutionary and messianic allure. It would be exposed in all of its puerile grandiosity. The pretension implicit in attempting a radical upheaval of *all* received ideas would collapse. As Bates (2005) has noted, the repeated flaws that Derrida diagnosed as central to Western thought are in part the result of his own penchant for repeatedly analyzing a relatively small number of classic philosophical texts. He was simply unaware of the philosophic traditions that addressed, and did not necessarily repeat, the flaws that he discerned.

If différance were understood as both a word and a concept, then the inflationary attitude of deconstruction and the correlate *negative* inflation of logocentrism—its compensatory bête noire and boogeyman—would both lose their affective charge. The belief that "time is out of joint" (Derrida & Kamuf, 1994 [2011], p. 20) as Hamlet claimed after visitation by his father's ghost, would be revealed as fallacious: It is not time that is out of joint, but the eternal youth's relationship to it. This is why, like Hamlet, he is riddled with indecision. When split from his senex self, a temporal lacuna exists where *the now* once was. Through the distorting prism of this lost moment, he perceives an abyssal rupture between time and eternity, but also signifier and signified, words and their meaning.

If différance were understood as both word and concept, then its errant logic, and the logic of the trace, could be clearly seen as a desire for something absent, something that is elsewhere. Derrida (1967 [1978]) tells us that "the trace is the erasure of selfhood, of one's own presence, and is constituted by the threat of anguish of its irremediable disappearance, of the disappearance of its disappearance" (p. 230). Could it be that all these disappearances in response to the threat of anguish are variants of the schizoid withdrawal, the strategy of disincarnation that forecloses the entrance into time and space reality? This erasure is "death itself" (p. 230), Derrida (1967 [1978]) tells us. But what kind? Is it one that comes to all of us, or a preemptive death that simply serves to evade life? And is this not the pothos that Plato refers to in Cratylus, the unfulfilled nature of which suggests death or a mourning so intense as to cause it? (Dollimore, 1998)

It is through the acknowledgment that différance is both a word and a concept that healing begins. It is an acknowledgment of the secret identity of puer-et-senex. When the archetype is internally divided, each fragment of the whole conceives itself by means of excluding its opposite. But perceiving identity at the heart of difference helps rejoin the two halves of an original whole, that of the eternal youth and father time, but also that of the manifest, formal, historically contingent aspect of différance—différance as signifier, as a word seen on a page, différance in its time-bound quality—and the ever transcendent, seemingly eternal aspect of différance as signified, as what it means. Without an acknowledgment of the identity of these two aspects of the sign, and of the archetype "eventually meaning declines into a philosophy of the absurd" (Hillman & Slater, 2005, p. 55).

Moving beyond such an absurdity involves, among other things, an acceptance of the more senex qualities of language, an acknowledgment that signs are not so slippery as we are led to believe. There is a certain fixity to them as well, a stubborn, leaden quality that seems to reside in something bedrock and speaks to cold hard facts that clash with dreams of infinite malleability. This allows for communication that need not last forever and always be called into question. Meaning requires that puerile instability be balanced by senex fixity. The two require one another, both philosophically and psychologically speaking. When the rationality of received ideas becomes reductive, unaware of its own limitations, puer rises to the challenge of pointing out those limitations and breaking through them. As Hillman (2005) notes

> The puer aspect of meaning is in the search, as the dynamus of the child's eternal 'why?', the quest, or questioning, seeking, adventuring, which grips personality from behind and compels it forward. All things are uncertain, provisional, subject to question, thereby opening the way and leading the soul toward further questioning."
>
> *(pp. 54–55)*

The quest is necessary, inevitable, and forms an essential part of what it means to be human but if "meaning expresses the invisible coincidence of the positive puer with the positive senex" (Hillman & Slater, 2005, p. 54), then the uncertain, provisional, and questionable require a sense of the unquestionable, settled, and certain.

So much in deconstruction becomes clear once we see within it a strategic desire or need to maintain this inner cleavage. If we are aware of the myth at work, it becomes evident that the archetypal imperative *requires* that texts be more indeterminate than they actually are, and that ethics must be more undecidable than necessary. From within the archetypal syndrome, seen through the eyes of the illness, such fundamental principles and philosophic universals as *essence* or *existence*, *consciousness* or *God*—the very principles that deconstruction aims to dismantle—appear to be mere *nomina*, mere names without substance, little more than the effects of a ubiquitous semiotic deferral. Yet the word that names this deferral is spared this same reduction. The *other* principles must be understood as constructs with scant reality beyond their (social, cultural) construction, mere names or designations, but this cannot be the case for différance, if we accept the premise that it is not a word at all. The *other* principles are assumptions, and prejudicial ones at that, accretions of a historical process that, by virtue of being historical, cannot speak to something that transcends history. Their deconstruction is an emancipating endeavor, a liberation from the violence of logocentrism (Derrida, 1976) or the regulatory fictions of an oppressive power regime (Butler, 1990 [2007]), both of which serve as philosophical stand-ins for the harsh imposition of an arbitrary senex authority.

Yet returning ideas to their complex roots allows for a revisioning of the primary tenets of deconstruction that casts them in a radically different light. From within the archetypal syndrome, the here and now—both presence and the present—warrant no privilege. Any metaphysic that construes otherwise suffers from an objectionable bias, one that is of enormous consequence because it establishes the conditions for all other privileging within the metaphysic in question. The exhaustive unraveling of metaphysical binaries that deconstruction attempts rests on the grounds of the ostensibly unwarranted privilege of presence. From within the syndrome, it can be asked: "Has not the entire history of philosophy been authorized by the 'extraordinary right' of the present?" (Derrida, 1982 [1986], p. 38), but it cannot be fully acknowledged that the extraordinariness of this right is warranted.

Yet seen from a perspective less beholden to archetypal machinations, it becomes self-evident that "the always-already present is the condition for *differance* [even] being thinkable" (Wood, 2001, p. 275). This fact is an embarrassing scandal no less scandalous than any and all of the aporias that deconstruction claims to elucidate. Furthermore, and more relevant for the work at hand, the seeming lack of warrant in this privileging of presence is merely the result of inhabiting the viewpoint of the eternal. From within the mythic perspective of eternal youth, to privilege one moment over another must be unjustified because this perspective is, precisely, that of eternity: Apprehended *sub specie aeternitatis*, all moments *are* equally determinant, all moments *do* have equal merit, and to privilege the present is "a matter of accidental perspective, a kind of unwarranted 'temporocentrism'" (Dillon, 1992, p. 207). The distinct prerogative of the present—the very prerogative that determines *being as presence*—is gratuitous. Presence can be accorded no priority over absence, and the *now* can be granted no value greater than the *yet to come*. All moments are essentially the same for the eternal youth when he is split from senex temporality. Yet seen from a perspective less enthralled by mythic conflict, the specious privilege of the present is specious because the archetype is split. Fictive immediacy is fictive because the now moment, in which time and eternity might be reconciled, remains estranged from itself, internally divided.

Yet if we allow for the senex perspective of time's unfolding without relinquishing puer's foothold in the eternal, what becomes evident is the absolute necessity of the vantage point of the present (Dillon, 1992). One cannot live any other moment in time. When the two poles of the archetype are reconciled, it is revealed that the bias toward presence is not so much bias as it is the expression of a primal experiential nexus: One is always already here, now. One cannot be in any other moment in time than the present. Its claim on us is unavoidable. This fact is faithfully reflected in a metaphysic that has been unduly chided for its privileging rather than extolled for this essential insight. The insight is twofold: First, it perceives that the nature of time's unfolding itself confines us to the present moment; the peculiar relation of incarnate human beings to time is that we can be nowhere else other than here, now. In this sense, there is always something truly special about the present. Second, it accurately perceives that it is only under the auspices of this moment that we can speak with an urgency that compels meaning. If we lose sight of it completely or are unable to return to it, all meaning is lost. What this insight alludes to is the essential relationship between meaning and presence. It is not différance that generates meaning, but the experience of being truly here, now.

Unsurprisingly, the eternal youth's liberation from hesitation, withholding, and indecision is through an embrace of the present, which is deconstruction's *lost moment*. Indeed, the hallmark of the positive puer, which is to say, the puer who is not split from his senex half, is his ability to live in the now, with all the *joi de vivre* of youth. The name for this youth within the Greek tradition is Kairos.

A deity depicted as a young man running tiptoed, with a single tuft of hair adorning his forehead, the winged figure that is Kairos, the rebellious grandson of none other than Chronos himself, represents the fleeting moment that is grasped, that is seized upon. Kairos is the mythic expression of the evanescent opportunity, the propitious moment that is recognized, not as something that has yet to happen, not as something that has always already passed, but as a moment that is present, recognized in its presence, and acted upon. As opportune moment, Kairos is the instant of undeniable immediacy. This divine youth is, in a sense, the mytheme of perceptual immediacy, and fittingly so: Such are opportune moments—they possess sufficient perceptual strength to press themselves upon us, at times with the force of revelation. Through Kairos one knows that the moment is now. The time has come. One makes the decision and takes the action. This is Kierkegaard's *leap*, what he called *the instant*, the point of contact between time and eternity.

Not the god of measurable, linear sequence with its demarcation of discrete units of definitive endings and beginnings, Kairos is, rather, the interruption of this sequence. It is also, simultaneously, the moment of the eternal youth's emancipation from Neverland. Yet, as the co-incidence of time with eternity, Kairos names the point of not only an interruption but also a conjunction. As interruption, it names the opportune moment of a breakthrough of the eternal into history (Tillich & Braaten, 1972). As conjunction, it is the fulfillment of both the temporal and the eternal (Mills, 2014), their rapprochement in the reconciling moment of the now—a moment that passes yet exists forever and always. Whereas previously time and eternity appeared absolute in their mutual otherness, by way of Kairos this otherness is resolved.

Most importantly for the present discussion, Kairos names the very moment that deconstruction attempts to render mute, the moment that Husserl's phenomenology rests its claims of veracity upon, the moment of "the presence of sense to a full and primordial intuition" (Derrida, 1973, p. 5). Insofar as Kairos represents the presence and instant of the now, it is also, according to Derrida, the moment that simply never comes, and cannot come, for it names the very possibility of self-presence that he repudiates (Agamben, 2005). It names the moment, or the aspect of each moment, that resides in the pure primordial perception, the full and simple presence that Husserl affirmed (Van Manen, 2017), the selfsame now moment that deconstruction displaces, defers, and delays forever and always. The moment of meaning in its plenitude, one of phenomenological insight, Kairos is the instant, or the aspect of each instant, in which the perceived world speaks with sufficient clarity and force as to compel a sense of meaning. In deconstructive terms, it is the name of an experience that is not indebted to an act of representation, or perhaps that aspect of each experience that is not so indebted. Kairos is the moment of meaning compelled and the compelling aspect of all moments, the moment of privilege and the aspect of each moment that is privileging.

In the presence of Kairos, the amniotic/semiotic sack that separates puer from the phenomenal world is torn asunder, so that reality is no longer once removed and held at a distance. Kairos is not the boy in a bubble, but the boy for whom the bubble has burst. In his presence, no longer does everything have to remain in the world of mental activity, in the realm of linguistic signs. Kairos is the image of a youth that no longer thinks his way out of immediacy and no longer suffers from nostalgia, which always "arises from a separation of halves, a missing conjunction" (Hillman, 1975, p. 52). Now, for him, unlike before, perception and affect can act as arbiters of belief, or exist as realities in their own right. Deferral is no longer his default. There is no pensive pondering, and therefore no reduction of perception to conception.

Kairos as opportune moment is also a moment of healing (Dohe, 2016), a historical moment into which eternity erupts and, in so doing, transforms the world or the individual. For existential therapists, Kairos was understood as the precise moment in which a decisive therapeutic intervention is called for (Ellenberger, 1970, p. 22). As such, it has affinities with Jung's belief that the healing powers of the psyche only appear when the patient is ready to be healed. It is only then that the unconscious produces the reconciling symbol to resolve the neurotic conflict (Dohe, 2016).

## II

When we first moved this discussion of ideas from the realm of thought to the realm of psyche and began to discern the myth at work within the theory, we explored the question of eros in its particular incarnation as pothos, drawing surprising parallels with the differing and deferring at work within sign systems. This was a first step in making the seemingly implausible case that deconstruction is not merely a doctrine or a technique but also an attitude, a disposition, a style of consciousness, one characteristic of youth, but more importantly a desire to remain too young for too long. So here, in evoking Kairos as the moment of therapeutic intervention, it is only fitting to acknowledge that the deferring desire of pothos is not love's only logic: Eros in its full complexity is not merely a desire for the absent and elsewhere; personifications of polymorphic amour are multiple because love has many guises. Within the Greek pantheon, there are three aspects of eros that have been classically distinguished: himeros, anteros, and pothos (Hillman & Moore, 1990).

In contrast to a love for what is absent, himeros is a love for what is present (Davidson, 2007 [2009]). It is love in all of its urgency, *imminent* love, in a dual sense that speaks both to the proximity of the loved one and to the threatening, menacing, impending quality of the desire itself. A seemingly foreign force that possesses one as if from the outside, it demands immediate fulfillment, at times, even at the expense of the desired subject, for the impetuous, possessive urgency of himeros can be so great as to inspire assault or attack. It seizes and possesses by force (Davidson, 2007 [2009]). Often sexual (Verstraete & Provencal, 2014), it is paroxysmal and convulsive by nature.

Anteros, in turn, is requited, reciprocated love. Literally transcribed, it means 'backlove,' love returned in kind by the beloved (Peirce, 2009). In contrast to the blind possessive urges of himeros, it has a reciprocal quality to it, and as such, it is a love both given and received, a love in which the beloved loves and the desired desires in turn. The current of anteros moves both to and fro, between lover and beloved. In this regard, it might also be understood as a reversible love in which the two people involved are both lovers and beloveds simultaneously. Because it suggests consummation, if not physical, then spiritual, this god of reciprocal affection is perhaps most dissimilar to pothos (Brumble, 1998). It is also most dissimilar to the false love that De Rougemont (1963) called passion or chivalric love because, on his account, "all true love is a reciprocal relation" (p. 160). As with the urgent immediacy of himeros, the requited nature of anteros suggests both a spatial and temporal proximity.

If presence is the funeral pyre of pothos, then one achieves presence when the desire for the absent and elsewhere dies, when it is either exhausted by the futility of its search or, conversely, when it is satiated, having encountered the object of its longing. Such a desire finds fulfillment only when, and if, the elsewhere becomes a here, when eternal longing meets temporal gratification. Then again, if one imagines pothos as the eternally renascent aspect of desire—for it will surely be born again, even from the ashes of its own pyric end—one might see presence not as the demise of this form of eros, but rather as evidence of a more fully developed eroticism. Just as Diotima concludes in Plato's Symposium that eros is the name given to the desire and pursuit of the whole (Plato, 1999 [2003]), in a similar vein, the erotic trinity of pothos, himeros, and anteros is desire in its wholeness.

But there are many possible ways of conceiving the issue, and the ancient Greeks differed in their responses to it, at times seeing pothos not as an aspect of eros at all but rather as something quite distinct. Tim Whitmarsh, in *Narrative Identity in the Ancient Greek Novel* (2011), contrasts philosophical and romantic views of the ideal relationship to pothos, noting that both, despite differences, were in basic agreement that pothos should be eliminated in order to attain happiness. The more philosophical view, which included that of the Stoics and Epicureans, sought to annul pothos through contemplation and self-sufficiency. In general, it is "treated from as early as Aristotle as a pathological mental state to be corrected by philosophical reflection" (Whitmarsh, 2011, p. 143). It was believed to have, inevitably, devastating effects on its subject.

The more romantic, narrative view, perhaps best epitomized in Homer's *Odyssey*, was far more ambivalent, in recognition of the fact that every plot of every great adventure required pothos. Without it, no plot is even possible: Odysseus neither leaves home nor yearns to return. Desire for what is far off and not yet attained is the *sine qua non* of every great adventure, the impetus to undertake every journey. Yet, in a similar vein, this desire's eventual satisfaction or demise is *required* to bring the story to an end. Without travel and travail, distance and discord, there is no romance. Without pothos, there is no great adventure or journey, yet if this is the only form of desire, and its supply is infinite, then there is no adventure at all because an endless plot is not a plot at all.

Whereas the philosophic approach was broadly pothophobic (Whitmarsh, 2011), attempting to bypass this desire as much as possible, the romantic view allowed for its necessity, while also acknowledging that it required limits. Only tragic consequences resulted for the heroes and heroines that did not heed them. As regards this dangerous desire, Whitmarsh (2011) notes that "in romance, the travels are the location for what Derrida would call difference: A deviation, both temporal and spatial, from the linearity that constitutes identity (in the root sense of sameness)" (p. 20). The present work suggests that there is a great deal of this tragic heroism in the deconstructive approach. Yet, like the romantic view that allows for the necessity of pothos, it recognizes that such a desire for the elsewhere cannot be eliminated. Without it, there is no adventure and therefore no evolution of understanding. But when it has no limits, or when it is the exclusive form of our desire or love, tragedy is at hand.

The tradition that Derrida has designated as the metaphysics of presence—one that is apparently encompassing of the entirety of Western thought—both in its clearly philosophic form and the more narrative (i.e., romantic, mythic) form is one that was in many regards deeply suspicious of certain forms of desire and well aware of their potential for destruction. This tradition is one in which, in many regards, desire is looked askance and oft understood as antithetical to happiness: Stoics, Epicureans, Aristotelians, and Greek romancers all developed their own complex vocabulary and ethics for discerning desire's benevolence and malevolence.

What Whitmarsh's reflections on pothos suggest to me is that, from the perspective of much of ancient Greek thought, both Derrida and Butler would have been considered dilettantes of desire, neither capable of putting forth functional, pragmatic philosophies nor telling coherent stories. They appear to understand little of desire's complexity or potential for destruction. Their eros is unidimensional, always directed elsewhere, and knows no limits. The latter point is critical and suggests possession by a particular archetypal narrative. Perhaps they have simply not mastered the art of quelling desire, or at the least, they have privileged one form of desire at the expense of all others. They understand little of the complexity of eros. Imagined from the perspective of the mythic and philosophic tradition that they themselves have inherited, they suffer from an errant desire. Enamored of a world of pure play or pure performance, ignorant of the demands of real life, they are fixated upon imagined villains with daunting names, 'logocentric' prejudices, and vile 'normativities.' This allows them to postpone the most obvious and self-evident conclusions, postpone confrontation with what is immediately *present*, in the dual sense of the word: that which is here and now, but also that which has been *gifted* by the past.

Hillman suggests that, at least in the West, we were once closer to a less fractured eros. Before Tristan, himself a figure of eternally unrequited love, in Greek antiquity *pothos* and *himeros* were not so divided from each other, though later, in the Renaissance, "Neoplatonists tried to restore the original interrelation between *pothos* and *himeros* and not fall prey to the Tristan complex of medieval man" (Hillman, 1997, p. 100, f. n. 122). Restoring this original interrelation, on his account, is a means of healing the puer-et-senex split and returning it to its original wholeness. The difficulty is that this complex, "refuses himeros and anteros in order to maintain the transcendence of pothos" (Hillman, 1975, p. 54), just as deconstruction strains credulity and logic to maintain the utter transcendence of the signified. To overcome this refusal is to heal an archetypal syndrome and enact an "archetypal therapy or therapy of an archetype" (Hillman & Slater, 2005, p. 36), which is what the present work itself is an attempt to do.

Just as the deferred desire of pothos is not love's only logic, différance is not the only logic of language. If the pothos that informs semiotic deferral requires that "the thing itself always escapes" (Derrida, 1973, p. 104), then the logic of himeros suggests that sometimes it does not: Language has the ability to grasp, possess, and conquer its object, albeit never fully. It does, in fact, reach that ostensibly mythical, mystical thing in itself 'outside' of language. Anteros, in turn, suggests that there is a reciprocal relationship between language and its other; The two fold back upon each other and mutually entwine as lovers do. Two become one as they possess one another. This is true because the logos of language is not merely one of eternal erotic longing, it is also one of erotic bonds. When signifier and signified no longer couple, bonds are broken and both life and language lose meaning.

Hillman's reading suggests that recognizing this complexity of eros forms part of the curative salve that heals the shared antipathy of senex and puer. This antipathy blinds them to their secret collusion, the identity at the heart of their differences. This antipathy, following the associative logic of the archetype, is one that extends to oppositional pairings like orthodoxy and heterodoxy, tradition and innovation, solidity and fluidity, consistency and capriciousness, nature and culture, entrenched order and its overthrow. It is manifest in the fierce holding to doctrines and dogmas and the blind defense of tradition, but also in the naive belief that the present is wiser than the past and that the future might be constructed upon fundamentally new ground. His reading also suggests that the two can flip at any moment. They can undergo what Jung often called an enantiodromia: a process by which something turns into its opposite. Thus, the revolution solidifies into a despotic regime, the liberatory impulse calcifies into a new rigidity, and the deconstruction of oppressive binaries manifests in its own no less oppressive binaries.

## References


Agamben, G. (2005). *The time that remains: A commentary on the letter to the Romans* (P. Dailey, Trans.). Stanford University Press. (Original work published 2000)

Bates, D. (2005). Crisis between the wars: Derrida and the origins of undecidability. *Representations, 90*(1), 1–27. https://doi.org/10.1525/rep.2005.90.1.1

Brumble, H. D. (1998). *Classical myths and legends in the middle ages and renaissance: A dictionary of allegorical meanings*. Fitzroy Dearborn Publishers.

Butler, J. (1990 [2007]). *Gender trouble: Feminism and the subversion of identity*. Routledge.

Caputo, J. D. (1987). *Radical hermeneutics: Repetition, deconstruction, and the hermeneutic project*. Indiana University Press.

Davidson, J. N. (2007 [2009]). *The Greeks and Greek love: A bold new exploration of the ancient world*. Random House.

De Rougemont, D. (1963). *Love declared: Essays on the myths of love*. Pantheon Books.

Derrida, J. (1967 [1978]). *Writing and difference* (A. Bass, Trans.). University of Chicago Press.

Derrida, J. (1973). *Speech and phenomena, and other essays on Husserl's theory of signs*. Northwestern University Press.

Derrida, J. (1976). *Of grammatology* (G. C. Spivak, Trans.). Johns Hopkins University Press. (Original work published 1967)

Derrida, J. (1982 [1986]). *Margins of philosophy* (A. Bass, Trans.). University of Chicago Press.

Derrida, J. (2007). Structure, sign, and play in the discourse of the human sciences. In R. Macksey & E. Donato (Eds.), *The structuralist controversy: The languages of criticism and the sciences of man* (pp. 247–265). Johns Hopkins University Press.

Derrida, J., & Kamuf, P. (1994 [2011]). *Specters of Marx: The state of the debt, the work of mourning, and the new international* (P. Kamuf, Trans.). Routledge. (Original work published 1993)

Dillon, M. C. (1992). Temporality: Merleau-Ponty and Derrida. In T. W. Busch & S. Gallagher (Eds.), *Merleau-Ponty, hermeneutics, and postmodernism* (pp. 189–212). State University of New York Press.

Dohe, C. A. (2016). *Jung's wandering archetype: Race and religion in analytical psychology*. Routledge.

Dollimore, J. (1998). *Death, desire, and loss in western culture*. Routledge.

Ellenberger, H. F. (1970). *The discovery of the unconscious: The history and evolution of dynamic psychiatry*. Basic Books.

Gilead, S. (1991). Magic abjured: Closure in children's fantasy fiction. *PMLA, 106*(2), 277–293. https://doi.org/10.2307/462663

Guntrip, H. (1992). *Schizoid phenomena, object relations and the self*. Karnac Books.

Hillman, J. (1975). *Loose ends: Primary papers in archetypal psychology*. Spring Publications.

Hillman, J. (1997). *The myth of analysis: Three essays in archetypal psychology*. Northwestern University Press.
Hillman, J., & Moore, T. (1990). *The essential James Hillman: A blue fire*. Routledge.
Hillman, J., & Slater, G. (2005). *Senex & puer*. Spring Publications.
Jung, C. G. (1970). Mysterium coniunctionis: An inquiry into the separation and synthesis of psychic opposites in alchemy. In *The collected works of C. G. Jung* (Vol. 14, 2nd ed., R. F. C. Hull, Trans.). Princeton University Press.
Kalsched, D. (2013). *Trauma and the soul: A psycho-spiritual approach to human development and its interruption*. Routledge.
Mills, C. (2014). *The philosophy of Agamben*. Routledge. (Original work published 1945)
Peirce, C. (2009). *Writings of Charles S. Peirce: A chronological edition, volume 8: 1890–1892*. Indiana University Press.
Plato. (1999 [2003]). *The symposium* (C. Gill, Trans.). Penguin Books. (Original work published c. 385–370 BC)
Tillich, P., & Braaten, C. E. (1972). *A history of Christian thought, from its Judaic and Hellenistic origins to existentialism*. Simon & Schuster.
Van Manen, M. (2017). Phenomenology in its original sense. *Qualitative Health Research*, *27*(6), 810–825. https://doi.org/10.1177/10497323176993
Verstraete, B. C., & Provencal, V. L. (2014). *Same-sex desire and love in Greco-Roman antiquity and in the classical tradition of the West*. Routledge.
Von Franz, M. L. (1970 [2000]). *The problem of the puer aeternus* (3rd ed.). Inner City Books.
Whitmarsh, T. (2011). *Narrative and identity in the ancient Greek novel: Returning romance*. Cambridge University Press.
Wood, D. (2001). *The deconstruction of time*. Northwestern University Press.
Yeoman, A. (1998 [1999]). *Now or Neverland: Peter Pan and the myth of eternal youth: A psychological perspective on a cultural icon*. Inner City Books.

# 8

# THE SERPENTINE CIRCLE AS IMAGE OF WHOLENESS

We find ourselves at a Kairos moment within the present work. The opposites personified by Husserl and Derrida have been constellated and a synthesis is needed. Now is the moment for a therapeutic intervention. The neurotic conflict under discussion, the puerile dissociation of language from primordial mother and temporal father, is ready to be healed. The Kairos is now, and the reconciling symbol goes by the name of *uroboros*, the self-consuming and self-generating serpent folding back upon itself (see Figure 8.1).

In *Mysterium Coniunctionis* (1970), Jung explores the meaning of the uroboros within alchemy, describing it as a preferred symbol of wholeness. Like the mandalas (i.e., magic circles) of other spiritual and religious traditions the world over, of which it is but one exemplar, it represents a sense of unity and completeness. Like Aristotle's circular line, it is an attempt to resolve the seeming contradictions between time and eternity, potentiality and actuality, origin and telos, as well as other metaphysical oppositions. Within alchemical symbolism, the uroboros expressed the restoration of an original state of wholeness (Jung, 1959, 1969). Jung considered this self-consuming serpent to be the earthly forerunner of his concept of the Self, just as he thought of the occult science of alchemy as the historic correlate of his own psychology (Jung, 2011). The Self, often written with a capital *S* to distinguish it from the self of the conscious ego, in his thinking, is both the center and circumference or totality of the personality.

He discerned in this particular serpentine circle the psychological process of 'eating' one's own substance. Such a devouring "means nothing less than the integration of those parts of the personality which are still outside ego-consciousness" (Jung, 1970, pp. 364–365) especially the shadow, which is far easier to project upon others than to assimilate into oneself. As alluded to in a previous chapter, confronting the shadow inevitably involves confronting one's own self-deception

DOI: 10.4324/b23321-9

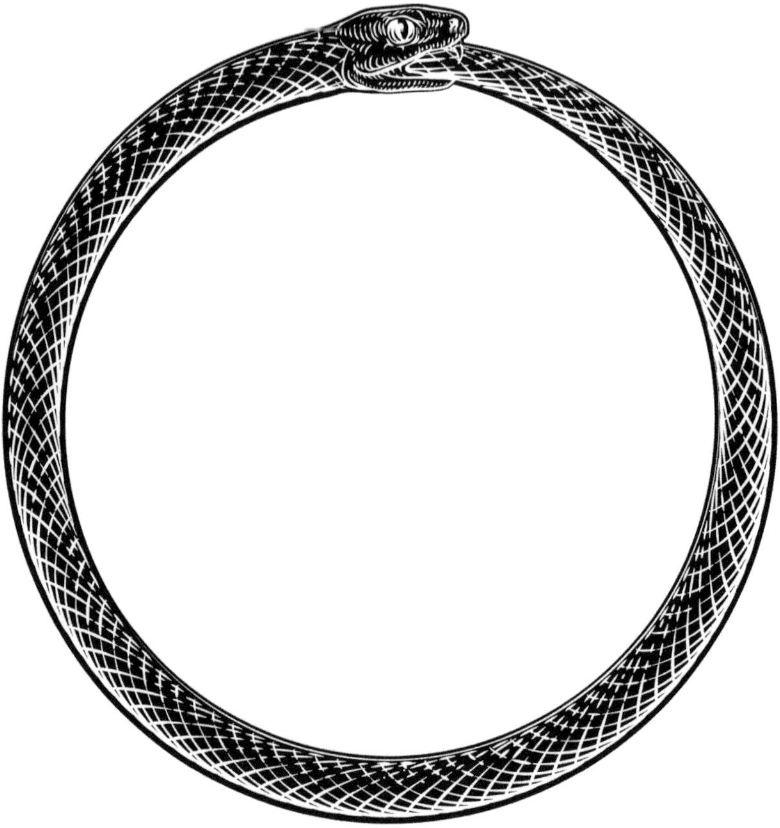

FIGURE 8.1 An uroboros, a self-consuming and self-generating serpent

and all of the dissociative and projective dynamics that make it possible. It presents the ego with the difficult moral challenge of recognizing aspects of one's own personality that one finds disagreeable or even repugnant. A confrontation with the shadow requires that one 'eat crow' and stomach the unpalatable. The moral challenge that the shadow presents is always one of identification: I am what I claim I am not. I am two people in opposition to one another. Confronting the shadow means confronting an inner cleavage, an underlying unity in apparent disunity. Without such a recognition, the splitting and projective dynamics of the psyche lead the ego to discern only in others what are, in fact, also negative qualities belonging to oneself. In such a state, I metaphorically bite my own tail believing that I am biting someone else's. Thus, Jung (1970) asserts that "the uroboros is one even though in the twilight of the unconscious its head and tail appear as separate figures and are regarded as such" (p. 294). In this twilight, a Neverland of sorts, the shadow, like Peter's own, detaches itself and appears utterly independent of the body that casts it. The two, body and shadow, like the head and tail of the serpent, appear as separate and are regarded as such.

But the self-consuming serpent is also self-renewing. The word *uroboros* means self-begetting. Its regenerative aspect is discernible to those who, in effect, move beyond this twilight state of unconsciousness and attempt "to integrate opposites that were previously projected" (Jung, 1970, p. 79). This is a challenge for the intellect, which is always tempted to see the head and tail only as separate. Yet when the challenge is met, the consumption is also a fertilization. The uroboros not only devours but also impregnates itself: "his tail is the masculine and his mouth the feminine organ" (Jung, 1970, p. 117). Thus, this sacred serpent possesses the quality of aseity, that is to say, that it is self-derived and self-originating, a quality it shares with the idea of God. In this, too, it shares attributes with Jung's conception of the Self, which often appears in psychic life as an all-powerful deity or through images of the divine.

Jung's reading of alchemy and the affinity with his own psychology are also found in the idea of a circumambulation: "The alchemists were fond of picturing their *opus* as a circulatory process, as a circular distillation or as the uroboros, the snake biting its own tail, and they made innumerable pictures of this process" (Jung, 1959, p. 264). Circular distillation, wholeness, self-consumption, and self-generation are all perhaps best summed up in the following paragraph, which describes a great deal of what is essential to alchemy and to Jung's (1970) understanding of individuation as well as the relationship that he believed existed between the two:

> In the age-old image of the uroboros lies the thought of devouring oneself and turning oneself into a circulatory process, for it was clear to the more astute alchemists that the prima materia of the art was man himself. The uroboros is a dramatic symbol for the integration and assimilation of the opposite, i.e. of the shadow. This "feed-back" process is at the same time a symbol of immortality, since it is said of the uroboros that he slays himself and brings himself to life, fertilizes himself and gives birth to himself. He symbolizes the One, who proceeds from the clash of opposites, and he therefore constitutes the secret of the prima materia which, as a projection, unquestionably stems from man's unconscious.
>
> *(p. 365)*

The idea expressed in the uroboros is, unsurprisingly, found within the Christian tradition in the image of Christ (also a Self image) as he who eats his own flesh and blood at the Last Supper. As Jung (1970) states, quoting Tertullian,

> In the same way the Lord applied to himself two Greek letters, the first and the last, as figures of the beginning and end which are united in himself. For just as Alpha continues on until it reaches Omega, and Omega completes the cycle back again to Alpha, so he meant to show that in him is found the course of all

> things from the beginning to the end and from the end back to the beginning, so that every divine dispensation should end in him through whom it began.
>
> *(p. 307)*

The motif of regenerative self-consumption, whether through the self-devouring serpent or the self-devouring son of god, is an ancient one. Unsurprisingly then, the uroboros is not only an image in medieval alchemy but also in ancient paganism. It is, in fact, "much older, and may ultimately go back to ancient Egyptian theology, to the doctrine of the homoousia [one being] of the Father-God with the divine son, Pharaoh" (Jung, 1970, pp. 307–308). The uroboros of Greek alchemy "is the symbol of the union of opposites *par excellence* and an alchemical version of the proverb: *les extrêmes se touchent*" (Jung, 1970, p. 504), the extremes touch one another. Such a union of opposites is both the goal of alchemy and in a similar vein, the goal of Jung's psychology, which seeks a reconciliation of opposing forces within the psyche.

This union of opposites within alchemy is also expressed through the more general idea that the beginning of the process is also the end: The goal of alchemy, the philosopher's stone or lapis also represents a new prima materia, the primary material or substance with which one starts: "That is why the *lapis*, as *prima materia*, stands at the beginning of the process as well as at the end" (Jung, 1959, p. 264). It was, in fact, rarely clearly defined what this *prima materia* was and it had no consistent name in alchemical texts. Alchemists often quarreled among themselves as to its identity:

> The names given to the *prima materia* show that it was not a definite substance at all, but rather an intuitive concept for an *initial psychic situation*, symbolized by such terms as water of life, cloud, heaven, shadow, sea, mother, moon, dragon, Venus, chaos, *massa confusa*, Microcosmos, etc."
>
> *(Jung, 1959, p. 155)*

*Mother* as a name for the *prima materia* is particularly important, given our past reflections on the term. We have already seen that there are deep, pervasive etymological and metaphysical associations linking *mother* to *matter* that traverse cultures and historical epochs.

It is not difficult to transfer alchemical modes of reflection, as inscrutable and opaque, as arcane and occult as they may be, onto more modern, familiar modes of phenomenological reflection. Both are, broadly speaking, processes of refinement, ways of distilling essences. The phenomenological method as envisioned by Husserl begins with a *return* to the things themselves, phenomena as they present themselves in their perceived immediacy are its prima materia. This return (an epoché) requires a setting aside of preconceptions, which is itself a purification of sorts, requiring an ascetic discipline of the mind. By way of a process Husserl called *free variation*, a sort of imaginative play that allows one to view something from multiple perspectives, one comes to grasp an *intuition* of the essence of the matter at hand. Then one furthers this distillation of essence into a description, a conceptualization that pretends to represent the fundamental nature of the matter under consideration. This is, in effect, the *lapis philosophorum*, the philosopher's stone that both alchemy and phenomenology seek.

Deconstruction takes issue with the prima materia of Husserl's phenomenology. Derrida and Husserl are a bit like two alchemists arguing over what substance to begin the work with. Husserl begins with perception, phenomena, self-evidence. Derrida begins with différance. The two philosophers are strikingly similar yet dissimilar, leading some to describe the latter figure as engaging in a sort of high-grade mimicry of the former (Wood, 2001). One seems to be the inverted image of the other. What this suggests, from a Jungian perspective, is that there are shadow dynamics involved. What Derrida critiques in Husserl may be a veiled version of himself. Is this, perhaps, why all of his critiques of primordiality and origins result in surrogate primordialities couched within quotes and non-origins that are somehow, nevertheless, originary? In this regard the image of the uroboros may be of use. On Jung's account, it involves an eating of one's own psychological substance, an integration of one's own inner other, the shadow self that one might deny in oneself while combating it through projections upon others. Consciousness of this process is an act of psychological integration, an overcoming or healing of dissociation. This is a conscious act of turning oneself into a circulatory process, or recognizing one's own circularity, recognizing that the head and tail of the uroboros belong to the same being (*homoousia*).

The image of the circular serpent is also useful in thinking through deconstruction in terms of its alpha and omega principles and the relationship between the two. Previously, I described this as the two bookends of Derrida's argument: One consists of the appeal to absolute priority, while the other consists of the appeal to an equally absolute inconclusiveness. Différance is at the unreachable beginning and the transcendental signified is at the unreachable end. The former is the source of linguistic differentiation: It is the common root of all oppositional concepts, a diacritical dynamic that makes possible such pairings as hot and cold, light and dark, up and down. The other bookend is a mystical, mythical realm, 'outside' of language, a thing in itself that is forever beyond our grasp, an opaquely termed 'other of language' that, on radically differing accounts, Derrida appears to either devoutly champion or utterly deny. Yet they would seem to be one and the same bookend, or bookends that touch one another, as the symbolic logic of the uroboros would suggest, which would mean, effectively, that the source of distinctions made in language is, in fact, the selfsame 'mystical' realm of the transcendental signified. This is, in effect, the view of Merleau-Ponty, as will be made clear in the following pages. Whereas Derrida, as if perceiving only through the twilight of unconsciousness, does not seem to understand that head and tail belong to the same creature, that they are of the same *flesh*, the French phenomenologist clearly does. In recognizing that différance and the transcendental signified belong to the same being, that they are like two extremes of a single serpent that touch one another, he assimilates the opposites, he confronts the shadow.

For Jung, the term used to describe the healing of dissociative splits is *integration*. The English word *integrate*, meaning to render whole that which was in parts, to form or blend into a larger unity, is rooted in the Latin *integratus*, which is the past participle of *integrare*: to make whole, from *integer* which means whole or complete. Its meaning parallels that of *individuation*, which is, for Jung, the hallmark of psychological well-being, a never fully realized state of becoming an individual. This, in turn, is understood as a never fully realized state of indivisibility. "Neurosis is self-division" (p. 20), for Jung (1953) "an inner cleavage-the state of being at war with one-self" (Jung, 1933, p. 236), and individuation represents an always relative transcendence of this division.

In contrast to the dissociative logic of deconstruction, Merleau-Ponty, who was deeply influenced by Husserl, offers a more integral view of language, one that, to my mind, reflects a greater psychological integration, the very integration called for by the Husserlian/Derridean split. Well-versed in Saussure's structuralism and Heidegger's *destruktion*, he took the linguistic turn that Derrida, Foucault, Lacan, Lyotard, and others also took, yet it led him in a different direction. Regrettably, his untimely death in 1961 prevented him from living to see the full influence of these figures' writings or address their major works. Still, one can read texts like *Consciousness and the Acquisition of Language* (Merleau-Ponty, 1973b), *Signs* (Merleau-Ponty, 1964b), *The Prose of the World* (Merleau-Ponty, 1973a), and *The Visible and the Invisible* (Merleau-Ponty, 1968) and marvel at his prescient ability to anticipate the directions that such thinkers would later take, as well as address their shortcomings as regards issues like the constitution of meaning and its exclusive location within the confines of linguistic signs.

Whereas "Husserl had to postpone, from one end of his itinerary to the other, all explicit meditation of the essence of language in general" (Derrida, 1973, p. 7), Merleau-Ponty did not and could not. The historical moment in which he lived would hardly have allowed it: The focus upon the formative power of language that has come to be known as the 'linguistic turn' (Levenson, 2011) was in his lifetime only growing in its influence upon continental philosophy and coming to deeply affect the entire intellectual milieu of a variety of disciplines in the humanities and social sciences. As heirs to his legacy, we are fortunate that this is the case. It forced him to understand the importance—later elaborated and taken in new directions by the aforementioned figures—of the undeniably critical and heretofore depreciated impact that language has upon both thought and perception. Yet he also understood early on the error inherent in grounding all meaning within a strictly semiotic domain.

His notions of *reversibility, chiasm, flesh, sedimentation, autochthonous organization, écart*, and a *tacit cogito* are all suggestive of an uroboric logic. Images evoked in his writings suggest and often even parallel the self-begetting, regenerative dynamics of the circular serpent. His thought attempts to discern a homoousia, a single being, an integrated whole, where others can only discern disconnected fragments. Put differently, he sought a non-dualistic ontology, and the terms italicized above serve as attempts to identify the excluded middle that such dualistic forms of thinking overlook. In this regard, they are mediating principles, much in the same way that for Jung the term *psychoid* was a way of suggesting that the human psyche is not ontologically separate from the rest of the world. This is a point that Roger Brooke (2015) makes in his masterful work *Jung and Phenomenology* in which he carefully draws parallels between the two men's attempts at overcoming similar forms of dualism: "Jung's analysis of the body's materiality as psychic depth and Merleau-Ponty's analysis of the body as flesh follow different paths" (p. 85) but arrive at the same integration, the same sense of the truth of the proverb *les extrêmes se touchent.*

Despite being profoundly impacted by Saussure, as was Derrida, for Merleau-Ponty perception and phenomena remain primordial, in the sense of taking precedence. He does not accept the premise that somehow everything *begins* by representation and in this regard he stays true to the understanding of phenomenology as a "philosophy of the Beginning" (Husserl, 2014, p. 18). This beginning resides in self-evidence, perception, an immediate 'seeing.' This is his prima materia, though it differs in important ways from Husserl's own.

But perhaps more important than taking perception as a point of departure are two related points. The first goes by the name of *reversibility* and will be addressed further on. The second point is that what is present to perception, the *matter* of perception itself is always "pregnant with its form" (Merleau-Ponty, 1964a, p. 15), or one might even say, laden with meaning: What we perceive is not merely a collection of sensations, an assortment of atomistic bits of sensory information without rhyme or reason. *Both rhyme and reason are already present in perception*, which possesses its own nascent logos, its own rationality (Merleau-Ponty, 1964a). One way of thinking of this is to understand that, for him, there are already both spatial and temporal *differences* present in the phenomenal world. Without these differences there can be no sense of form. This inherency of form is not of a conceptual order, one imposed upon otherwise unintelligible sense data; Phenomena manifest relations among themselves that transcend human projection, or cannot be reduced to it (Dillon, 1997). This is the case whether projection is conceived of in terms of Kantian categories, Derridean signifiers, what Butler might call regulatory powers, or by any other name. Both form and meaning are not merely imposed upon perception, as if from the outside, as something that is brought to it by way of some ancillary process. They are already there. The perceived world carries with it and serves as the ground of every *Sinngebung*, every meaning (Merleau-Ponty, 1962 [2002]). Because what is perceived is already pregnant with form, form is not simply superimposed upon perception by virtue of some preexisting reason.

Because this is the case, "I do not look at a chaos, but at things" (Merleau-Ponty, 1968, p. 133). There is always a certain perceptual genius at work that *precedes* the thinking subject or cannot be reduced to it. Perception itself is an irreducible sensemaking, a coordination and synthesis of disparate sensations and moments. Merleau-Ponty (1964a) writes:

> We observe at once that it is impossible, as has often been said, to decompose a perception, to make it into a collection of sensations, because in it the whole is prior to the parts—and this whole is not an ideal whole. The meaning which I ultimately discover is not of the conceptual order. If it were a concept, the question would be how I can recognize it in the data, and it would be necessary for me to interpose between the concept and the sense data certain intermediaries, and then other intermediaries between these intermediaries, and so on.
>
> *(p. 15)*

Such a statement expresses both his deep commitment to Gestalt psychology, for which the whole is the fundamental unit of perception, and his disagreement with such empiricist philosophers as Hume and Locke, for whom the smallest possible perceptual atom was the most fundamental.

This coordinating, synthesizing quality of perception and the way that it organizes itself into wholes takes place between the senses: hearing, sight, touch, smell, and taste form gestalts that already carry significance for us. Our senses synthesize into the coherency of perception: If I touch with my hands the unseen side of a lamp, I also anticipate that this unseen side will be visible from another standpoint, just as the side that I currently see is. Touch and sight work in conjunction with one another to give me a coherent sense of the lamp before me. If I reach gropingly to turn its switch, I understand the subsequent clicking sound to be the result of my hand's movement, which has also caused the room to darken. What I sense with my sight, touch, hearing, and even smell is synthesized into a gestalt, the perceptual whole that forms my sense of inhabiting the room. This is the root meaning of perception as a gestalt: The whole is greater than the sum of its parts and the relationships between the parts determines the meaning of the whole.

This perceptual synthesis, or sense making takes place independently of any need to express or conceptualize it in language (Merleau-Ponty, 1962 [2002]). Yet perception is not meaningless. It is, metaphorically, an original text, carrying its meaning within itself. In this sense, the perceived world is itself a prior speech. It speaks to me, to all of us, in a prose of its own and I, in turn, respond in a silent conversation carried on with my surroundings: If for example, while crossing a busy street, I quicken my gate to move out of the way of an oncoming vehicle, I am responding to a significant statement from my perceptual field, one that I myself also inhabit. Lifting my leg to step upon the curb before me is evidence again that the curb *indicates* or *signifies* to me a need for a particular form of movement. Such perceptions possess their own nascent logos, their own emerging sense. What we call *meaning* does not reside wholly within words.

One name that Merleau-Ponty gave for this inherency of meaning and form within the perceived world is *autochthonous organization* and two of the primary elements of this organization were theme and horizon, a focal point and background context, something upon which our attention is directed and a milieu within which it appears: the lamp in the previous example and the room that contains it. This theme/horizon structure constitutes for the Gestalt psychology that so deeply influenced his work one of the most fundamental forms with which the matter of perception is 'pregnant,' one of the most fundamental elements of *autochthonous organization*. This theme/horizon structure is, furthermore, *diachronic*: it is not static but continually emerging and evolving through time. Theme and horizon, figure and ground are primary differentiations always already present in perception. The figure is *different* from the ground and this difference is present before, or independent of, words like *figure* and *ground* or *theme* and *horizon*.

Closely related to this matter of figure and ground is the fact that perception is always partial. A perceived object is never perceived completely. Some elements are revealed, while others are concealed. Some are present while others are absent. Merleau-Ponty conceives of these issues in terms of immanence and transcendence, a within and a without, a quality of being indwelling and a quality of surpassing. This immanence and transcendence is for him a central, one might even say foundational aspect of perception:

> There is a paradox of immanence and transcendence in perception. Immanence, because the perceived object cannot be foreign to him who perceives; transcendence, because it always contains something more than what is actually given. And these two elements of perception are not, properly speaking, contradictory. For if we reflect on this notion of perspective, if we reproduce the perceptual experience in our thought, we see that the kind of evidence proper to the perceived, the appearance of 'something,' requires both this presence and this absence.
>
> *(Merleau-Ponty, 1964a, p. 16)*

Returning to the image of the lamp to make these observations clearer, I can only see one side of it at a time, depending on my perspective. Likewise, I can only touch one portion of it. I can only perceive part of it at any given moment. At any given moment some of it will be within, or *immanent to* my sight and touch, while other portions of it will be outside of, or *transcendent to* them.

Figure and ground, immanence and transcendence, as well as proximity and distance, originate within the very order of perceptual experience. The matter of perception is pregnant with their form. This is important because, as explained in Chapter 1, the attribution of such oppositional pairings to différance serves Derrida's strategic intent to erode the very foundation of the Western philosophic tradition, with all of its metaphysical assumptions, biases, and baggage, the greatest of which is logocentrism itself: The ostensibly erroneous belief that language is an expression of some fundamental reality, be it objective, phenomenal, or otherwise. This undermines the possibility that inherited *pre-conceptions* might also be, in a sense, *post-perceptions*. It undermines the possibility that the linguistic distinctions of the metaphysical heritage might be the echoes of what prior generations perceived and what present generations continue to perceive. Merleau-Ponty's thought suggests that perception is not merely the *result* of a metaphysical heritage, but its *source*.

In *Phenomenology of Perception*, he conceives of the primacy of perception in relation to thought and language by way of what he called a *tacit cogito*, a term that he would later abandon, in part because he had his own misgivings about the particular way that Husserl conceived of consciousness. This term is best understood in relation to the Cartesian dictum *cogito ergo sum*: I think therefore I am—which was intended to establish an absolute certainty, a fact above and beyond all logic, upon which Descartes might found his philosophy.

Two related aspects of the tacit cogito distinguish it from the Cartesian cogito: The first is clearly alluded to in the word *tacit*, meaning without words or speech. Whereas Descartes' dictum is a *spoken* cogito—a reflection formed in words stating that my thinking proves my existence—the tacit cogito is silent. The term refers to an originary, primordial consciousness without language, a prelinguistic self of pre-reflective experience. The former says 'I am' while the other does not. The Cartesian cogito is a form of explicit self-consciousness, as well as an act of self-objectification, an act of thematizing oneself as an 'I.' But the tacit cogito, most simply put, refers to a pre-reflective subject, one that exists before, and makes possible, a reflective subject capable of making statements. "Behind the spoken *cogito*, the one which is converted into discourse and into essential truth," he tells his reader, "there lies a tacit *cogito*" (Merleau-Ponty, 1962 [2002], p. 469). In this sense it is "anterior to any philosophy" (Merleau-Ponty, 1962 [2002], p. 470).

Thinking in terms of a tacit cogito is an attempt to conceptualize a primordial consciousness, the type required by the phenomenological reduction—the setting aside or bracketing of inherited theoretical and philosophical preconceptions. But it is also a means of conceiving an awareness of, and genesis of, language itself. For him, there can be no Cartesian cogito, no articulated reflection, 'I think,' without a tacit or unspoken cogito that precedes it. This is because, "language presupposes nothing less than a consciousness of language, a silence of consciousness embracing the world of speech in which words first receive a form and meaning" (Merleau-Ponty, 1962 [2002], p. 469). For him, it is clear that in order for a person to think and be able to articulate in words the fact that he or she thinks, there must be a consciousness that is subordinate to neither of these processes. Consciousness is the condition of possibility for both thinking and speech.

The second distinguishing aspect follows from the first. Because it is unspoken, the tacit cogito is also, in a sense, pre-personal. It is anonymous. Thus, "if I wanted to render precisely the perceptual experience," he writes, "I ought to say that one perceives in me, and not that I perceive" (Merleau-Ponty, 1962 [2002], p. 250). The 'I' is a subject that arises after the fact, as a *result* of reflecting upon perception. I am always already perceiving, even before I have the thought 'I perceive,' in fact, it is only upon attempting to render the perception in words, to explicitly thematize it that an 'I' arises. Perception is, in this sense, pre-personal and anonymous.

Importantly, the difference between the tacit cogito and the explicit cogito of Descartes is that the former conceives of consciousness as incarnating *through* a sensate body, whereas the latter is more conducive to conceiving a ghost in the machine, a consciousness alien to and alienated from all other objects, even the body itself! This is a consciousness that has been made unworldly, a fact that Merleau-Ponty, the great philosopher of the body, could not abide by. Such a consciousness is a pure intelligence without any corporeal involvement, or what he also termed a *kosmotheoros*, a contemplator of the world that, paradoxically, does not inhabit it (Merleau-Ponty, 2003). Such a conception has been described as a Cartesian split, a dualism that divides the world into a *res cogitans* or mind and a *res extensa* or matter (Bordo, 1987). Many writers from a variety of disciplines (Berman, 1981; Brooke, 2015; Johnstone, 1992; Kleinberg-Levin, 1988; Spretnak, 1999) are critical of this split and have sought to overcome it. Merleau-Ponty, through the idea of a tacit cogito, also attempted to overcome this alienation fostered by Descartes (Dillon, 1997), who was, in fact, something of a philosophical nemesis for him, one that he critiqued quite often. But *attempted* here is the operative word, for the tacit cogito is a failed attempt by his own account, one that he explicitly rejected in his later work (Merleau-Ponty, 1968) in which he reaches toward a language more adequate to the intuition he sought to express.

This rejection is best understood as part of his effort to save phenomenology from the idea of a transcendental ego as handed down by Husserl. 'Transcendental' is here best understood to mean *preceding any experience*. For Husserl, all things, all bodies, all other minds, absolutely everything could be thought of only as constituted by this ego (Nakhnikian, 1964). The problem with the tacit cogito is that it is a cogito; it still reflects a form of thought confined within the limits established by Husserl's transcendental ego. It may not put the *ego cogitans*, a thinking subject in the place of an ultimate ground of truth and being, but it puts *an* ego there, one no less vulnerable to accusations of solipsism than is Descartes.' It still grounds philosophic truth *within* individual experience, which ultimately is no less isolated, no less self-contained than the Cartesian subject. Because, as M. C. Dillon (1997) states and Merleau-Ponty would agree, "solipsism is intrinsic to Cartesian thought" (p. 113), Husserl's transcendental ego would seem, likewise, to suffer from solipsism. It is difficult to see the 'lived experience' that it grounds itself upon as taking place anywhere other than *within* a subject. Husserl's phenomenology as the study of *phenomena*, that is to say, things in their appearance, is a study of how things appear *within* our experience, and it is this sense of within-ness or immanence that renders it vulnerable to critique. This is, arguably, its original sin, one that Merleau-Ponty (1968), Heidegger (1927 [1967]) and others sought to remedy by de-emphasizing consciousness and subjectivity.[1]

For the Merleau-Ponty of later works, especially that of *The Visible and the Invisible* (1968), consciousness and subjectivity are no longer constitutional in the way they had been for Husserl. Like Derrida, he takes issue with Husserl's origin story, not only regarding consciousness but also the issues of presence and the phenomenological reduction. The three issues, and his approach toward them, are intrinsically entwined. As regards the first issue, both men reject grounding their thought in a constituting subject, but one does so in a way that intends to preserve phenomenology as a discipline that still privileges perception and phenomena, yet without evoking the specter of subjectivism or solipsism, to which any form of thought grounding itself in the idea of consciousness is potentially vulnerable.

The abandonment of the tacit cogito and the phenomenological reduction is less an abandonment of the project of phenomenology than it is a radicalization and rehabilitation of it (Dillon, 1997; Hamrick & Veken, 2012). It is a further exploration of what is meant by the word *perception*, which is best understood as not merely something that takes place *within* a subject but, rather, as something that opens a subject to a phenomenal world. In Merleau-Ponty's mature thought it is not a subject, ego, self, or consciousness that is constitutional, it is relationship, and the relationship for him goes by the name of *reversibility*. This radicality was already implied in his earlier work but had not yet found adequate form. In later works, perception will still remain primary in relation to thought, but the way of conceiving of this primacy, the place in which it might be located, will change. Perhaps this is why Derrida's engagement with Merleau-Ponty was notably scant, given his sustained critique of phenomenology as a discipline, which relies so heavily upon undermining the viability of a transcendental ego: Said critique addresses, conveniently, Husserl while leaving Merleau-Ponty aside. When Derrida (2005) did manage to not leave him aside, as is the case in *On Touching—Jean-Luc Nancy*, he criticizes him, unsurprisingly, for privileging immediacy and continuity, over rupture and distance.

At times in a manner surprisingly similar to that of Derrida, Merleau-Ponty also took issue with Husserl's conception of time and its spatialization, his construal of moments in terms of points on a line (Al-Saji, 2009). Yet his response to this misconception was remarkably different: For him, the foundation or source of space and time was not différance, but the body, or what he referred to as a *corporeal schema*, a close synonym of which might be *body image* (Merleau-Ponty, 1968). This schema included an element analogous to différance, a temporal and spatial gap, what he called écart, but this gap was not, first and foremost, simply a question of sign systems in the strict sense.

Briefly, as to the similarities, he discerned comparable issues regarding the now as point and the now as duration, its divisibility and continuity. He too understood that the present moment as conceived by Husserl required a certain fullness that was, nevertheless, subverted by an alien element that made this impossible. In words that might just as well belong to Derrida, he stated that, "the present itself is not an absolute coincidence without transcendence; even the *Urerlebnis* [primal experience] involves not total coincidence, but partial coincidence, because it has horizons and would not be without them" (Merleau-Ponty, 1968, p. 195). The assumption of a full and primordial presence with its sheer immediacy as conceived by Husserl was therefore mistaken: In construing such a full self-presence one encloses the present as if it were sufficient to itself and fully independent of other moments. Yet this cannot be. Such a moment would not seem to even pass into other moments, and in this regard, it would be an absolute present. Interrogating this temporal logic, he asks, "Is it the new present, in its individuality, that pushes the preceding one into the past, and that fills a part of the future?" (Merleau-Ponty, 1968, p. 190).

Yet in a manner that, to my mind, is quite alien to the deconstructive approach, he observes that the present "is ungraspable from close up, in the forceps of attention, *it is an encompassing* [emphasis added]" (Merleau-Ponty, 1968, p. 195). The now is not a point on a line, or a duration on a line, because it is not on a line at all. It is that which always already surrounds us. It is a milieu. The present is unlocalizable insofar as it cannot be considered an isolated 'point' in time. Points are perceivable only within a field. They are, in effect, *figures* upon a *ground* or *themes* within a *horizon*. The now as point, by virtue of being a point, is already something that exists within a perceptual Gestalt. Furthermore, such lines and points are abstractions, mere geometric idealizations. To conceive them as such tacitly assumes a point of view of absolute contemplation, an observer outside the temporal flux, capable of observing past, present, and future simultaneously.

Like Derrida, Merleau-Ponty also took issue with Husserl's transcendental reduction. As early as *Phenomenology of Perception* (1962 [2002]), he tells his reader that "the most important lesson which the reduction teaches us is the impossibility of a complete reduction" (p. xv). The two men concurred that we cannot set aside or momentarily bracket our preconceptions in the hopes of attaining perceptions cleansed of all cultural and linguistic antecedents. Our cultural, linguistic history is too deeply sedimented within us. Our perceptions are too inextricably intertwined with a history of representation, too embedded within a culture, what Derrida would call a metaphysical heritage. No such return to the things themselves purified of any linguistic contamination is possible but, importantly, neither is it necessary (Merleau-Ponty, 1968).

Yet, if the reduction is not possible for either, this is so for different reasons and has different consequences. Throughout Merleau-Ponty's work, perception is taken to be epistemologically primary (Dillon, 1997; Merleau-Ponty, 1964a, 1968). For him, the perceived world continues to be "the always presupposed foundation of all rationality, all value, and all existence" (Merleau-Ponty, 1964a, p. 13). Whereas Derrida casts a skeptical glance at the very notion of phenomena, Merleau-Ponty places great faith in it. Throughout his work, phenomena were held to be ontologically primary, although he did not explicitly thematize the question of ontology until shortly before his untimely death (Dillon, 1997).

Yet, more importantly, Merleau-Ponty refuted another reduction that Derrida did not: The semiological reduction that would later become the grammatological reduction—the thought that separates language from its non-linguistic milieu and later brackets perception to envision a world of signs without fault, truth, or origin.

Husserl's brackets become quotation marks, parentheses, and crossings-out in Derrida, but they function in a similar manner. One reduction is simply the inverse of the other. One seeks a perception purified of preconceptions; the other posits a purity of linguistic play in which perception has been nullified. Each attempts to bracket out, to exclude from consideration, the foundational term or grounding concept of the philosophical opposition. The problem with both is the need for purity. This is, perhaps, the problem with every reduction, and if Merleau-Ponty refutes them both, it is because he prefers synthesis to purity, prefers to accommodate *both* the insights of phenomenology *and* those of the budding linguistic turn that would later blossom into the approaches of Derrida, Foucault, Lacan, and others.

In Jungian terms, he sought to withstand the tension of the opposites in search of a transcendent third position that would incorporate both. He gave this third position various names, among them *flesh* and *reversibility*. Both can be seen as attempts to incorporate and transcend the extremes represented by the aforementioned reductions. Both terms are attempts to speak of the "one that proceeds from the clash of opposites" (Jung, 1970, p. 365). Both are means of acknowledging that, as in the image of the uroboros, *les extrêmes se touchent*. The extremes touch. But how?

To answer this question, one must think of perception not as something merely taking place within consciousness but as a relation between an *embodied* consciousness and a world in which both are understood to be of the same *flesh*. It is tempting for those who possess a passing familiarity with Merleau-Ponty's thought to assume they know exactly what is meant by the term *flesh* without quite realizing the particular sense with which he imbues it. Certainly, the great philosopher of the body, as he is known, is referring to the embodied, perceiving subject, not flesh as mere matter, a physical body, but sentient flesh, a locus of perception through which the world is perceived. And, in fact, there are times when he uses the word in this way. But there is another sense of the word that did not appear in print until the posthumous publication of the unfinished work *The Visible and the Invisible* (Merleau-Ponty, 1968), which is far more relevant to understanding his mature thought. There, his use of the term is a means of articulating that which subtends or precedes the body-subject/world-object divide. It is a means of discerning that the two sides of this divide are of one being, a homoousia, an uroboric whole in which both head and tail belong to the same serpent, metaphorically speaking. Flesh, in the sense that he wishes to grant the term, is not a substance, not a body, not a spirit but an *element*, a "concrete emblem of a general manner of being" (Merleau-Ponty, 1968, p. 147).

Just as the ancients sought in earth, air, fire, or water the fundamental constituents of all things, the rudimentary first principles or simplest components of being in all of its complexity, Merleau-Ponty sought a component, an elemental first principle. The simplest component was flesh: an underlying unity to the apparent disunity of body-subject and world-object. Like the head and tail of a serpent turning back upon itself, the two may appear to be separate, yet ultimately, they belong to the same scaley creature. Head and tail may appear utterly different, but they are not, insofar as they both belong to a greater whole. The idea of *flesh*, as he uses the term, is an attempt at the restoration of an original state, an integration of opposites. Flesh, in this work, is synonymous with a sense of *reversibility*, which he describes as "the ultimate truth" (Merleau-Ponty, 1968, p. 155).

The prototype for this notion of reversibility is the phenomenon of touch. *Les extrêmes se touchent*—the extremes touch one another, and one can learn a great deal through reflecting upon that fact. If I consider my hands, I notice that, felt from within, they are also accessible from without. A hand is both a means by which I touch and is itself touchable. In other words, the touched/touching relationship is reversible. It is not possible to touch something without being, in the act, touched by it. The point of contact is a point of reciprocity. My hand is both a means of investigating the palpable world and forms part of this world. It can be touched by others. Perception of tangible objects is only possible because I am myself as tangible as they are, and in this regard, we are kindred. I, as body/subject, am only this on condition of also being an object. I am able to perceive worldly things through touch, sight, smell, taste, and hearing only on the condition of being a worldly thing myself that can be likewise perceived. If I touch my hands together, patting, stroking, rubbing, one with the other, I have an even greater sense of this reversibility. Each hand is both sentient and sensible, subject and object, ambiguously entwined. The touching and tangible crisscross and incorporate themselves one into the other, and it is at this point of crisscross where what we call perception is born.

These are such simple, elementary observations. Yet this is the point, and their simplicity serves an important purpose in Merleau-Ponty's thought: In his earlier work, despite its emphasis on bodily perception, in some ways it replicated faults inherited from Descartes via Husserl. In his more mature work, he reflected that "the problems posed in [The Phenomenology of Perception] are insoluble because I start there from the 'consciousness'-'object' distinction" (Merleau-Ponty, 1968, p. 200). This is, in effect, the mind/matter distinction made by Descartes. By choosing a different point of departure, that of the reversibility of touch, he does not start from this distinction. After all, consciousness cannot be touched, but a truly incarnate subject most certainly can, and it is by starting here that Merleau-Ponty is able to overcome some of the undeniable flaws in Husserl's thought.

Understanding the phenomenon of touch leads to a recognition of the reciprocity of the sentient and the sensible that is applicable to other senses as well. Consider the phenomenon of vision: "He who sees cannot possess the visible unless he is possessed by it, unless he is of it, unless . . . he is one of the visibles, capable, by singular reversal, of seeing them—he who is one of them (Merleau-Ponty, 1968, pp. 134–135). Just as the touching hand can be touched, the seeing eye can be seen. I perceive a visible world and I am myself, in principle, visible to it. I encompass within my gaze a world that is capable of encompassing me within it. Through this mutual encompassing, I sense that for a world outside of myself I am an object within it. The recognition of this world-body relationship is the recognition of "a correspondence between its inside and my outside, between my inside and its outside" (Merleau-Ponty, 1968, p. 136). He writes:

> [Flesh] is the coiling over of the visible upon the seeing body, of the tangible upon the touching body, which is attested in particular when the body sees itself, touches itself seeing and touching the things, such that, simultaneously, as tangible it descends among them, as touching it dominates them all and draws this relationship and even this double relationship from itself, by dehiscence or fission of its own mass.
>
> *(Merleau-Ponty, 1968, p. 146)*

The surface of my skin, which marks the limits of my corporeal self, is the meeting place of the within and the without. Here, at the point of contact, the two ambiguously entwine and intersect in a complex interplay of inside and outside, subject and object: When I touch an object with my hand, let us say an unfinished table of still rough, grainy wood, I feel not only its gritty, dry texture but also my hand itself. Through perceiving the sensations on my hand, I perceive what is not my hand. When I glance at a far-off brook, I sense not only its distance from me but my distance from it. In locating it with my eyes, I also locate myself within a greater spatial field. I sense myself by way of otherness, so deeply interwoven are the two at the perceptual level.

Such observations not only offered Merleau-Ponty a way to overcome trenchant dualisms, it should be noted parenthetically that they also offered him a means of critiquing his colleague and friend Jean-Paul Sartre. For the existentialist philosopher, the body-subject (what he would call *my body-for-me*) can touch, and the body-object (what he would call *the body-for-others*) can be touched, but the two remain essentially different orders of reality. They are different ontological dimensions, remaining mutually exclusionary, philosophically disjunct, and unreconciled (Sartre, 1943 [2021]). Yet this makes as much sense as to think that a glove turned inside out and then back again is two different gloves, rather than one glove seen in two different ways.

What Merleau-Ponty draws our attention to is that such an absolute disjuncture is not possible, nor is the more general disjuncture between what Sartre calls the *in-itself* and the *for-itself*. Such a conception lacks a "living bond and communication between one term and the other" (Merleau-Ponty, 1964c, p. 72). As early as the *Phenomenology of Perception*, he wrote:

> The thing is inseparable from a person perceiving it, and can never be actually in itself because its articulations are those of our very existence, and because it stands at the other end of our gaze or at the terminus of a sensory exploration which invests it with humanity. To this extent, every perception is a communication or a communion, the taking up or completion by us of . . . our body with things.
>
> *(Merleau-Ponty, 1962 [2002], p. 373)*

This fundamental inseparability, this sense of homoousia transcends the two extremes of perceiving subject and phenomenal object or, put in a more metaphoric idiom, it reflects the way in which the head and tail of a circular serpent touch one another. In that point of contact, the world perceived is invested with humanity and *in turn invests us with itself.* This sense of investment only deepens as his thinking unfolds throughout his career. In his final work, he writes:

> One can say that we perceive the things themselves, that we are the world that thinks itself—or that the world is at the heart of our flesh. In any case, once a body-world relationship is recognized, there is a ramification of my body and a ramification of the world and a correspondence between its inside and my outside, between my inside and its outside.
>
> *(Merleau-Ponty, 1968, p. 136)*

Such passages evoke Jung's writings on the alchemist Paracelsus: "everything without is within, everything above is below. Between all things . . . reigns 'correspondence'" (Jung, 1956, p. 9). But in reading Merleau-Ponty, one is struck even more so by a sense of the irreducibly interwoven, the inextricably entwined. Being is made of a single fabric, albeit composed of infinite threads. He extended these reflections on themes of reversibility, flesh, and entwinement to questions of language, which we will now turn our attention to.

In Chapter 1, while explicating the idea of 'spacing' according to deconstruction, it was noted that because the repetition of a sign is always dependent upon a (spatial) gap or (temporal) interval, it is never quite the same sign twice, much like the repetition of a piano chord will never have the same aesthetic effect if it is played within a different measure of a song, at another tempo, or within another melody. It is the composition of words in relation to one another that makes them make sense and gives each word its ever-changing meaning. This is an idea with which Merleau-Ponty (1968), influenced by Saussure no less than was Derrida, agreed, and he made the point by way of an analogy with music: "Language as well as music can sustain a sense by virtue of its own arrangement" (p. 153). Just as words acquire meaning by virtue of how they are arranged in relation to one another, notes acquire an aesthetic sense by virtue of a similar arrangement. Place a word in a different location in a sentence or place a note in a different location of a melody and in both cases something of their sense will be altered.

Yet it is also by way of the analogy with music, and more specifically musical notation, that it is made clear the profound *disagreement* with the direction in which Derrida would later take Saussure's thought. Musical notation is a facsimile of the perception of sound, and without it, without reference to notes played upon an instrument and heard by human ears, the notation is meaningless, little more than random scratches upon a sheet. The scratches acquire their value by virtue of their relation to the primary experience of sound. This experience is not dependent upon the notation; a person who cannot read a musical score can, nevertheless, perceive pitch, duration, rhythm, and other musical qualities. They can recognize a melody and notice if it is played at a different tempo. They may even be able to perform or sing an entire song without being able to read a single note, if they have learned to play or sing 'by ear.' The notational system replicates a primary phenomenon—a song or melody—that even those who do not understand the notation can nevertheless perceive. There are skilled musicians who cannot recognize a caesura, clef, bracket, or brace, yet they are able to distinguish and replicate all of the sounds and silences that these symbols represent.

In a similar vein, a person skilled in transcribing musical notation may be able to listen to a composition played on an instrument that they do not master themselves and still be able to faithfully replicate that composition on a page. "Musical notation is a facsimile made after the event," Merleau-Ponty (1968) observed, "an abstract portrait of the musical entity, language as a system" (p. 153). Yet this system would be meaningless without the music itself, without the experience of sound to which the notation corresponds. If sounds were not first perceived, there would be no way of creating their facsimile and no need to. Similar observations are likewise relevant concerning the words on the page before you: "For the linguist language is an ideal system, a fragment of the intelligible world. But . . . if my words have a meaning, it is not because they present the systemic organization the linguist will disclose" (Merleau-Ponty, 1968, p. 154). Rather, it is because they disclose the autochthonous organization, the perceived world pregnant with form that we inhabit. They would be meaningless otherwise.

With this analogy in mind, the importance of semiotic spacing takes on a different tenor. We are reminded of the fact that gaps, intervals, differentiation, deferral, spacing, temporalization, and repetition, all of the dynamics that make up this strange non-concept known as différance allude to fundamental *experiences*, fundamental *perceptions* of primary phenomena. For example, I sense an interval between the drips of two drops from the kitchen sink. I defer my arrival home by slowing my gate. I repeat a phrase to ensure that it is just the right one. Spacing and associated dynamics may be the root of all oppositional concepts, as Derrida contends, but in a very different sense than intended because they are all undeniably aspects of the phenomenal world that we inhabit, just as metaphors of 'reaching' a referent or 'sailing' outside of a dictionary rely upon primary experiences. All of the aforementioned characteristics of différance can be viscerally sensed in something as simple as a three-note melody heard by a child who cannot understand the meaning of musical notation or words on a page. The very concept of différance, Derrida's philosophic stratagem, is dependent on the perception that, on his account, does not exist or is not 'primordial' in the sense of coming first.

Another sense of spacing explored early on refers to a gap between language and its other. In speaking of this gap, we quoted Caputo's insistence that one will never find in the dictionary a word that might detach itself from its relations to other words and send a person sailing toward some mythical thing in itself 'outside' of language, a 'transcendental signified.' Yet this is a false framing, and musical notation offers a simple means of demonstrating its falseness. Yes, each note on a sheet exists in relation to other notes, and their relative placement within a series will determine the scale to be played. Yes, the meaning of each one changes by virtue of its placement within this series. Yet both note and scale would be but meaningless inkblots on a page if they did not, in effect, send the pianist's fingers sailing to the particular black and white keys that correspond to sounds that will reverberate in the eardrums of the listener. The meaning of the note depends not only on intralinguistic relations (relations between notes) but also on extralinguistic relations (actual sounds).

Yet this latter relation is precisely what is denied, or made exceedingly difficult to comprehend by a deconstructive understanding of language, so much so that it has inspired a fierce interpretive tribalism, as described in Chapter 4 as regards the shibboleth *il n'y a pas de hors-texte*. It is this latter relation that is called into question by the passage through deconstruction's magic portal. What exactly is the relation between words and what they ostensibly refer to, or correspond to? Even the simplest of words like *sunrise* or *sunset*, we are told, are only meaningful because of some endless semiotic deferral, or because they exist within a ceaselessly shifting series of other words. But what of those crimson and amber extravaganzas that creep over and disappear beneath the horizon? What of those events that I see with my eyes? Do they not also have a say in the matter?

The thing itself, if there is anything at all to it, slips away, we are told. But does it? If I say to you, 'Look at the beautiful sky today,' are you sent down an endless interpretive rabbit hole, never able to truly fathom the ultimate meaning of my request? Or is it more likely that you will simply bend your neck and look to the heavens? Some will inevitably argue that this is not what is meant by phrases like 'thing in itself' or 'transcendental signified.' More arguments can always be mustered, and the latter of the two phrases has such an intimidating ring to it, suggesting that perhaps one needs to study more continental philosophy, or worse yet, that one is simply too obtuse to fathom the profound issue at hand. Perhaps, but it is hard to escape the sense that something, somewhere, somehow has been left out of the account of language and meaning that deconstruction puts forth.

Earlier in the present chapter, I stated that différance is at the unreachable beginning of the deconstructive argument and that the transcendental signified is at the unreachable end. The former is the source of linguistic differentiation, the common root of all oppositional concepts. The latter exists in a seemingly mythical realm, 'outside' of language, a thing in itself that is forever beyond our grasp. I also suggested that the two are one and the same, as the symbolic logic of the uroboros—the serpent that folds back upon itself—would suggest, and that Merleau-Ponty knew this to be the case. That which, for Derrida, is never reached, for Merleau-Ponty, is always already reaching through us. This means, effectively, that the source of distinctions made in language is, in fact, the selfsame 'mystical' realm of the transcendental signified. This is, in effect, his argument: The things themselves, those very things that we perceive as embodied subjects, the sensual world and our inhabitance within it are both the origin and end of our language. In alchemical terms, they are both its prima materia and its lapis. They are both alpha and omega.

The analogy with music clarifies what deconstruction renders obscure. Musical notation is a replica of sounds heard—not a carbon copy, but a replica in its root sense. As the etymology of the word attests, a replica is a repetition. From *re*, meaning 'back, again' plus *plicare*, meaning 'to fold,' its Latin cognate *replicare* means 'to repeat' as well as to 'fold or bend back.' This is relevant for at least two reasons, the first of which is, as was articulated in Chapter 2, it is through the notion of an (originary) repetition that Derrida renders problematic notions like representation, retention, and recognition. He claims that repetition is itself originary as opposed to being the repetition *of* an original something. This is a muddled logic that leads to so many oxymoronic phrasings, so many impossible possibilities and surrogate primordialities. It leads to cognitive dissonance precisely because it lacks this sense of 'folding back.' This lack is, in a nutshell, the entire problematic regarding the question of representation described at the outset: Because the 're' of representation conveys the sense of *back to the original* or *to return once more*, it is difficult to think of it as an origin at all. In contrast to this, Merleau-Ponty understands repetition (and representation) in this sense of folding back, and consequently his meaning is congruent with the terms he uses. He is aware of the serpentine, uroboric logic of Being, aware of the way in which language is a replica and a reply to the perceived world. There is a gap (an écart) between the two, yet they belong to the same flesh. Figuratively speaking, he understands that the head and the tail of the snake belong to the same creature. They are not identical, nor are they so different as deconstruction would have it. Thus, he (1968) writes, "there is not identity, nor non-identity, or non-coincidence. There is inside and outside turning about one another" (p. 264). For Derrida, this is not the case. He sees the gap between head and tale—signifier and signified, presentation and representation, language and phenomena, etc.—and he imagines their union to be forever deferred, forever unbridged. He construes the gap as absolute without realizing that head and tail are always already one being, two aspects of a single body. In this sense, his is a dissociated logic.

## Note

1 Husserl himself addressed this as well, particularly in his final great work, *The Crisis of European Sciences and Transcendental Phenomenology*. Dermot Moran (2012), in his introduction to this work, writes "Husserl's understanding of phenomenology evolved and changed over his life, and the Crisis represents the mature expression of his transcendental phenomenology. Initially, he focused on individual processes of consciousness—perception, imagination, memory, time-consciousness, and so on—understood as 'lived experiences' (Erlebnisse), mental episodes. But gradually he came to recognize the need to address the manner in which the flowing, connected stream of conscious experiences is unified into a life, centred around an ego but interconnected with other egos in a communal life of what Husserl calls broadly 'intersubjectivity,' leading, finally, to the shared

experience of a world as a whole (primarily experienced as the familiar 'life-world'). This turn to the ego especially, led Husserl's phenomenology in a transcendental direction (and Descartes is for Husserl the father of transcendental philosophy). The Crisis revolutionized phenomenology with its introduction of the life-world understood as the historical world" (pp. 4–5).

## References

Al-Saji, A. (2009). An absence that counts in the world: Merleau-Ponty's later philosophy of time in light of Bernet's "Einleitung". *Journal of the British Society for Phenomenology, 40*(2), 207–227. https://doi.org/10.1080/00071773.2009.11006682

Berman, M. (1981). *The reenchantment of the world*. Cornell University Press.

Bordo, S. (1987). *The flight to objectivity: Essays on Cartesianism and culture*. State University of New York Press.

Brooke, R. (2015). *Jung and phenomenology*. Routledge.

Derrida, J. (1973). *Speech and phenomena, and other essays on Husserl's theory of signs*. Northwestern University Press.

Derrida, J. (2005). *On touching—Jean-luc Nancy* (C. Irizarry, Trans.). Stanford University Press.

Dillon, M. C. (1997). *Merleau-Ponty's ontology* (2nd ed.). Northwestern University Press.

Hamrick, W. S., & Veken, J. V. (2012). *Nature and logos: A Whiteheadian key to Merleau-Ponty's fundamental thought*. State University of New York Press.

Heidegger, M. (1927 [1967]). *Being and time*. Blackwell Publishing.

Husserl, E. (2014). *Ideas: General introduction to pure phenomenology*. Routledge.

Johnstone, A. A. (1992). The bodily nature of the self, or what Descartes should have conceded Princess Elizabeth of Bohemia. In M. Sheets-Johnstone (Ed.), *Giving the body its due* (pp. 16–47). State University of New York Press.

Jung, C. G. (1933). *Modern man in search of a soul*. Harcourt.

Jung, C. G. (1953). Two essays on analytical psychology. In *The collected works of C. G. Jung* (Vol. 7, R. F. C. Hull, Trans.). Princeton University Press.

Jung, C. G. (1956). Symbols of transformation. In *The collected works of C. G. Jung* (Vol. 5, R. F. C. Hull, Trans.). Princeton University Press.

Jung, C. G. (1959). Aion: Researches into the phenomenology of the self. In *The collected works of C. G. Jung* (Vol. 9.2, R. F. C. Hull, Trans.). Princeton University Press.

Jung, C. G. (1969). The archetypes and the collective unconscious. In *The collected works of C. G. Jung* (Vol. 9.1, R. F. C. Hull, Trans.). Princeton University Press.

Jung, C. G. (1970). Mysterium coniunctionis: An inquiry into the separation and synthesis of psychic opposites in alchemy. In *The collected works of C. G. Jung* (Vol. 14, 2nd ed., R. F. C. Hull, Trans.). Princeton University Press.

Jung, C. G. (2011). *Memories, dreams, reflections*. Vintage.

Kleinberg-Levin, D. M. (1988). *The opening of vision: Nihilism and the postmodern situation*. Routledge.

Levenson, M. H. (2011). *The Cambridge companion to modernism*. Cambridge University Press.

Merleau-Ponty, M. (1962 [2002]). *Phenomenology of perception* (C. Smith, Trans.). Routledge.

Merleau-Ponty, M. (1964a). *The primacy of perception: And other essays on phenomenological psychology, the philosophy of art, history, and politics* (J. M. Edie, Trans.). Northwestern University Press.

Merleau-Ponty, M. (1964b). *Signs* (R. C. McCleary, Trans.). Northwestern University Press.
Merleau-Ponty, M. (1964c). *Sense and non-sense*. Northwestern University Press.
Merleau-Ponty, M. (1968). *The visible and the invisible: Followed by working notes* (A. Lingis, Trans.). Northwestern University Press. (Original work published 1964)
Merleau-Ponty, M. (1973a). *The prose of the world* (C. Lefort, Trans.). Northwestern University Press. (Original work published 1969)
Merleau-Ponty, M. (1973b). *Consciousness and the acquisition of language*. Northwestern University Press.
Merleau-Ponty, M. (2003). *Nature: Course notes from the Collège de France* (R. Vallier, Trans.). Northwestern University Press. (Original work published in 1994)
Moran, D. (2012). *Husserl's crisis of the European sciences and transcendental phenomenology: An introduction*. Cambridge University Press.
Nakhnikian, G. (1964). Introduction. In E. Husserl (Ed.), *The idea of phenomenology* (pp. ix–xxii). Springer.
Sartre, J. (1943 [2021]). *Being and nothingness*. Simon & Schuster.
Spretnak, C. (1999). *The resurgence of the real: Body, nature, and place in a hypermodern world*. Addison Wesley.
Wood, D. (2001). *The deconstruction of time*. Northwestern University Press.

# CONCLUSION

## A Return to the Present

On February 23, 1931, Jung (1973) wrote in a letter to the German author Oskar Schmitz the following:

> I consider the *puer aeternus* attitude an unavoidable evil. Identity with the *puer* signifies a psychological puerility that could do nothing better than outgrow itself. It always leads to external blows of fate which show the need for another attitude. But reason accomplishes nothing, because the puer aeternus is always an agent of destiny.
>
> *(p. 82)*

What are we to make of Jung's claim that the attitude of the puer aeternus is both evil and unavoidable? Is Jung's statement made nearly a century ago true now and potentially so for future generations, or is it merely a dead historical artifact? The archetype's unavoidability, I believe, betrays its necessity: Archetypal attitudes are, on Jung's account, adaptive and essential. This is precisely why they have become *archaic* and *typical*; they are evolutionarily advantageous (Jacobi, 1959). It is only when we become too enthralled by a given archetypal pattern and fully possessed by its dictates that the human psyche becomes out of balance and at odds with itself. The archetype's necessity and adaptiveness is important to remember when speaking of its potential for malevolence. If there is any merit to the framing of deconstruction as a form of the eternal youth myth, and I believe that there certainly is, then it follows that something we might call a 'deconstructive attitude' is both necessary and potentially destructive.

More than merely a method of philosophical and literary analysis originated by Jacques Derrida and furthered by Judith Butler and many, many others, deconstruction is also, broadly speaking, a contemporary style of thought that aims to

DOI: 10.4324/b23321-10

challenge what seems obvious, self-evident, universal, or natural. Far from being confined to the cloistered halls of the academy, this style of thought has come to pervade the broader culture, fostered by the institutional legitimation conferred by its academic bona fides. Yet this contemporaneousness does not belie the fact that it is, in a sense, also perennial and the result of a recurrent "readiness to produce over and over again the same or similar mythical ideas" (Jung, 1953, p. 69).

Eager to point out the contradictions of accepted wisdom and dispel commonly held beliefs, this readiness is keen to discern the seeming absurdity of received wisdom. It seeks to erode all orthodoxy in the name of the new, although this does not prevent it from establishing, perhaps unawares, its own orthodoxy, its own set of unquestionable tenets. Nevertheless, it undermines norms or 'normativities,' in the belief that this is, by definition, a liberating and beneficial endeavor. Such a style of thought will always be needed, just as there will always be a place for pointing out the historical and cultural underpinnings of ideas to call their seemingly eternal or universal validity into question. Each generation needs to interrogate the received wisdom of its mothers' and fathers' generations. This is an archetypal imperative that requires one to jettison the weight of a historical legacy and attempt to fly toward the brave new world that awaits just over the horizon, just over the rainbow. Driven by this imperative, one sails with seemingly limitless freedom into the bright beyond and toward a utopia that beckons one ever forward. No longer tied to anything bedrock, anchored or tethered to the ground, now fully unfettered, one is free to define the world and oneself anew and also free to believe that the act of defining is not subject to limitations given by the nature of things. Definition becomes a matter of self-definition and a fully creative act, an abracadabra of sorts, a belief that 'I will create as I speak.'

The potential for malevolence of this puerility is perhaps best thought of in terms of its limitlessness. The eternal youth does not do well with limits and does not know when to stop. Peter Pan teaches Wendy and her brothers the art of flying and ever more acrobatic maneuvers, but he does not teach them how to stop. Perhaps this is because he does not know well enough himself, and the same can be said of other figures like Icarus and Phaeton. Stopping implies limits to absolute freedom and this is what the eternal youth scoffs at. Limits chafe his spirit, which must be freed of all restrictions of both time and space. Perhaps this is why he can only conceive of such restrictions as being arbitrarily imposed by adults, rather than, simply, by the nature of things. Perhaps it is this belief in the arbitrariness of restrictions that leads him to the external blows of fate alluded to by Jung, the blows that show the need for another attitude. Yet reason, apparently, accomplishes nothing. It rarely does when one is gripped by a supraordinate idea, an archetypal imperative that drives one relentlessly forward.

Hillman (2005) claims that the eternal youth's dilemma manifests itself "all about us outside in the historical field" (p. 31) and it is, to my mind, current debates regarding both sex and gender that most clearly epitomize this. The historical moment in which I write these words will be seen as an inflection point concerning both, regardless of the direction that this inflection takes. These debates display multiple themes typical of eternal youths, one of which is their peculiar aversion toward binaries: "Two is the beginning of the end" (Barrie, 1911, p. 1) laments Wendy's mother, and with this lament Wendy becomes aware that she cannot remain young forever. She has, like Eve, tasted fruit plucked from the tree of knowledge, and this knowledge has a binary aspect. It is not only knowledge of good and evil but also knowledge of female and male. Two is the beginning of the end because it represents our fall into time and the finitude of human form. Eternal youths would rather be 'non-binary' in the broadest sense of this term.

Other themes present in current debates regarding sex and gender that are also typical of the eternal youth are *limitlessness* and a *generational divide*. Writing on what might be considered such a divide within feminism, one more commonly articulated in terms of successive 'waves,' Holly Lawford-Smith (2022) writes in her book *Gender Critical Feminism*:

> Pointing to the fact of social construction when the meaning of a thing is pernicious, or hurts people, is often a first step in finding a way to deconstruct it. This is exactly what the second-wavers were trying to do when they first made use of the sex/gender distinction. This strategy makes sense when it's deployed against things like money and universities (although once made, it is not necessarily easy to unmake). But it's absolutely hopeless against things like rocks and trees.
>
> *(p. 43)*

Deconstruction, broadly speaking, has a certain value within the realm of the strictly cultural, although 'strictly cultural' is perhaps a distinction not easily held to in practice, given the mysterious entwinement of culture and nature. Pointing to the historical and cultural dimensions of what it means to be a woman and differentiating them from the purely biological aspects—in short, making the distinction between sex and gender—is an approach that served one generation of feminists (those of the second wave) in their attempts to articulate sex-based oppression and discrimination. The strategy makes sense within a given context, within certain limits. It makes sense if it knows when to stop. But it is hopeless if one fails to understand that "sex is like rocks and trees" (Lawford-Smith, 2022, p. 42). It is a universally human, self-evident binary that, like rocks and trees, is not merely the result of social construction. No amount of linguistic play, muddled allusions to 'materialization,' or parodic 'performativity' can change this, and second-wave feminists hold fast to this fact. Biological sex is a foundational difference, easily perceptible to those who do not live entirely in "a world of signs without fault, without truth, and without origin" (Derrida, 1967 [1978], p. 292). It is easily recognized by those who acknowledge "the blind and involuntary logic of things perceived" (Merleau-Ponty, 1973, p. 36), who acknowledge that signs *do* have origins and *can* speak to a world that transcends them, those who appreciate the self-evident.

It is easily perceived by anyone who cannot only enter through the magic portal of deconstruction but also return through it.

For second-wave feminists, unlike those of the third wave to which Butler belongs, the sex/gender distinction has not become *absolute*, in the root meaning of this word. As Jung comments in a footnote to *Two Essays on Analytical Psychology*, the word *absolute* means cut off or detached. If something is absolute it is unconnected. Thus, an absolute god "would be of no consequence at all" (Jung, 1953, p. 235 f. n. 6) because it would be utterly disconnected from human affairs. In a similar vein, when the sex/gender distinction is made absolute, when one term is dissociated from the other, the terms lose their meaning, becoming, paradoxically, conflated, confused, and confusing. Second-wave feminists acknowledge the sex/gender distinction, the difference between the two, but in a way that is not made limitless by the logic of deferral, and it is this logic that has split one generation of feminists from the other. Those of the second wave are able to recognize that although the content of female socialization varies across time and place (Lawford-Smith, 2022), the category of humans known as female does not, not in any comparable way. Put differently, because the denotation/connotation distinction as it relates to the word 'female' has not been thoroughly deconstructed, this word still has a denotative meaning that is indisputable, yet all of the culturally imbued connotations of what it means to be female can still be meaningfully addressed. In the words of Lawford-Smith (2022):

> Sex is a necessary ingredient in gender, because it tells us what it is that the social meanings are attached to. There is no way to eliminate or displace sex—as some of those committed to gender as an identity want to do—without a massive loss of explanatory power.
>
> *(p. 47)*

Yet the aforementioned attachment is precisely what deconstructive approaches undermine. They have, as it were, attachment issues. They detach and displace linguistic/cultural meaning from the logos of life, that is to say, biology. For them, in a sense, life is elsewhere.

But *logos of life* should not be taken merely in this limited sense. Deconstruction detaches itself from something much broader than this. Two notions that Merleau-Ponty (1968) adopted from an unlikely source, the philosophy of the Stoics, are worthy of mention here. These ancient philosophers spoke of a *logos endiathetos* and a *logos proforikos*. The first term of this pairing, the logos endiathetos is the "logos of the natural, aesthetic world," which can also be described as the fundamental, inherent sense of the world, its shape and texture, its mute meaningfulness, yet before we have translated this meaning into our own human idiom. It is what he calls the logos of "brute or wild Being" (Merleau-Ponty, 1968, p. 170), or the "logos that pronounces itself silently in each sensible thing" (p. 208). It is the pregnant form of the world as perceived. The later half of the pairing, the logos proforikos, is the human articulation of "meaning first held captive in the thing and in the world itself." He also states that "the description of the perceptual logos is a usage of the logos proforikos" (Merleau-Ponty, 1968, p. 179). In other words, it is signs, language, and with them culture, which are all understood to be an elaboration of the former. This means that the two *logoi* are linked by way of a founding to founded relationship (Dillon, 1997; Hamrick & Veken, 2012) characterized by an asymmetrical reciprocity. The movement from the intrinsic meaning of the phenomenal world to the meaning put into words is a question of translation: "to understand is to translate into disposable significations a meaning first held captive in the thing and in the world itself" (Merleau-Ponty, 1968, p. 36).

The *absolute* dissociation of these two logoi is what the second wave and oft-described 'radical feminists' reject. Sex and gender, nature and culture cannot be entirely detached from one another lest the terms lose all meaning, lest they suffer a "massive loss of explanatory power" (Lawford-Smith, 2022, p. 47). This second wave includes such luminaries as Germaine Greer, Mary Daly, Susan Griffin, Monique Wittig, Andrea Dworkin, Adrienne Rich, Audre Lorde, Sheila Jeffreys, and many others (Lawford-Smith, 2022). Ironically, part of the radicality and what differentiates these women from their third-wave counterparts lies in something that, at first glance, does not seem radical at all, if by this term what is meant is something of extreme change or measure. On the contrary, much of their radicality resides in the fact that they still base their thinking on a primary differentiation, a fundamental difference that is not différance but rather, a difference that is, shall we say, nakedly self-evident. I refer to the simple distinction between two forms of sexed bodies that, until recently, appeared quite indisputable and easily perceived, the distinction between female and male. Holding firm to this distinction is now, apparently, a radical position, as odd as it may seem. Yet from another perspective, this makes perfect sense if we remember that the word *radical* comes from the Latin *radix*, meaning *root* or having an origin in the ground. In this sense, these women most certainly are radical because they fiercely defend the root, foundational meaning of terms like 'female' and 'woman.'

As a result of the aforementioned generational split, on Lawford-Smith's account, much of the groundbreaking work of the second wave has been either forgotten or misremembered by third-wave feminists eager to differentiate themselves from their foremothers. For the second generation, much of the third generation's work amounts to a form of female erasure, given that terms like 'female' and 'woman' are no longer understood to refer to biological givens. When "discourse produces the effects that it names" (Butler, 1996 [2011], p. xii), and sex does "not qualify as a prediscursive anatomical facticity" (Butler, 1990 [2007], p. 11) as Butler would have it, women are easily erased. When sex is no longer observed but 'assigned,' it is merely penciled in and something just as easily scratched out. As a consequence of this erasure, words like 'mother,' and with it, all of the adjacent meanings and associations that have come to surround this word suffer a similar erasure.

Perhaps such erasure exemplifies the sort of evil to which Jung referred to above. The reader will come to her or his own conclusions in this regard. But taken too far, ignorant of its own limitations, and playing out a mythic narrative never made fully conscious, deconstruction wreaks havoc, as can any ideology left unchecked, leading to the "loss of meaning and materialism of our time [that] are the offspring of lost contact with traditions and ancestors, the outcome of an unquestioned falling in with 'progress'" (p. xiii) as Glen Slater notes in his introduction to Hillman's *Senex and Puer* (2005). This loss of meaning is inevitable when progress is conceived of as a mere looking back at what seemed natural or universal, so as to reconceive it as nothing more than a set of cultural constructs blind to themselves. Meaning is inevitably lost when cultural construction and natural givenness are understood to *absolutely* preclude one another. The dimensions of this lost meaning are manifold: It is a loss of historical continuity, as well as an understanding of what words meant to prior generations; it is a loss of our sense of consanguinity with these generations as well as a loss of our moorings in the immediacy of perception.

Dispossessed in this way, language falls apart and descends into gibberish and cacophony, fracturing the cultural and political spheres with rhetoric that is no longer grounded in the shared meanings of words. In such a Tower of Babel, narratives are scarcely subject to any empirical proof or disproof and they direct our attention to no consensual reality. Yet they gain persuasive power, compelling us with the mythic tenor of their incantation and the invocation of absolute good and absolute evil, fostering "tyrannical, obsessive, intoxicating ideas and delusions" (Jung, 1964, p. 212), enticing us "to believe the most absurd things, just as the possessed do" (p. 212). When such is the case, ideology can easily trump even the evidence of direct perception, leaving a profound sense of cognitive dissonance in its wake. Perennial stories parade themselves in clever disguise and possess the imagination. When language no longer grants a sense of continuity, consanguinity, and a mooring in perception, it is easy for consciousness to become dominated by an intrusive, irrational, autonomous fragment of the psyche.

Yet because language itself reaches back into the haze of prehistory, even when it is falling apart, it offers us bounties of ancestral insight if we allow it the opportunity. The words themselves have something to teach us. Despite this, their deeper meaning is often lost to ardent reformers and linguistic zealots who, in the rush to usher in a more just future and with remarkable shortsightedness, attempt to institute reform by fiat. Such is the hubris of the current historical moment. The method of the present work demonstrates the folly of such an approach. Throughout its entirety, I have attempted to retrieve the root meanings hidden in words and follow an associative logic based on these meanings with the intent of discerning the "tissue that word or image is embedded in" (Jung, 1977, p. 84). This continued reflection upon etymology and the drawing of parallels has been an example of what Jung called *amplification*: a search for analogies and correspondences in the most varied sources. This is a technique he used not only to diagnose and heal patients, but one that he brought to bear in his attempts to diagnose and heal the collective psyche (Jung, 1964, 2012), and Jungians have followed in his footsteps (Singer & Kimbles, 2004). For him, amplification was a means of broadening a patient's understanding of his or her own personal neurosis so that it could be recognized as a more general, perhaps even universal affliction hardly unique to any one person. In a similar vein, I have tried to amplify the meanings of a contemporary form of literary and philosophical analysis so as to recognize within it a universal problematic hardly unique to the current moment. The method has been largely one of following the historical meanings, the ancestral insight sedimented within words.

As if elaborating the meaning of a dream image or teasing apart multiple aspects of a psychological complex, I described parallels between the *dif* of différance and the *dis* of dissociation and displacement. By following the implicit logic in this cluster of ideas, an interpretation and an argument were formed. This, in turn, led unexpectedly through Dante's inferno toward the demonic lord Dis. But the reader and I also traveled to imagined utopias made possible through displacement. Arguments of primacy and sequence inspired reflection upon words like *primordial* and its relationship to the idea of *mother*. Parallels drawn to this latter figure then suggested the idea of matter, which, in turn, hinted at the possibility that deconstruction has both an issue with the maternal and an issue with the material world. This also led—like a form of Freudian free association, yet one not so free as to lead us too far from the theme at hand—to reflections on *gender* and its deeper meaning, its relation to birthing and begetting, as well as that which is natural, natal, nascent, and native. The point here is not to recapitulate an argument or a chain of associations but to draw attention to a method: By amplifying meanings sedimented in words over millennia, I have attempted to articulate the deeper sense of an ultramodern, even postmodern form of thinking that is, paradoxically, far older than it imagines.

The fact that such a method is even possible is testament to what Merleau-Ponty referred to as *sedimentation*. Because he believed in the primacy of perception, for him, what Derrida would have called the metaphysical heritage is not an obstacle to perception but an outgrowth of it and a means to further elaborate upon it. Words that we have inherited are not merely arbitrary constructions. Language is a repository of crystalized experience and perception. Its structure, grammar, and syntax, though immensely varied from one language to another, nevertheless mirrors and echoes a world perceived. There are loose parallels one can draw between the idea of sedimentation as described by Merleau-Ponty and Jung's understanding of the archetypal. Both are the result of "the archaic heritage of humanity, the legacy left behind by all differentiation and development and bestowed upon all men like sunlight and air" (Jung, 1956, p. 178). Like Jung's (1953) conception of the archetypal, sedimentation is to a great degree the result of "recurrent impressions made by subjective reactions" (p. 69). It is such recurrent impressions, recurrent perceptions that Merleau-Ponty alludes to in his idea of sedimentation. It is always the settling in of "a primary differentiation which . . . precedes without any doubt the relation of sign to signification, since it is what makes the very distinction between signs possible" (Merleau-Ponty, 1973, pp. 32–33). Sedimentation, unlike the metaphysical heritage as conceived by deconstruction, is grounded in a perennial experience of self-evident differences, and such differences are not subject to deconstruction.

## References


Barrie, J. M. (1911). *Peter and Wendy*. Charles Scribner's Sons.

Butler, J. (1990 [2007]). *Gender trouble: Feminism and the subversion of identity*. Routledge.

Butler, J. (1996 [2011]). *Bodies that matter: On the discursive limits of sex*. Routledge.

Derrida, J. (1967 [1978]). *Writing and difference* (A. Bass, Trans.). University of Chicago Press.

Dillon, M. C. (1997). *Merleau-Ponty's ontology* (2nd ed.). Northwestern University Press.

Hamrick, W. S., & Veken, J. V. (2012). *Nature and logos: A Whiteheadian key to Merleau-Ponty's fundamental thought*. State University of New York Press.

Hillman, J., & Slater, G. (2005). *Senex & puer*. Spring Publications.

Jacobi, J. (1959). *Complex/archetype/symbol*. Princeton University Press.

Jung, C. G. (1953). Two essays on analytical psychology. In *The collected works of C. G. Jung* (Vol. 7, R. F. C. Hull, Trans.). Princeton University Press.

Jung, C. G. (1956). Symbols of transformation. In *The collected works of C. G. Jung* (Vol. 5, R. F. C. Hull, Trans.). Princeton University Press.

Jung, C. G. (1964). Civilization in transition. In *The collected works of C. G. Jung* (Vol. 10, R. F. C. Hull, Trans.). Princeton University Press.

Jung, C. G. (1973). *C. G. Jung letters: Vol. 1—1906–1950* (G. Adler & A. Jaffé, Ed., R. F. C. Hull, Trans.). Princeton University Press.

Jung, C. G. (1977). The Tavistock lectures, lecture III. In *The collected works of C. G. Jung: The symbolic life: Miscellaneous writings* (Vol. 18, R. F. C. Hull, Trans.). Princeton University Press.

Jung, C. G. (2012). Answer to job. In *The collected works of C. G. Jung* (Vol. 11, R. F. C. Hull, Trans.). Princeton University Press.

Lawford-Smith, H. (2022). *Gender-critical feminism*. Oxford University Press.

Merleau-Ponty, M. (1968). *The visible and the invisible: Followed by working notes* (A. Lingis, Trans.). Northwestern University Press. (Original work published 1964)

Merleau-Ponty, M. (1973). *The prose of the world* (C. Lefort, Trans.). Northwestern University Press. (Original work published 1969)

Singer, T., & Kimbles, S. L. (2004). *The cultural complex: Contemporary Jungian perspectives on Psyche and society*. Psychology Press.

# INDEX

For Product Safety Concerns and Information please contact our EU
representative GPSR@taylorandfrancis.com
Taylor & Francis Verlag GmbH, Kaufingerstraße 24, 80331 München, Germany

www.ingramcontent.com/pod-product-compliance
Ingram Content Group UK Ltd.
Pitfield, Milton Keynes, MK11 3LW, UK
UKHW020008200926
475702UK00015B/2533
* 9 7 8 1 0 3 2 4 5 5 3 2 7 *